Praise for *Expectin*

"Alexis Marie Chute, tasked with living as she mourns the death of her child, writes vividly and honestly about loss and grief. *Expecting Sunshine* records a journey that proves to be revelatory for reader and writer alike. This is a brave, memorable book."

—**Jane Brox**, author of *Brilliant: The Evolution of Artificial Light*

"In *Expecting Sunshine*, the Edmonton-based writer and artist Alexis Marie Chute writes about loss—the most primal loss we can experience, the loss of a child—in such luminous prose and with such clear-eyed insight that the beauty of the text brings the reader to the edge of tears. Tears of sadness for her family's loss, yes, but more profoundly, tears of release and healing as we witness the cathartic powers of art and the scope of a young family's love. This is a beautiful, honest, important book that makes death a starting point for the continuation of life—literally, as the book chronicles Chute's first pregnancy after the death of her son Zachary—and grief, the catalyst from which joy is born."

—**Pamela Petro**, author of *Sitting Up with the Dead: A Storied Journey through the American South*

"Honest, raw and vulnerable—Alexis Marie Chute opens her heart to share her journey of love, loss, transformation, and rebirth. Her message that love binds us together even beyond death, resonates deeply with me as a bereaved mother; it is also a consistent message I heard in my research with bereaved families who experience perinatal death. This is an important, engaging book for bereaved parents, especially those who are considering a subsequent pregnancy."

—**Christine Jonas-Simpson**, RN, PhD Professor of Nursing, York University, Toronto, ON Canada

"Alexis Marie's honest, unflinching memoir reads more like a novel in its elegant use of prose and narrative structure. But there's no mistaking its truth—that losing a child at any age can cause a shift in a parent's universe. Alexis Marie's struggle to move forward and heal, and still honour baby Zachary, is an inspiration."

—**Janice Biehn**, Editor, *ParentsCanada* magazine

"This memoir is a moving journey of infant loss and the pregnancy that follows in the midst of a society that does not understand the dynamics of perinatal loss. The book explores the different ways men and women process grief, suppressing grief while wanting others to remember a baby no longer physically present, and how to find a new normal. The pregnancy that follows brings multifaceted feelings of continued grief, memories of the previous pregnancy along with anxiety and fear for the safety of the much-wanted new sibling. This is a book for parents, professionals, and families and friends wishing to support someone who has suffered a loss."

—**Joann O'Leary**, PhD, Parent-Infant Specialist, author of *Meeting the Needs of Families Pregnant and Parenting After the Loss of a Baby*

"*Expecting Sunshine* is an exquisite book for all those who have lost a child and those who need to understand and cope with untimely grief. It is one woman's heart-rending story of a mother' loss which confounds ideology, faith and any of the prescribed cures for mourning. Its pain and wisdom are as old as time, the simple truths of nature, nurture and the bonds of mother and child. It is also an uplifting lesson in redemption."

—**Rachel Manley**, author of the Governor General Award–winning memoir *Drumblair: Memories of a Jamaican Childhood*

"Wow! The story of Alexis Marie Chute and her precious pregnancies was almost impossible for me to put down. I know that this book will be so helpful for families living through subsequent pregnancies—a chance to validate their varied emotions and know that whatever they are feeling is 'normal.' Thank you for sharing your story so that others can learn from your journeys. Thank you, Zachary, for helping your mother tell yours and Eden's stories."

—**Lori Ives-Baine**, RN, MN (CPB), Perinatal and Pediatric Grief Support Coordinator, Toronto, Ontario, Canada

"*Expecting Sunshine* is a brave book, walking the reader through the deep grief that accompanies the loss of a child and moving beyond immediate pain to recovery. Alexis Marie Chute speaks honestly of all the areas of life that are threatened by the death of a child: the relationship of the parents, and their faith, creativity, and belief in themselves and one another. At the same time, *Expecting Sunshine* acknowledges the myriad support systems that exist to help bereaved parents heal from this kind of trauma and emerge together, altered but vital. Part memorial, part celebration, this is a striking book."

—**Jenna Butler**, Lieutenant Governor of Alberta Award winner and author of *Profession of Hope*

"An amazingly moving and emotional story that any woman—or any parent—can easily relate to."

—**Jennifer Hamilton**, Editor, *CanadianFamily.ca*

"An honest and tender memoir about the complex and difficult emotions of grief and joy a mother goes through during a pregnancy that follows a death of a child."

—**Lindsey Henke** LICSW, founder of Pregnancy After Loss Support

"When a baby dies, too many parents suffer alone in silence. While grieving the unexpected death of her son, Zachary, Alexis Marie courageously gives powerful voice to a mother's primal heartbreak as she searches for renewal and rebirth in her own healing while carrying her next son, Eden. In her enthralling memoir, for those of us bereaved mothers who share similar memories, Alexis Marie helps us to honour our own lives."

—**Shari Morash**, Founder of Josiah's Journey and author of *Loving Your Baby: A Gentle and Practical Guide to Parenting Through Miscarriage, Stillbirth and Infant Death*

"In *Expecting Sunshine*, Alexis Marie allows you to accompany her on the tumultuous journey of pregnancy after loss. While navigating the complex emotions during this time, she is vulnerable and allows the reader to witness her most private moments. This is a beautiful story filled with love—both for the baby who has passed on, as well as the one she is expecting."

—**Kiley Krekorian Hanish**, occupational therapist, founder of the Return to Zero Center for Healing, and bereaved mother to Norbert

Expecting Sunshine

Expecting Sunshine

A Journey of Grief, Healing and Pregnancy After Loss

Alexis Marie Chute

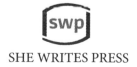

SHE WRITES PRESS

Published 2017
Printed in the United States of America

ISBN: 978-1-63152-174-4 pbk
ISBN: 978-1-63152-175-1 ebk
Library of Congress Control Number: 2016960233

Cover design by TK
Interior design by Julie Valin

For information, address:
She Writes Press
1563 Solano Ave #546
Berkeley, CA 94707

She Writes Press is a division of SparkPoint Studio, LLC.

With the exception of the names of my husband and children, and the babies listed in the Walk to Remember chapter called "Seasons," all the names and places in this story have been changed to protect individuals' privacy. I would also like to acknowledge the role of memory in the telling of personal histories. Suffice it to say that anyone who has endured parental sleeplessness will understand the shortcomings of such recollections.

In loving memory of
Zachary Jonathan Chute

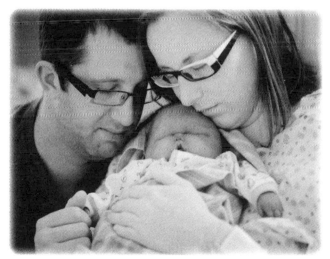

Not Until I Met You
By Suzy Kassem

Not until I felt your sunshine,
Did I realize that I had been in the shade.
Not until I saw all your colors,
Did I realize that mine had faded.
Not until I heard your dreams,
Did I realize that I was still sleeping.
And not until I experienced my life with you,
Did I realize that I was barely
Breathing.

Contents

PART 1

FIRST TRIMESTER

PART 2

SECOND TRIMESTER

PART 3

THIRD TRIMESTER

Conception

It was September 2011 and the last photography job in my Year of Distraction. Nearly twelve months before, my second child, Zachary, had been born and, without even a breath, had died in my arms. As I stood in the hundred-year-old Greek Orthodox church as wedding guests slowly seated themselves for the upcoming ceremony, I could not allow myself to think of Zachary; I was the photographer and had a job to do. Yet, as I aimed my hefty Nikon up to the gold-leaf dome that buttered the walls and marble altar in an unearthly sunshine, all I could see was Zachary's face.

The light refracted into my eyes, and for a moment I could see nothing at all. Then my son's face returned. His smooth, taut skin. His purple lips.

On the day of Zachary's birth, his swollen cheeks were freckled with the telltale marks of Tuberous Sclerosis Complex. The doctors assured my husband, Aaron, and me, after nine wearisome months of genetic testing following Zachary's death, that randomness, not an inherited gene, was to blame. Still I crucified myself with guilt and survived only by stepping into my Year of Distraction intentionally, working like an addict to curb my brain from wandering to the god-forsaken randomness.

During that year I booked wedding photography gigs for every Saturday and Sunday and filled the weekday evenings with portrait sessions and commissions. I snapped thousands of photographs in that time, filling the visual palette of my mind with

1

grinning families, brides with lash extensions and parasols, couples entwined in love and others in lust, and the living babies with marble-round eyes who smiled at me and smacked pink gums as I crowed like a rooster to earn their attention. All the while I was also *Mother* to my firstborn, my spirited and charming Hannah, as she approached and passed her first birthday.

Look, I said to myself. *You are in control. This can't touch you.* With the goal of distraction, I was relentless. There was no time for sorrow.

The carpeted aisle of the church muffled the *click clack* of my work heels, but I wouldn't have heard them anyway. My breath was loud in my ears. Blinking hard, I reviewed the list of family portraits to be taken following the bride and groom's *I do*s. I thumbed, rolled, and folded the paper nervously until it became smooth as fabric. The bride was still en route, so I lingered among the guests, waiting for genuine flashes of emotion and perfect angles—the *decisive moment*, as famed photographer Henri Cartier-Bresson termed it. My muscles were tense and ready as I slowly strolled the aisles past sixty rows of glossy oak pews.

"Maybe you should slow down," Aaron had said months before as the stress of work fractured my sleep each night. "Just in case." He looked down at my chest as if seeing through my blouse and freckled flesh and wide ribs to my heart. An unforeseen result of the genetic testing was the discovery of my enlarged heart, which, like Zachary's condition, was diagnosed as random. There was no treatment plan, no next steps, no answers; the cardiologist simply fanned through my test results and shrugged. I would have accepted the diagnosis of a broken heart, but that would have required an examination of my soul.

At the beginning, I ignored Aaron's concerns about my health, barely hearing him above the anger that deafened me to his voice. He returned to his teaching job one week after our son died, just a

2

few days after Zachary's memorial. "I can't stay, I have to go back to work," he yelled as I cleaved to him.

"I need you. Please. I can't handle this. Please stay with me," I begged through the lightning-sharp storm of sorrow.

The memorial flowers thrived in vases throughout our home for weeks until they, too, died, and still Aaron was a ghost to me. His side of the bed was cold when Hannah called me from sleep each morning. His breakfast dishes were put away, the counter wiped; he left no trail of crumbs for me to follow. He stayed late at the high school where he taught, coaching volleyball and texting me the score of each game as his team approached the championship.

Most evenings he did not arrive home until after nine and then eagerly recounted the events of his workday and the volleyball game in the same gonging baritone as his father. But to me it was the monologue of a mime. I watched his lips, but there was no sound. Sitting motionless I became like the wall, the hunched lamp in the corner, the stained rug, as I too disappeared into myself. I'm sure my breath did not even ripple the air between us.

Focus, Alexis Marie. Focus. Be professional, I huffed while exhaling, shaking my head lightly. Thankfully no one at the wedding seemed to notice—except for two small blue eyes that met mine and did not look away. A flaxen-haired baby boy snuggled on his mother's lap stared at me, a bottle of frothy formula between his plump lips. I took a step in his direction. As I smiled at him he turned his pudgy body toward me, forfeiting his suction, and appraised me, full-faced like the harvest moon.

The boy's gaze drew me another step toward him, and I was startled when he raised his tiny hands in my direction. The gesture was unmistakable: *Pick me up*, he cooed. His mother excused herself from a conversation to look at me, confused. "He never does this," she said, letting me collect her baby in my arms. His features were fair, like Hannah's. He had her gem-blue eyes, pearl-colored hair, and creaseless skin flushed with curiosity.

"He's beautiful." I cradled him on my hip. "How old?"

"He will be one in October."

My large heart swelled. "Wh . . . when in October?" I gulped and closed my eyes.

Just a few weeks before that wedding, my Year of Distraction had fulfilled its purpose: busyness. I was dog-tired and no further along in my grief than the day I'd left the hospital with empty arms. When Aaron again suggested a slower pace, the inky-black bags beneath my eyes spoke up without permission. I gave in, imaging quality time with Hannah and starting to paint for myself—an act I had outlawed after Zachary's death for fear of what anguish might subconsciously take form on the canvas. I was ready to end my Year of Distraction and canceled each upcoming booking, returning every deposit and cloaking my calendar in a crusty layer of White-Out.

Just get through today; just get through today. I steadied myself and opened my eyes to the voice of the little boy's mother at the wedding.

"October 24," she answered loudly as the sanctuary echoed with the laughter of boisterous guests parading in their suits, autumn dresses, and polished shoes.

Zachary would have been two weeks older than the child in my arms. *Is this what my son would have looked like?* I passed the baby back to his mother, and he hungrily resumed his lunch. An usher touched my arm and whispered, "The bride has arrived."

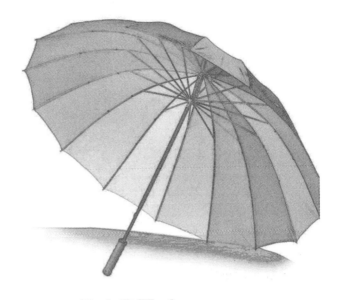

PART 1

FIRST TRIMESTER

Week 1: Baby Shower

Everyone was surprised when I volunteered to co-host Theresa's baby shower. It was less than a year since Zachary died, but Theresa was my best friend and had organized a party for me when Hannah was born. Since I would be in attendance either way, I figured it would be easier to host than to be a guest. The hostess is a busybody, refreshing the punchbowl with crackling ice, bringing out more paper plates, and tracking down extra pens for the party games. A guest has to ogle over the swaddled infant and applaud the gifts. Theresa had a baby boy; at the time of the shower he was three weeks old.

My co-host, Lisa, arrived early, trailing candy-apple-green and periwinkle-blue helium balloons behind her. One particular balloon was extra large and shaped like a cradle, boasting *It's a Boy!* in baby-blue swirls. Lisa tied the balloons to a frilly weight and put them in the corner of the living room beside the couch and extra chairs Aaron had hauled in before taking Hannah to McDonald's for ice cream. Lisa and I hung metallic swirly streamers from the kitchen light and put our two gifts on the table as a cue for the other guests. We scattered milk-bottle-shaped confetti across the coffee table and sprinkled it around the snack plates in the dining room.

Guests began to arrive, toting large teddy-bear and rocket-ship gift bags, boxes wrapped in superhero paper with blue ribbons and sport-themed cards. Ladies beamed at Theresa's sleeping newborn, rocking him and bickering over which parent the child most resembled.

"Good for you for hosting," an older woman whispered in my ear, nodding with approval as if I were a pillar of strength.

"I am so happy for Theresa," I replied with a lopsided smile.

I fidgeted once my hosting duties were checked off the list. With the main floor of my house looking like a pastel wonderland, the plastic wrap removed from the plates of snacks and Lisa leading the shower games, there was nothing left for me to do but sit in the circle of women. Theresa held her child lovingly to her heart, standing and swaying, stroking his smooth, glossy brown hair that matched her own. *You will not make a scene*, I warned myself, looking away.

That was the first party for Theresa's son, and in the years that followed I expected I would celebrate many more milestones with their family. Zachary, on the other hand, had no such future. There were no cradle-shaped balloons to announce his arrival, no baby shower to welcome him; there would be no report cards, stamped passports, caps and gowns, wedding rings, or bags of outgrown clothing as he wore the wardrobe of an expanding life. All I had were minutes with my baby before he died, and the hours I held him against my skin afterward, rocking him back and forth, willing his lungs to suck in air and his heart to beat.

Zachary's ashes, which lived in a heart-shaped metal urn, were all that was left of my son.

On the morning of the baby shower, Hannah chirped for breakfast at six. I let Aaron sleep and carried my girl on my hip downstairs to our kitchen. "Eggies," she squealed. As I slid the egg carton from the top shelf of the fridge, I happened to read the words printed between my fingers. *BEST BEFORE OCTOBER 14.* My breath wheezed through my throat.

October 14.

The trigger.

A trigger is an event, image, or person—anything, really—that reminds you of the moment you ceased to be you and became someone else. A memory, loaded and cocked, fires, annihilating your carefully monitored composure, spilling sadness like blood. The force of impact sends you backward into another time, which you relive in anguish as wounds are unstitched.

October 14 was Zachary's expiration date. I don't know how long I stood motionless at the fridge door, my feet rooted deeply to the grey-blue kitchen tile. I clutched the refrigerator handle with one hand while the egg carton hung limply in the other. Cold white light leaked out and made my skin glow and goosebump. Hannah's high, happy voice rang out, but I could not understand. Her words were a murmur. Everything was static, a hum.

"Thank you for the gifts," Theresa said as some of the ladies stood to leave. I must have been staring but abruptly snapped back to the baby shower, jumping to my feet to retrieve their coats. Guests thanked Lisa for the gift bags and me for hosting, a few women offering me long glances of a silent sympathy before heading out the door.

"That was a success," Lisa said when we were alone. She began unhooking the swirly streamers as I vacuumed up the confetti. We stacked all the salvageable decorations, and I put them away quickly in my purple bin of party supplies. Lisa didn't want them, nor did Theresa. I refused to let myself wonder if I might have a use for them one day.

During that time, I recalled reading that the earth balanced upon a perfect axis—that, if tilted even a degree away from the sun, we humans would freeze; a degree in the opposite direction and we'd burn. It was obvious to me that I had been thrown off my balancing point, despite my outward appearance of functionality. *Am I burning? Or frozen? Or both?* What was abundantly clear, though, was that I was hopelessly, frustratingly lost within my own life.

Caught in a cycle beyond my understanding of how I survived

the last day or what my place was in the present one, I could not worry about the impending tomorrows. I couldn't see even that far ahead and chose not to dream. The future was dead to me. *How did I get here?* And yet there I was; there we all were. My parents still fed Hannah too much vanilla ice cream and too many Smarties. My house needed cleaning. The stack of books I wanted to read gathered dust.

How did I get here? The question haunted me. Every night it peppered colorless dreams. Someone important was missing—*has everyone forgotten?* All things moved forward, shifting, changing, growing, and dying all around—and yet there I was, like a frozen burning being in the midst of an eerily familiar life. There were those who said, "Move on." But how could I? I was lost and didn't know the way.

In the quiet absence of party guests and my home mostly back to normal, I took a breath. A deep breath. I didn't want to think about baby boys anymore. Not that day. Aaron and Hannah returned home from McDonald's, and my girl instantly fell in love with the balloons I had forgotten in the corner. I cursed myself for not immediately puncturing the helium-filled reminders of my son's absence.

"Get rid of them, please," I whispered to Aaron. He released the balloons from our back deck as Hannah wailed in protest inside. "When will this get easier?" I wondered aloud. Aaron did not answer.

Week 2: Seasons

The leaves were yellowing, falling to the earth like physical shards of sunshine spent on long summer days. "Mommy! Look!" Hannah kicked a pile of leaves on the wilting grass, and they roared to life in the wind. She laughed, turning back to see my face. I smiled, and she ran on. We collected colorful leaves with interesting shapes and filled our red wagon to the brim.

Almost one year before, at the beginning of October 2010, our family had lived in anticipation of Zachary's death. "There is nothing we can do," the doctors had told us. The autumn scene out our hospital window was just like that within, an evolving landscape of diminishing and dying color. The six months that followed were miserable seasons; a wicked-cold winter followed by a reluctant spring.

"How about this one, Hannah?" I asked, holding up a leaf that looked like fire in my palm.

"Yeah!" she nodded with authority, her eyebrows pinched into one as she carried out her inspection. Her blonde curls bounced at her ears.

"Are you cold?" I asked for the fourth time, but she pretended not to hear and smiled mischievously before bolting down the path. I sprinted and caught her around the waist, lifting her upside down so her feet ran upon the clouds. We grew breathless in a wriggling war of tickles and squeals.

"More," Hannah giggled, but she'd grown dizzy. I steadied her on the ground and zipped her coat to her chin before we continued along the path just south of our home.

In early summer 2011, almost nine months to the day after Zachary's death, Aaron and I got a phone call from the hospital. "Good news!" the genetics counselor began. I had pestered the woman relentlessly, calling multiple times a week, impatient to hear those very words from her mouth. "After all the extensive testing we've done, and the results from the lab in the UK, we are certain, Alexis Marie, that Zachary's condition was only a randomly occurring genetic abnormality."

"Does that mean we can have more children?"

"Yes. You and Aaron do not have Tuberous Sclerosis Complex. The alteration of the gene occurred spontaneously after conception. You can have more children." I repeated everything the counselor had said, sentence by sentence, to Aaron, who lay beside me on the bed. We celebrated silently: our hands stretched open, smiles spread across our faces like skydivers.

"There is a chance, though"—I held my breath—"that it could happen again." I was too startled to repeat the woman's caution to Aaron. Worry grew in my gut like a stone. "Couples who have had a child with TS Complex may have a very slight chance of it happening again."

My response was slow, each word weighted. "How slight?"

"It's really nothing to worry about. The statistical reoccurrence is almost back to the chance of it randomly appearing in the general population. I just need to make you aware."

She said *almost.*

Almost.

I shuffled my feet through the leaves, remembering that conversation. "How 'bout this one, Han?" I held up the skeleton of a leaf, but Hannah scrunched her nose at it.

Autumn was macabre. I found myself drawn to the sickly-looking leaves, the pale ones, raw sienna and umber-shaded with holes and veins, clearly homesick for their tree. Delicately, I folded those skeletons into my pocket. My mind saw beauty in their sadness and in the flora so dry it crumbled or burst to dust within my grasp. I wished to capture that visual, as it was a picture of where my grief and Year of Distraction had left me.

When Hannah began filling the wagon with wet grass, dirt, and sticks, I tossed in the collection from my pocket. Her lips quivered in the chilly air. "Home time," I announced.

Once we were warm indoors, I spread out the flawed and perfect leaves to create a pattern, overlapping them across a three-foot-square primed canvas covered in acrylic gel. I bathed each leaf in the flowing medium as well, securing and layering the collage. Hannah paid no attention to me or my artwork as she made a pasty tower of princesses from a Disney sticker book.

A few days later Hannah, Aaron, and I drove downtown to the provincial legislature grounds for the annual Walk to Remember for families that had lost a baby. It was Saturday, October 1, 2011. My parents were to join us, along with Aaron's parents, his siblings, and their spouses. The walk took place two weeks before what would have been Zachary's first birthday.

The large grassy park beneath the steps of the legislature buzzed with parents, grandparents, and children, yet despite the candy-colored checkered flags and teddy bears, the mood was not festive. The commonality of those gathered, the bond that formed our community, was the absence of a child or, for some, multiple children.

The year before, Aaron and I had attended the memorial event while I was still pregnant. Though Zachary's death was imminent, we still wondered if it was faithless to grieve while he continued to kick inside of me. As we were about to leave, a woman approached and asked me, "Can I touch your belly?" She stared longingly, eyes welling, and added, "You must be so excited to be pregnant again."

"Actually," I choked as I cradled my midsection tenderly, "this is the baby we are losing." She told me that on the morning of her daughter's dedication at church she discovered her child had died in the night of SIDS—sudden infant death syndrome. "Why do these things happen?" we echoed each other. There were no answers. Only randomness.

At my second Walk to Remember I shared the longing of that woman to touch life. While randomness was unable to satisfy the *Why Zachary?* and *Why us?* questions, it did provide hope that we could again conceive a healthy child. It was a hope we eagerly accepted with the genetic counselor's news, throwing our condoms in the trash and fucking our brains out for months.

My focus took a dramatic shift from seeking answers to baby-making, and I bought ovulation tests in bulk at the pharmacy. The stress of waiting for the results of the genetic testing had been so debilitating that, once free of it, all I could imagine was having another child—and, hopefully, healing in the process.

That July, I used seven ovulation tests to track my hormone levels, stalking my ovaries' release of that one precious egg, but the six pregnancy tests that followed revealed our timing had been off. The next month, another four pee-sticks confirmed we were still unsuccessful. "Be patient," Aaron had told me. I tried to mellow, although I still insisted on the missionary position. After sex I tipped my pelvis toward our stipple-covered ceiling with my hips on our headboard, letting gravity do its part. I was careful not to spill even one drop of semen.

Only weeks before our second Walk to Remember, I had felt confident. By that point, I could sense my body's ovulation. When my nipples were tender and my stomach thick, Aaron and I made love several times a night. "You are going to break my penis," he joked, but the pregnancy tests again displayed only one lonely pink line. I wept on the floor, holding myself, wishing Zachary were in my arms.

On the nippy October morning of the Walk to Remember, Aaron's words blew white clouds into the air when he spoke. "Keep your hat on," he told Hannah as she squirmed beneath a blanket in the red wagon. The wind had the smell of winter, the coolness of the mountains to the southwest, and I tugged Hannah's toque down over her ears, kissing her peach-colored cheeks.

"Go, go!" Hannah screamed merrily. She was the light of our trio, pulling us toward life, pulling me specifically out of bed each day and into the rhythm of being. Without her I would have died in my flannel pajamas. Once all our extended family had gathered, we spread a red-and-blue quilt made by Aaron's mother onto the crunchy frost-covered grass and ate cupcakes and chocolate-chip cookies distributed by volunteers.

As a patchwork family, we wrote notes to Zachary on small squares of paper, which we then tied to the white ribbon of a single blue balloon. The notes fluttered in the breeze like the last remaining leaves on the trees. We carried the balloon with us as we joined the Walk in a loop around the park, somber as a funeral procession though young children darted off the path to splay themselves on top of raked leaf piles and play hide-and-seek behind the oak trees.

The sidewalk was lined in chalk with the names of dead babies, names written in coral script, tangerine block letters, and apple-green squiggles. Families paused when they arrived upon their child's name, took pictures, cried, and then walked on.

Holly Grace Cochrane, Taylor Dewald, Angel Baby Semchuk, Olivia Grace White, Xavier Grey Thompson, Lars Michael Collins-Hood, Peanut, Trouble, Sweetpea, Sprout, Ernie Walker, Perry Walker, Suzanne Washington, Peyton Lisa Hall, Jayden Maximus Lopez, Brooke Catharine Harrington, Tessa Isabel Vladicka Gue, Ethan Alexander Dzikowski, Morgan Avery Dzikowski, Sebastian Isaiah Schroder-Smith, Bretton-Elijah Lucas Roberts, Ciara-Rose Kennedi Roberts, Cadence-Raven Lyric Roberts, Berkeley-Fionn Kings-

ton Roberts, Beau-Harper Levi Roberts, Cambria-Sage Kassady Roberts, Bentley-River Kai Roberts, Cabriola-Ireland Lacey Roberts, Avery Deanne Hiscock, Beck Thomas Coyle, Bentley Aaron Coyle, Ethan Arthur Cyr, Hope Anne Marie Cyr, Wesley Parker Hughes, August Hughes, November Hughes, March Hughes, Matilda Grace Hewitson, Finn Donald Brooke Millar, Emree Jane Forget . . .

My dad touched my arm when he spotted Zachary's name. Our family regarded the blue dusty script at our feet. *Zachary Jonathan Chute.* My tears speckled the sidewalk like rain.

Once all the families had returned to the field, a woman stood on the stage at the bandshell and began, "When you hear your child's name, you may release your balloon." It was a long list for brief lives, humble and secret lives—babies that were the dreams for futures that would never be— disappearing along with the balloons as they reached higher elevations.

Zachary's name . . .

Our balloon floated quickly into the dusty-blue sky. I locked my gaze on the place it disappeared as if it might change its mind and return.

Week 3: Mourning Together

At the beginning of September I had noticed the Presbyterian church near the grocery store advertising a course on grief called Mourning Together. Aaron and I had not attended church since Zachary's death, not counting those times we visited when photographing weddings. Aaron had grown up in a Christian family; he had never known life without religion's overture. I on the other hand had found faith at a Pentecostal summer camp when I was a lonely and somewhat-existential thirteen-year-old. In the time leading up to Zachary's birth, we prayed and believed. Referencing Matthew 17:20, we said, "Even if our faith is as small as a mustard seed, it can move mountains." In that time we gave our son a name that reflected our hope. *Zachary*: remembered by God.

When Zachary died, I was lost, grieving not only my son but also my faith, the pillars of which crumbled like sand. Searching for a guiding truth or at least to make sense of my absent savior, I called and signed up for the twelve-week Mourning Together course. Aaron opted out. "I don't think I need it," he said.

The first meeting was September 14.

The church glowed from within like a beacon in the dark autumn evening. I found my way through the labyrinthine hallways to the church library. A table with books on loss and a scattering of nametags greeted me at the door. Only one other person entered after me. Aaron and I had visited a support group in the initial months after Zachary died, but it was specific to parents who had experienced a miscarriage, stillbirth, SIDS, or early infant loss. Mourning Together was anything but specific.

"Welcome. Thank you all for coming. My name is Tania," said a rosy-cheeked blonde who stood as she addressed the group. She looked to be about fifty and wore sparkly blue eye shadow. "Let's start by saying our names, who we lost, and our favorite snack." Tania nodded, agreeing with herself. "Tania. My mother died of breast cancer in 2009. And I love Smarties."

Tania gestured to the brown-haired girl sitting next to her, who couldn't have been over twenty-five. "Hi, my name is Eliza. My husband died three months ago. I like doughnuts."

"I'm Mike, and I lost my wife, Lane. Popcorn." Mike slouched down into the dated upholstered chair and crossed his arms. His green eyes were fixed on the table, his face expressionless.

"Hello and welcome. I'm Bruce, a leader here along with Tania." Bruce's voice was deep, like rumbling thunder. He straightened his comb-over of copper-colored hair. "I lost my father and mother in the span of four months back in '05." He paused. "And I like pretzels."

"I am Joe, and this is my wife, Rita." Joe spoke with a French accent and gestured to the tired-looking woman with cropped black-and-silver hair beside him. "Our daughter, Simone, was hit by a distracted driver while riding her bicycle. That was six months ago." Joe leaned back in his chair and looked just as exhausted as his wife.

"And your favorite snack?" Tania chirped.

Joe shook his head and looked at Rita. "Wine gums. We both like wine gums."

"I'm Alexis Marie. My son, Zachary, died just after birth. Peanut M&M's."

"And do you have a partner, Alexis Marie?" Bruce asked. I nodded. "And, so, why did you come alone?"

"I, uh, I don't know exactly. Aaron and I haven't really clicked since, well, you know."

"We would strongly encourage him to come," Tania smiled at

17

me, clasping her hands. I did wish Aaron had joined me, that we could at least grieve conjointly in some manner instead of living emotionally estranged. I promised Tania I'd ask him when I got home. "All right, last but not least . . ." Tania lightly touched the shoulder of a hunched, white-haired granny.

"My name is Martha McLoider, and eight months ago my husband, Ralph, succumbed to congestive heart failure after we'd been married for fifty-four years—but the Lord is good and his grace has sustained me, though many days I am lonesome in my old house. It's much too spacious for one, really."

"Thank you, Martha," Tania interrupted politely. She distributed workbooks, and we watched a short video from a church in Australia.

The tanned video host promised God would heal; I hoped he was right but was not consoled. The promise seemed incompatible with the stories the group had shared moments before, the losses, which irked me as I pictured Hannah and Aaron and my parents. *What if something happens to them?* As the first meeting came to a close, all I could think about was speeding home to check on Hannah while she slept and being so close to Aaron I could feel the warmth of his body thaw my own.

Aaron reluctantly agreed to attend Mourning Together the following week. "I want to support you," he had said, and I introduced him to the group. Everyone was quiet, apart from Joe, who proved to be quite chatty, as we sat around the misshapen rectangular table formed by pushing many smaller tables together. Unconsciously most of us were grouped by our losses. Aaron and I sat beside Joe and Rita. Eliza and Mike sat opposite us. Just like the tables, our group proved a mismatch of personalities and cultures.

"Thank you all for coming tonight," Bruce smiled through his dentures. "You are brave for being here."

Tania cleared her throat. "God says, 'I will turn their mourning into gladness; I will give them comfort and joy instead of sorrow." Jeremiah 31:13." Everyone bowed their heads as she prayed. Aaron knew the heat of my anger toward God and at the idea of a master plan. He glanced at me, and I grimaced back at him while Tania droned on.

✕⊃

At our third meeting, on the last Wednesday in September, the Mourning Together participants gathered again around the hodgepodge tables. "Grieving people expend a huge quantity of energy resuming life's activities," Tania began, reading from her notes. "They embrace busyness to avoid stillness. In stillness we have time to think and feel and acknowledge our loss and its impact on us." Eliza nodded, and Martha sighed loudly.

"I don't want to be still!" Rita barked suddenly, tipping her head in punctuation. The rest of us sat up, startled; it was the first time Rita had spoken since the meetings began. "When I am still I look at pictures, I look in the mirror. I don't want to eat. The world is not real to me." Rita shook her head, lost in thought. Joe put his arm around her.

The room was silent for a moment before Bruce's voice boomed in response. "Your feelings are natural. We have all felt like that. Maybe some here still do."

"I do," I nearly whispered. As I left my Year of Distraction behind, it was the stillness that terrified me.

About fourteen months before that meeting I was happily naive in my pregnancy with Zachary, although we had not yet named him. At my twenty-week ultrasound, everything was perfect. We learned we were having a boy, and Aaron beamed with fatherly pride as he imagined all the sporting gear we'd require. His daydreams were uninterrupted by Hannah, who squirmed in his arms as she grew bored in the darkened exam room. We called our parents over celebratory burgers at Brewster's and took silly family pictures in a photo booth at the mall, holding up a sign that read, "It's a boy!" That was July 23, 2010, and one of the last happy memories during that time.

"God is here for you, Alexis Marie. And for you, Rita," Tania said sweetly.

"But can God decode this mess inside me?" I snapped, doubtful.

"It is okay to be angry, Alexis Marie. God can take it." Bruce was calm. "Would you be comfortable telling us what happened to your son?"

"Yeah, okay." I took a breath, replaying the chronology of my pain. "At the end of August 2010, when I was about twenty-five weeks pregnant, we visited a private ultrasound facility called Baby Before Birth Portrait Studio. It was supposed to be fun." My words choked me, and Aaron took my hand under the table. "The technician said, 'Your baby has Daddy's chin and your blonde hair, Alexis Marie'—but he never said anything about Zachary's heart. At my next prenatal appointment a few days later, my doctor broke the news."

My mind triggered that day: "Hello there, hi," Dr. Stilles had said, entering the patient room swiftly. He seemed distracted as we went through the normal routine, his eyes never meeting mine. His responses were curt and to the point. "Weight, good. Blood pressure, yep. You're measuring about twenty-six weeks now. Okay, okay." His demeanor shifted as he closed my file and tucked it under his arm. He cracked his knuckles. "Baby Before Birth called, Alexis Marie," he said slowly. *That's strange*, I thought; they never phoned Dr. Stilles after I had pictures taken of Hannah.

"I didn't speak with them," Dr. Stilles continued, raising his eyebrows and wiping a hand through his thinning hair as he spoke. "But in their message they said that Baby has an irregular heartbeat."

I couldn't respond right away, although my lips moved in search of words. "An irregular heartbeat," I repeated. "An irregular heartbeat? That's something we can fix, right?" Dr. Stilles did not respond.

"I have booked you in for an ultrasound tomorrow at River Valley Medical Center on the west side. You need to be there." He passed me the exam requisition he'd already typed. "Bring Aaron." I nodded.

Once in my car I called Mom and told her what the doctor had said. "I'm sure everything will be okay," she replied. "They just want to double-check."

⚬

I couldn't meet eyes with anyone at Mourning Together as I continued speaking. "We had another ultrasound the next day. The doctor told us there was extra fluid building up in our son's abdomen, in his lungs and around his heart, where there was a large tumor."

Aaron took over for me. "We were referred to the high-risk clinic at The Arthur Memorial Hospital downtown. They confirmed Zachary's tumor was causing cardiac failure and fluid in his body since his heart was not pumping properly."

"Aaron and I spent every day at the hospital for a month and a half, trying to find a way, but—but there was nothing we could do."

"What caused the tumor?" asked Eliza.

"Zachary had a genetic condition called Tuberous Sclerosis," Aaron answered. "Basically, the gene that prevents tumor growth was altered."

"There was really nothing you guys could do?" Bruce probed. "Surgery? Heart medication?"

"But did you pray to the Lord?" Martha interrupted.

"We did pray. We never stopped praying," I answered bitterly. "And the pediatric cardiologist told us that surgery would be like grating cheese; Zachary's heart muscle would be minced."

"The other option," Aaron began, "was termination—but that was not a road we wanted to go down."

"Praise God," Martha chanted. I ignored her.

Tania's eyes blossomed and reflected the light. "No parent should be faced with those options," she said.

I shrugged and nibbled the skin on my lower lip. "They told me my baby would be stillborn," I sighed heavily.

"We eventually had to induce." Aaron stretched his fingers, which had been clenched into tight balls. "Alexis Marie's health was getting worse. It was like her body was mimicking Zachary's. Scared the crap out of me."

"I was thirty weeks but measuring forty because of all the extra fluid building up in me, just like in Zach. They call it mirror syndrome."

"Alexis Marie was scheduled for induction, but—what I think is pretty cool—she went into labor all on her own the night before."

"Praise God," Martha repeated, tipping her head in a nod that bobbed her scraggly bun like a bird's nest in the wind.

"And Zachary didn't die in the birth canal like the doctors predicted. He moved a little in my arms." I was crying and feeling rather deflated. As always, I ached for my baby as if for a ghost limb. Aaron again took my hand and this time did not let go.

"Zachary didn't cry," Aaron reminisced. "He did not open his eyes—but I peeked. They were blue."

"Blue like our daughter Hannah's eyes, and with her blonde hair, too. Zachary's tiny features were so swollen. His ears were like little sausages," I recalled. "I held him and repeated, over and over again, 'I love you; I love you, Zachary.' He looked so peaceful. I rocked him and sung to him Hannah's song."

"'Twinkle, Twinkle, Little Star,'" Aaron pursed his lips. "Hannah's favorite."

"We bathed him and put him in pajamas. He was already gone. Aaron took Zachary to the window and let the sun shine in on his little body. And he said, 'This is the world.'"

Martha spoke in a crackling voice. "Even if you don't understand, move toward God." She said this not only to Aaron and me but to everyone around the table. "It's too scary not to." I bit my tongue until it throbbed.

Bruce and Tania praised and affirmed Martha words. I couldn't keep quiet. "I was so faithful to God," I said louder than I intended. "Then my son died, and where was he? I felt nothing from any higher power. All I wanted was comfort, love, to feel like there was something more—but nothing. If this is supposed to be a *relationship* with God, then I think he should do something—but all I found was nothing. *Just nothing.*"

"Turn around and you will see the face of Jesus!" Tania's voice quivered.

"Jesus?" I scoffed, no longer crying. "Where was Jesus in any of this?" Martha covered her mouth.

"Alexis Marie, it's okay," Aaron said, always the peacemaker.

"No, Aaron." I gave him a look, and he leaned back in his chair. "How can Christians be so arrogant as to say there is only one way to God? My son never accepted Jesus. What does that mean for him, considering the Christian version of original sin?" I looked at Bruce but didn't give him or Tania or Martha a chance to respond. "And for all those people not born into a Christian culture, you're telling me they just get booted down to hell? Maybe all religions are worshiping the same God."

"That's what I believe," Eliza said evenly.

Joe interjected and began grumbling to Martha while Eliza avoided Tania's cautionary words and probing stare by doodling in her workbook. Bruce spoke over everyone, although no one was listening. I leaned back in my chair like Aaron and whispered, "Oh, shit; what have I done?"

Week 4: Planting and Building

Pine Landing Greenhouse was not busy, despite their autumn sale advertised roadside by a wooden scarecrow holding a sign. Aaron, Hannah, and I wandered the tree nursery for quite some time. My senses were lost in the smell of the place, as if I were retracing my childhood steps through the creek-lined forest of my aunt and uncle's Okanagan acreage.

It was October 14, 2011—what would have been Zachary's first birthday. At Mourning Together the week prior, Eliza had suggested Aaron and I plant a tree in our son's memory. It turned out her family owned a tree farm outside of the city. "Make sure you ask for a hearty tree," she advised. "And blanket it over the winter." Aaron and I agreed on planting two trees: one for Zachary as our son, the other for Zachary as Hannah's brother.

While I couldn't decide what kind of tree I wanted, I could very well articulate what kind I disliked for our backyard. "Not to sound picky . . ." I began, but I stopped when Aaron made a loud sigh. I scowled in his direction, and he looked away to read a tag tied to the arm of a wild-looking bush. "I don't want anything ugly—even if it is rated to minus a million degrees Celsius or it will stand up against a bark-chomping beetle or rocky soil." Aaron did not respond, and Hannah was growing fussy as her naptime approached. He picked her up and perched her on his shoulders, where she squirmed and yanked on his hat.

"We just need to make a decision," he said firmly, and I could read the frustration on his clenched jaw through his stubble. "I think I want an evergreen," he added. "I wouldn't like a plant that lost its leaves and looked like a skeleton all winter."

"Agreed."

A spunky white-haired gentleman in a greenhouse apron shedding soil and pine needles led us down an aisle under the late morning sun, our quickly disappearing shadows struggling to keep up. He stopped us in front of two short evergreens in black plastic pots. *Columnar Dwarf Mugo Pines,* their tag read. "They're perfect," we decided, and, before paying, we snapped a family photo in front of our trees.

Back at home, I put Hannah down for her nap. While Aaron made two trips hauling the trees, I spent a quiet hour alone scrapbooking the Walk to Remember photographs onto zoo-themed pages. Burning beside me was an ivory candle I had decorated with blue ribbon on Zachary's original due date, December 20, 2010. Its shape began to slouch and hollow out as the wax melted and its scent of daisies hung in the air. I wondered how many more birthdays before the candle disappeared entirely.

Once Hannah awoke, the three of us labored in the backyard, sweating under the fall rays in our warm work clothes. Using Aaron's hatchet, I chopped the grass into two large circles on either side of the back gate. Aaron dug deeply with the shovel while Hannah struggled to wield the nozzle on the whipping hose, spraying Aaron and me more than she succeeded in dampening the carved-out holes. The water fight lasted another hour after Hannah got the hang of the nozzle.

"Doesn't that just make you smile?" I said to Aaron and our girl as we peered over the balcony railing at our newly planted pines. "A brother tree and a son tree." In an experience where much had been taken from us with so little visual evidence left behind—besides a few scrapbooks, the hospital teddy bear, and my stretch marks—we suddenly had something that lived.

Zachary's birthday had been spent happily, but as the daylight crept beneath the freshly planted trees in the yard, our sadness slipped into bed with us. We flipped through the photo album of Zach's birth, going back there in memory. We slid our fingers over the photographs, tracing our son's puffy eyelids and the blisters of excess fluid on his chest from his struggling heart. I covered myself in Zachary's fleece blanket, the one we had wrapped him in at the hospital. I wished Mom hadn't washed it; maybe then I could have smelled him on its fibers.

"I miss him so much." Aaron choked up as he wiped his eyes hard with the heel of his palm. I leaned into him and bawled, but rage, too, blazed in my chest. The emotions were dense, esoteric, and the two of us fell silently to sleep.

The next day we were again in the yard, and I found myself glancing at the trees every few seconds. Aaron and our friend Jake were building a shed we had bought four months before in June. Putting the simplistic-looking structure together had proven to be a Herculean endeavor, but Aaron promised to get it constructed before it snowed.

Jake's wife, Megan, and Hannah and I went for a long walk to stay out of the men's way while they oozed perspiration. I had met Megan only once before. Jake had moved to Manitoba to court her while Aaron and I were living in New Zealand, and they had just recently moved back to Edmonton. On our walk, Megan nervously asked about Zachary, and I told her our story and that Aaron and I were trying for another baby—without success.

Megan asked, "If you don't mind, can I see the photographs of Zachary?" Back at the house, with Hannah down for her nap, Megan and I sat on the carpet and flipped through the solitary photo album.

"I think I've given up on finding answers to the *Why* questions. There's no point wondering why bad things happen to good people," I blurted. Until the words were out of my mouth I hadn't realized

I felt that way, but it was true in that moment. "I do wish that God would reach out to me, though," I continued. "All I want is peace."

"What does peace look like to you?" Megan asked, leaning against the wall, her long legs stretching out across the hall.

"Good question," I sighed and paused. "Feeling loved and hopeful, I guess; not feeling alone, knowing everything is going to be okay because God is with me."

"Your idea of peace sounds very nice," Megan said. She was a Christian and was about to say more on the matter of faith when the men began hollering from the yard. They had finished and wanted us to applaud their handiwork. Megan headed out, but I hung back. I had felt a little off the previous few days, thicker somehow, my body sensitive, my nipples sore. *Maybe it's the flu? Or my period—or a baby?* I thought anxiously, then cursed myself for jinxing it.

Don't get your hopes up, I said to myself. *It's too early to check. Why throw away another test at ten dollars a pop?* My nonchalance was a facade. Even though it often took well over a month for pregnancy hormones to show up on a pee-stick, I'd grown addicted to testing. *Screw it! No one has to know.* I tore open the crunchy plastic packaging and plunked myself down on the porcelain, letting myself go. Placing the test facedown on the counter, I washed my hands slowly. More soap. Slather, rinse. *How long has it been? Oh, whatever!* I flipped the test.

Are my eyes playing a trick on me? There were two pink lines: one strong, the other barely visible. When I stared at them too long I thought my desire must be projecting the second, but when I looked away and then back again, it was still there. Two lines. Two tiny pink lines.

I dashed through the house, skipping stairs, and ran onto the balcony that overlooked the backyard. The shed was built, and everyone was standing on the grass admiring the grey plastic structure.

"Aaron!" I shouted, holding the test behind my back. "You guys, I have an announcement to make." Aaron, Jake, and Megan looked up at me, squinting in the sunshine. "I'm pregnant!" I whooped. Aaron's face wore one distinctly complete emotion after another. Confusion. Acceptance. Relief. Elation.

I revealed the positive test, and Aaron yelled, "Toss it down!" He caught it tenderly. "It's faint, but I see two lines. We're pregnant!" He laughed, breathless, and staggered drunkenly in the grass. In that moment we did not worry about our slight risk of another genetic abnormality.

That would come later.

Week 5: Camaraderie

After announcing the pregnancy to our family and most of our close friends, there was one more person I needed to call. "Hey, Christine," I said.

"Hi, Alexis Marie. Are you all ready for our plans this weekend? I'm excited."

"Christine, I have to tell you something." Silence. I took a deep breath. "I'm pregnant." In the summer, Christine had miscarried her second child, which was then followed by an invasive DNC, the scraping of the uterine wall to remove remaining tissue that had not passed naturally. My friend had always been one to use humor as a decoy, poking fun at others through sarcasm, diverting attention from herself—but after her miscarriage, she wept.

"Hello? Christine?"

Three weeks earlier, at the birthday party of our mutual friend's toddler, we had talked about our losses. In hushed voices to avoid terrifying the children playing at our feet, we had confessed our common anger and made plans to visit a gun range. The goal was to release the feeling of helplessness through pulling the trigger, feeling the kickback and seeing the silhouetted paper target punctured and torn. I would have aimed for the heart. It was supposed to be cathartic.

"Oh," Christine said finally.

"Are you okay?"

"You can still shoot if you are pregnant—as long as you are not too far along," she replied.

"What?"

"I'm on the website." She read me the pertinent gun-safety information. "Lead is expelled as the gun fires. When it's breathed in by a pregnant woman, there is the *possibility* it may be passed from mother to baby—but," she added happily, "if you are early in the pregnancy, it should be fine." Her tone was pleading, although she would never admit it, and I reluctantly agreed.

Arriving early, I paced the gun shop, reading and re-reading the waiver printed on flimsy paper. I asked the young tattooed man behind the counter about my situation. "You'll be okay," he mumbled, polishing something he pulled from the display case with a linen square. He checked out my breasts.

"I can't do this. I can't," I said under my breath while loud blasts echoed through the store from the indoor range behind the counter. A father was teaching his ten-year-old son how to aim. More blasts. Each was like a defibrillation to my chest. My heart pounded in my throat, and I rubbed my sweaty palms on the fronts of my jeans and cracked every knuckle. A biker in full leathers entered and pointed to something in the glass case, and the young man reached in. I couldn't watch.

When Christine arrived she looked at my face, and hers instantly fell in disappointment. "You're not gonna do it, are you?"

I panted and shifted from foot to foot. "If anything happened . . . to my baby, anything that I caused and could have prevented, I don't know what I would do . . ." I was unable to stand still, nearing panic.

Christine sighed loudly, not meeting my eyes.

"You can still go," I offered.

"No, no, it's fine."

Christine and I spent the afternoon loitering around the mall like teenagers. We climbed through a ropes course and got strange massages from a kiosk with machines that looked like giant condoms. "It wasn't the same as shooting a gun," Christine said, "but the third level of the course really got my blood flowing." She smiled as we drank Cokes in the lounge of a restaurant on Gateway Boulevard.

"Thank you," I said, and she shrugged.

"So, you're pregnant. How does *that* feel?"

"Like it's going to be the longest nine months of my life."

Christine nodded. "It's going to be so different for me next time too. I'll never feel relaxed. It's gonna be hell." She paused and took a sip. "I was so excited to have another baby. I lost it just before we were going to tell people. A few days later one of my coworkers announced her pregnancy. Of course I didn't want to be Debbie Downer, so I didn't say anything. Now I have to endure this woman's endless gibber-jabber, her pregnancy stories and her baby talk. She's starting to show now, too. If I see her coming down the hall, I avoid her. It sucks. I keep asking myself, *Why me?* You know?"

"I *do* know . . . Aaron and I are going to this church grief group. Mourning Together. The session just a few days ago was about that very question."

"And what was the answer?"

"The leaders sort of skirted it, actually. They tag-teamed a preachy Bible message, and this one woman, Martha, kept shouting, 'Amen.'"

"Oh, God; that sounds like torture. Did they say anything helpful?"

"Well, the evening went kind of like this . . ." I shifted my weight from side to side and changed my voice, enacting Tania and Bruce's script and using Martha's *hallelujah*s as commas. "They said: 'There is no point in asking *Why me?* Instead ask, *Why not me?*'" I mimicked Bruce's baritone. "'Have faith,'" I said in Tania's chipper squeak. "'Death is inevitable because of the fall of Adam.'"

"Oh, man!"

"There's more: 'God has a plan,'" I continued. "'Everything happens to bring him glory.'" Christine shook her head. "'You don't have to know where God is leading you—just follow.'" I took a swig of my Coke.

"They probably said that God doesn't owe us answers."

"Were you there?" We laughed. "Needless to say, I booked it out of there at the end of the night. Aaron and his long legs could barely keep up. I'm not looking for platitudes."

"Some people find religion when life sucks, but it sounds like you're losing it, instead."

I paused. "Yep. And now I'm just a disgusting sinner like everyone else."

"You said it, not me," Christine said slyly.

"I became a Christian as a teenager because I felt like there was something more to life . . . I still do."

"I feel that way too."

"And for a while faith filled that void, you know? But religion muddies it. I want to believe, but when I look at things objectively, there are no answers to prayer."

"That's how my husband feels." Christine swooshed the ice around at the bottom of her cup. "Even if I wanted to go to church he wouldn't go with me. What about Aaron?"

"He grew up Christian. Both his grandfathers were pastors. Aaron's mom is a church secretary. She was babysitting for us that night we went to Mourning Together. When we got home, I asked her to tell me why Christianity is real, to convince me. All she said was that I have to figure it out on my own."

"There is nothing to figure out. You have to take care of yourself, you hear me? We have to take care of each other; that's what's real." I reached across the table and held Christine's hand. "Stop being such a loser; you're making my eyes leak." The waitress refilled our drinks. "So, you've booked in with that high-risk obstetrician this go-around?"

"Um, well, I did schedule prenatal appointments with Dr. Barker—but I'm not sure I want to go with her. Yes, she specializes in high-risk pregnancies, but she kept forgetting to read my chart at our appointments. Aaron and I often headed directly to her from an ultrasound at the hospital where the docs there told us it was any day now for Zach—and then Dr. Barker would do a Doppler exam and hear there was still a heartbeat and say something like, 'Sounds all right to me.' Then she'd check our record on the computer and have to backtrack."

"Brutal."

"So I also booked in with Dr. Stilles . . . just in case."

"Cover your bases. That's good. Seriously, though, I don't know how you are so calm right now. I'm going to be a fricken basket case next time."

"If only you could feel my heart racing." I lifted my hands into the air in front of me. They trembled.

As I drove home after my afternoon with Christine, I nearly skidded onto the shoulder as a torrent of emotion suddenly overshadowed my excitement of having another baby. The landscape of my joy darkened like the prairies to the south along the Anthony Henday Highway beneath the ever-shifting cloud cover. I shivered.

Nature, be good to me, I whimpered as I drove on autopilot. *God—or whatever your name may be—please help me get through this pregnancy. Give me strength. Calm my heart. Protect my child. Please, be with my baby. Please . . .*

Week 6: Get Me Out of Here

Aaron drove to Mourning Together while I leaned against the passenger door and watched snow-covered suburbia blur beyond my window. The storm pond behind our yard had iced over; the shimmering golden-orange reflection from the path lights that lined the trail were unmoving as if frozen in the sudden chill. Winter had begun.

Mourning Together had morphed into weekly penance I begrudgingly paid to the god of grief. I once thought I'd find strength in the presence of shared sorrow—and faith to go on—but that was before the theological debates began and my growing restlessness in religion was left unredeemed by clichéd spiritual jargon. Aaron honored his commitment to attend despite my failing resolve.

"This week our topic is the grief that follows the suicide or murder of a loved one," Bruce began, and he read a Psalm. I understood the course must account for all causes of death, but if I had realized the topic before leaving the house I would have persuaded Aaron to stay home with me to cocoon on the couch and watch *Big Bang* reruns instead.

"Hello, Alexis Marie," Martha said, smiling so that her eyes were barely visible behind her wrinkles. "Have you picked out a baby name yet?"

"Not yet." I feigned a grin and sat down in my usual spot.

"She's only a month along," Tania chimed. "Lots of time."

Martha was not the only one who spoke of my pregnancy as if it were a certainty. Since announcing I was expecting, I had people ask all kinds of definitive questions. "Are you excited to have another baby in the house?" "How are you going to handle the lack of sleep?" "Are you going to breastfeed?" "Are you hoping for a boy or a girl?"

There was a part of me that didn't believe I was actually pregnant, and another part that wondered how long it would last. I was not thinking about first or middle names, Pampers versus Huggies, or even gender; I wondered how life could endure within me in the presence of my history. The Passover had come, but the blood on my door was not enough. Was not my body consecrated for death? My genetic helix a distorted and unsteady ladder? I could not see into the future; it was a blackout.

Bruce and Tania reenacted their weekly bit, fumbling with the sound in the darkened room while the lips of the video host moved along silently. "Can I help?" Aaron asked, and in less than a minute the audio blared from the speakers. Rita covered her ears. The people featured in that week's video had alarming stories about their children being accidentally shot in the head or a spouse who overdosed on drugs.

My mind wandered. I thought of my younger self back as a hypersensitive teen and young adult, fighting through suffocating stretches of clinical depression. I would rub my wrists with a butter knife and hold my breath underwater in the bathtub, testing myself, searching for the narrow line between dead and alive. Thankfully, I never found it. *You are a fucking coward*, I would tell myself back then, as the realization of physical pain was more terrifying than the release from it.

Suicide is a way to be heard, I had reasoned. Yet I never thought about the true depth of heartbreak I could inflict. Not until having a child of my own. Then I understood.

As the Mourning Together video continued, I began to think of Hannah, who was a few weeks away from turning two. What if she grew up to be like me, with a tendency toward melancholy? What if her thoughts ran black and she used something sharper than a butter knife? My notes in the Mourning Together workbook were few, only random scribbles that bled together beyond readability through the tears I could not dam.

I can't lose Hannah.

I can't lose any more children.

I cannot lose Hannah.

I cannot lose this baby.

I can't lose another child . . .

The first-trimester illness had begun a week before. My stomach heaved like white-capped sea curls in a squall; each day I was nauseous, agitated, and fatigued. Yet I actually relished the semi-torturous state. It was my one evidence, the solitary external demonstration of my internal workings—but what I experienced while watching the screen at Mourning Together that night was not morning sickness.

The video ended, and as Tania rose to flick on the lights, I was already partway out the library door. I sprinted to the end of the hall to the single unisex bathroom and turned the lock with a *thwack* behind me. Stumbling around in circles in the tiny porcelain-tiled space, my body lurched forward as my mind was ravaged by fatal premonitions. My shoulders jerked up with each erratic breath, and I bounced off the walls while my thoughts ping-ponged off the inside of my skull.

I cannot lose any more children!

I held my head, rocking forward. The mother in me wept, wanting to protect, but since Zachary's death I had known all too well that such control was a dangerous illusion. It danced seductively, taunting, tempting. My dread turned inward. I wondered how I was going to survive my pregnancy without knowing—at any point, with any amount of certainty—if my child was going to live or die. *And then what if he or she does live but chooses to jump off the High Level Bridge?*

I wrapped my arms around my midsection and leaned over the toilet, gagging painfully, my tongue pressed to the back of my throat. Fevered tears and sweat washed my flushed cheeks; saliva dripped from my chin. My eyes strained to focus as I shuffled drunkenly at the foot of the toilet.

"Alexis Marie?" Aaron asked through the door. *Bang, bang, bang.* "Let me in." I did somehow.

Aaron held me like a child, letting the door slip shut behind him. His large arms encompassed my trembling body, and my breathing decelerated. I calmed, like a swaddled baby. *Where was this man after Zachary died?*

"I can't take this," I said. "This is too much. Please get me out of here."

We left the bathroom and headed up the long hall past Bible-verse posters and Sunday-school rooms. We had to pass the library door to exit the church, but before we did, Aaron leaned in to my ear. "Just keep walking. I'll grab our stuff. I'm taking you home."

Week 7: Waiting Rooms

It was an unpleasant morning in which I was a puppet, string-bound in the reenactment of fatal memories. The alarm screamed, and Aaron and I showered in shifts with our eyes half open and hustled to feed Hannah before Mom arrived to babysit. Aaron and I then set off on the familiar drive to the hospital at sunrise.

The shop names along the way were imprinted in my mind, and I could list a string of them from home to hospital. I knew which buildings were brick and which were stucco and weathered, which curb the hobo with a shopping cart full of sticky bottles had made home and where the Catholic Social Services building sat at a perfect cross in the road.

While I saw all these things, I was by then blind to them as well: a passenger disillusioned by the predictable shuffle of urban life on a well-worn route. The activity of the city, its multi-textured facades, and even the very shadows on the street were the same that day as they were every day of the month and a half leading up to Zachary's death. *Are we then or now? What day is it? Am I dreaming?*

Aaron and I chitchatted in the car as he drank a Tim Horton's half-and-half and I sipped a hot chocolate. Mom had brought them for us, along with a box of Tim Bits for Hannah, which always angered me.

"Stop it, Mom," I had said every morning as we left for our daily ultrasound of Zachary's heart. "She's not even a year old; give it a rest." Every morning. Why should I expect anything to be different fourteen months later?

The drive took forty minutes through rush-hour traffic, and I was cold in the brisk fall air that slipped in between the seams of our car. My wet hair that I hadn't had time to dry sat coolly against my neck. My purse was propped on the floor between my feet, spilling medical records, a worn notebook, water bottle, snacks, and the gloves required in the wintery chill of that November morning. Our appointment was in the boxy Huntington Medical Facility across the street from The Arthur Memorial Hospital, and we slipped down its icy drive into the expensive underground parking.

Ding! The elevator doors opened. Aaron and I rode to the twelfth floor to see Dr. Barker, the high-risk obstetrician who had delivered Zachary. Already her waiting room was full. My knees wobbled as we entered and checked in; I wished I were anywhere else. The air was stale, almost as if the dust of death lingered in its air-conditioned circulation—but we were not there to discuss death. Life, the early bud of life, had brought us back to that place.

Dr. Barker's standard procedure with pregnancies that followed losses such as ours was to begin with an ultrasound to inspect early fetal development. We had booked the appointment with Dr. Barker's nurse over the phone. I was more than eager to have a quick peek at my baby.

"What do you think they are going to see?" I whispered to Aaron, who sat beside me in the waiting room, passing the time with Stickman Golf on his phone. He shrugged and shook his head. He seemed so calm, as if our errand were normal. A tall technician in a shrunken white coat and similarly tight pants called my name, and Aaron and I followed him silently through a winding hall.

"This way," the technician said, directing us with his broad hand.

The washroom-sized exam room had a patient table in the corner; a monitor mounted to the wall across from where I lay, midriff bare; and a wheeled cart holding the ultrasound keyboard and devices. The technician neither smiled nor apologized for the temperature of the gel he squeezed messily onto my belly.

"Oh m' gosh!" My skin goosebumped instantly, but he was already digging into my abdomen with the wand as if scooping freezer-burnt ice cream. He paid no attention to my shudder. As Aaron and I watched the monitor, black-and-white abstractions twirled and morphed like lead flecks pulled to and fro by a magnet. We squinted, attempting to decipher a hidden-image puzzle, yet there was nothing familiar.

"I am going to do an internal ultrasound now," the technician barked. "Take off your pants and underwear; cover up with this." He tossed me an onionskin-thick paper blanket. "I will be back in a moment."

Aaron saw panic shadow my face. "Um, why do we need that?" he asked, the technician already a step out the door.

The tall man turned slightly. "I cannot see enough; she is too early." His eyes flashed to me as if it were my fault.

"But it can't be good for the baby to have something poked around in there . . ." I interjected slowly.

"It's fine." He turned again to leave.

"Wait, please, wait . . ." I almost cried; the technician turned back toward us, blinking slowly as if humoring children. "Are there any risks?" I asked.

"Well, everything has risks," he sighed as he swiveled on his heel back into the room and closed the door. "All I can see externally is the gestational sac in the uterus."

Oh, that's what we saw; the gestational sac. It had looked like a short alien robot with a large base, probably concealing wheels for mobility, I imagined, and a rectangular screen for a face. The technician wanted to get closer to that face, to see within its four walls to the nearly invisible embryo I carried.

"What risks specifically?" Aaron probed.

"There is a very small risk of miscarriage," the technician said plainly, as if a miscarriage was like missing the bus. No big deal. Just catch the next one.

I shook my head. "No. No way. My answer is no."

"We are so early on," Aaron reminded me.

I finished his thought. "We can wait."

"Fine. I'll book you back in ten days," the technician said curtly as he left the room. Aaron helped me wipe the sloppily applied gel from my skin. Despite not seeing my baby, I was not jaded by the appointment, although I too, like the technician, wished to probe deeper for certainties. Instead, I was content, proud at defending the balance of information and patience. At defending my child.

Aaron and I rode the elevator to the ground floor of Huntington Medical Facility and crossed the street to The Arthur Memorial Hospital. One blood test remained outstanding to conclude what had begun as genetic testing following Zachary's death. The discovery of my enlarged heart had confused the cardiologist, and he'd referred me from one specialist to another, and finally to Dr. Ellison, whose specialty I could not pronounce. I had put off Dr. Ellison's blood work for over a month, and I would have put it off forever, but I had an appointment booked with him at the end of the week. He was my last referral. After Dr. Ellison, the cardiologist would confirm his suspicion: I was a small woman with a mysteriously large heart.

I hated The Arthur Memorial for its unchanging appearance, and its effect on me was palpable. My stomach acid grew sour, though my mouth was dry and chalky. I avoided touching the hospital's buttons and handles, using my sleeve instead of my fingers. The sterile-smelling hallways under florescent lights, the droopy-eyed patients in faded blue hospital gowns towing IV drips as they retraced their steps a thousand times; it very well could have been the year before.

We found the hospital blood clinic and waited in another room overflowing with people. Aaron pulled out his phone and resumed his game as I flipped through dated magazines, their pages so worn they fell from their spines. My name was called, and I followed a stout female technician to the back room, where I sat down for the test, turning away so I did not see the blood sucked out my bulging vein vial by vial. I was surprised I had anything left to give.

My adrenaline continued to buzz days after the ultrasound at Dr. Barker's office. Standing up to the technician was a balm to the sting of helplessness, awakening in me the empowered voice of advocate. No longer would I blindly trust that others looked out for my best interests. As Mom always said, "No one cares as much about your children as you do."

Ring! I held the receiver tightly in my sweating palm as I waited for someone to answer.

"Good morning. Dr. Ellison's office. How may I help you?"

"Hi, my name is Alexis Marie Chute. I'm supposed to have an appointment with Dr. Ellison tomorrow. About some bloodwork. I was really hoping I could get the results over the phone."

"Um, okay, well, we don't do that." The receptionist paused. "If the doctor says he needs to see you—"

"So my son died—and I have seen so many doctors—I just can't . . ." I pulled off my chunky glasses and wiped my eyes. I had grown to loathe waiting rooms, doctors' exam tables, blood tests. By then I was reading between the lines of medical reports and interpreting the creases on the foreheads of the technicians as I was being examined. I sighed, wishing to be naive to that reality. "I just can't bring myself to come in . . . Please . . ."

"Okay, okay." I could tell the receptionist was pondering how to relay my request to her boss. "I'll talk to Dr. Ellison. I don't know what he'll say. I'll call you back."

"Thank you so much. I really appreciate it." Blowing my nose, I rested back in my desk chair.

Ring! Ring!

That was fast. "Hello?"

"Hi, I'm calling from Dr. Ellison's office. I spoke with the doctor, and he reviewed your test results. He said everything is good. You don't need to come in."

"Thank you." I hung up quickly, as if the doctor might change his mind.

Week 8: Gummy Bear

Ten days had passed, and it was my follow-up ultrasound at Huntington Medical Facility. There were nine people in the large square waiting room. Seven women, two men. My eyes traced the arcs of the round bellies. Were the babies cocooned within waiting for death? Maybe those mothers-to-be were still praying for a miracle, as I had been with Zachary, and as I was in secret every day of my pregnancy that followed. No one in the waiting room met my eyes.

"So what is life really all about?" I asked Aaron. "Remember what you wrote in my journal a few months ago?" Aaron wrinkled his brow, reluctantly looking away from his game.

"Remind me."

"You basically said there is more to the human experience, more than just being born, working, having a family, dying." He nodded but didn't seem to recall.

"What's on your mind?"

"I don't know. I'm stuck in this birth-to-death-to-birth-to-death cycle—accelerated. We have a baby and lose a baby in the same breath. I don't know. I just need something to ground me, to look forward to."

"Well, isn't that what you have now, with this pregnancy?" I did not answer. "There is a lot in life that is not guaranteed, Alexis Marie."

"I know! Don't you think I know that?" Again I counted the bodics in the waiting room, grumbling under my breath. Three women were asleep; one snored and bobbed her head. "Maybe we shouldn't talk about this here. I don't want to be in a bad mood for the ultrasound. This should be a happy time. Fuck. I'm just so fucking scared."

"Don't swear."

"What does it matter?"

"Let's keep talking," Aaron said, and he straightened his hat. "There is a lot of love in the human experience. That is something worth thinking about." He was right. Even though Zachary's death weighed me down like a heavy rain, stronger still was my love for my children, which rainbowed over all the heartache.

A nurse called into the room. Every woman wished it were her name on the manila-colored chart. The snoring woman got up slowly, her belly weighty; she had the thirty-plus-week waddle. All eyes in the waiting room watched her go. Another name was called, another eager departure. Five women were left, and two men.

The day of the ultrasound was also Hannah's second birthday. Aaron and I planned to meet Mom and my stepdad, Ken, and the birthday girl at The Keg for a steak dinner. An owl cake with rich chocolate icing applied like feathers awaited Hannah back at our house. Her birthday party would be the following Saturday.

I was antsy to celebrate my girl—and what I hoped would be a healthy check-up of Baby Number Three. When I thought of Hannah, I couldn't help but smile, even as I waited in that clinic where dreams for unborn children were torn from parents' hands. My love for Hannah was the one certainty in that place of constant flux. If I had the slightest possibility of mothering another little life, as I had with Hannah the previous years, all the vulnerability to heartache would be worth the risk.

Still, I wished I had been left untouched by so intimate a death as Zachary's, for Hannah's sake. "You'll be an even better mother for Hannah," Mom frequently told me. "And for

Baby Number Three—because of all the things you've been through, all the things you've survived."

Is Mom right? I wasn't sure. Whenever Hannah saw me cry, a look of concern would spread across her brow; she understood more than her words allowed her to express. *Don't grow up too soon, my girl!*

"I'm okay, Hannah. Happy tears!" I would feign a goofy grin and lie to my daughter—because I had no idea how to protect her. I hoped to one day embody Mom's words, to one day understand the benefit of such a turbulent road. My heart ached to be the got-it-together mother who could give Hannah a childhood free of worry, but I was not that person anymore.

ᛉ

"I need good news today," I told Aaron without looking at him. "I need it." With that thought, a short, round woman appeared at the waiting-room entrance and called for me.

"Alexis Shoot." She pronounced my name incorrectly, but I leapt from my seat with pleasure, eager for the appointment and also delighted to have a different technician from the time before. Aaron and I entered the familiar exam room. The technician was shadowed by an intern, to whom she explained every monochrome detail on the screen with added narrative and medical depth as she maneuvered the wand across my skin.

"There's your baby!" she pointed to the screen. "A cute little gummy bear."

The ultrasound showed a tiny, pixilated silhouette with arms and legs that popped out in the shape of stubby cartoon append-ages. The robot of the week before had expanded itself for us. The nurse recorded measurements. "Baby is about eight weeks," she said cheerfully. "About the size of the tip of your finger, with a heart rate of 151 beats per minute. Everything looks good, normal."

"Normal?" Aaron and I both repeated, then looked at each other. The technician didn't realize the significance, but in a word she had delivered the news I craved.

Week 9: Birthday Party

Hannah's first birthday party had been three weeks after Zachary's memorial service. Our house was crowded with family and friends. Hannah opened her presents; the sound of ripping paper signaled a thrilling game, and all the toddlers shuffled over to play. I'd catch the eye of a friend or one of my parents from across the room, and we'd smile faintly at each other for a full five seconds before turning away.

A few asked outright, "How are you doing?" I appreciated their concern, but I stumbled over my response.

"Fine. Good. Well, yeah. Um, okay." What could I say at the party without flooding the house with salty tears and then drowning in them?

After Hannah's first birthday party, the streamers stayed up for weeks and the balloons wilted and wrinkled, drooping a little more each day until they hung from the walls like rotten bananas. We baked pre-made lasagna every night, food gifted to us around the time of Zachary's death. I was thankful for Hannah's presents, the new toys and books; they were a welcome distraction for us both.

Hannah's second birthday party was altogether different. We lived in a new house, and I was expecting a baby instead of being just weeks past the death of one. The compassionate glances and sympathy smiles of the year before were replaced with chipper catches of the eye and relieved expressions. I was still asked how I was, but the question was accompanied by a downward gaze at my belly and the addition of the word *feeling*.

"How are you *feeling*?" friends and family asked, referring to my first-trimester morning sickness with Baby Number Three.

"Good. Yeah, *feeling* good." I gave them the same awkward head bob as the year before. "Nauseous," I added, but I did not mention my secret fears. After losing a child, there is no naivety, no easy pregnancy; not a day that goes by without heart-stabbing, headache-inducing, make-you-go-crazy fear—fear of what some days seemed an inevitable death. Two deaths, actually, for I did not think I could survive it again.

An hour after Hannah's party, the Happy Birthday banner and streamers were put away. We stored the extra cupcakes in the freezer. *Hannah is two years old.* In some ways it did not make sense. I had a distorted perception of time; it seemed immaterial, liquid, some moments thick while others were thin and fleeting. My days were mysterious. While I taught Hannah to count to ten and ride her princess trike, I also possessed, in tandem, a collection of dreams for my son as he grew and was a part of the world. His absence took on its own presence in our family, and its shadow was long and dense.

Week 10: Baby's Cry

Birth. A baby's instinctual gasp for air and startled cry. The first time it knows its own voice. The air is cold. The light is bright and fires arrows into the brain. Many hands, skin to skin. Stretching. Sound: loud, sharp, soft, sweet. Baby wails at it all. Recollection did not serve me well. It seemed so long ago since Hannah was born that I could not remember the sound of her first cry.

Zachary did not cry. Not one sound. His delivery seemed silent to me—all voices, every audible noise, muted in unimportance. The doctor and nurses must have spoken, Aaron and I both wept, our camera clicked in Mom's hands, yet none of it registered. I have the photographs but no memory of how they were taken. Everything moved in half-speed as there was nothing to rush for. Those were the only moments we had, and they labored themselves. That experience became my point of reference, and I could not envision Baby Number Three's entrance unfolding in any other way.

My first prenatal appointment at Dr. Stilles's office began with the standard weight documentation and pee test for sugars. As I obeyed the nurse's instructions—*Step onto the scale now. Pee into this cup. Bring the test strip back to your room when you are done*—I wondered if she knew my history. The procedures seemed trivial. I was onto larger issues with a bigger vocabulary. *Rhabdomyoma. Hydrops fetalis. Tuberous Sclerosis. Mirror syndrome. Cyst. Tumor. Fetal echocardiogram. New normal.*

Hannah and I did not wait long before Dr. Stilles entered the patient room smiling. He likely weighed no more than a hundred pounds, but his presence and demeanor were encompassing. He had short cropped grey-brown hair and wore a fitted olive collared dress shirt beneath the long white coat. "I'm glad to see you! How are you feeling?"

I nodded, taking a deep breath before answering. "Okay. Nauseous—and nervous."

He pulled out a multi-layered paper wheel, spinning the front level of stiff cardstock to determine my due date. "June 25, 2012. A summer baby. That will be nice." His confidence made me jittery. "Do you want to hear Baby's heartbeat?" he asked.

"Please." I pulled Hannah close to me, both of us sharing the narrow exam table. Hannah had been playing a *Dora the Explorer* game on my phone, but it held no interest once Dr. Stilles squirted a generous glob of translucent blue gel onto my relatively flat stomach.

"Mommy?" Hannah stuck her hand in it. "Ewww! Yucky," she gasped as she pinched the sticky substance between her fingers and thumb, disgust twisting her face. I wiped her hand clean in mine.

"It's pretty rare to hear a heartbeat this early," the doctor warned as he searched around my lower abdomen with the wand. "But it's worth a try!" Hannah and I listened quietly.

Bah bum, bah bum, bah bum.

Hannah's face lit up and she clapped her hands. Dr. Stilles held the angle of the wand steady, and we listened to the baby's heartbeat through the single speaker. The doctor's shoulders eased as he exhaled fully and nearly chuckled, looking as relieved as I felt in that moment. Hannah turned and looked to me to match her enthusiasm at such an alien yet wondrous sound, but her expression fell as she noticed the tears running from the edges of my eyes and across my cheeks and trickling into my ears.

"It's okay, Hannah. Listen! There's a baby inside Mommy's belly," I said. *Hold it together!* "Hannah, do you hear that? It's our baby."

"It's a good, strong heartbeat," Dr. Stilles said as he used the wand to wipe most of the gel from my abdomen. Sitting up, I dabbed my face dry on my sleeve, and Hannah and I exchanged a silly glance before she reached again for my phone.

The doctor was about to leave, but I could not bridle myself any longer. "How am I supposed to do this?" I blubbered, beginning to cry. Dr. Stilles passed me a tissue box. "I am so stressed. This is terrifying!"

He nodded, staring at me with authority in his brown eyes that held my gaze. He gestured as he spoke, using my chart as a prop. "You do it by taking a cognitive approach and speaking positively to yourself. You have a 50 percent success rate with your pregnancies thus far. Hannah is alive; she counts for 50 percent— more than 50 percent." I didn't debate the doctor's math. "Your genetic testing gives us the best possible platform to move forward. I have been delivering babies for twenty years, and I've never before seen a case like Zachary's. You and Aaron and Hannah are all fine. Trust me. It would be very unlikely for this type of thing to happen again. Unlikely."

"As unlikely as being struck by lightning?" The odds of a fetus having Zachary's condition shared the same probability.

"Look at your daughter; she is perfect." Hannah peeked up from her game, giving what I could only describe as a *Yeah, Mom* look. Dr. Stilles said all the right things, all the words I needed to hear, but I was too far gone. My hands trembled, so I sat on them, my wedding ring digging into my ass. My large heart played hard against my ribs, but not in the soothing rhythm we had heard with Baby Number Three. *Fuck, get it together*, I yelled in my head.

As I rambled through tears and snotty tissue, I somehow stumbled upon the fact that I had visited Dr. Barker's office. "You know you don't have to go with her, right?" Dr. Stilles looked me squarely in the eyes. "I have access to the same resources she does. The choice is up to you. You decide what your healthcare will look like. That's the beauty of living in Alberta."

"I'll talk to Aaron about it," I said, but once the words were out of my mouth I realized that talking to Aaron presented its own challenges.

$\wp$

After the previous week's Mourning Together meeting I had asked him, "Want to talk about tonight?"

"What is there to talk about?"

"Actively pursuing our healing, the subject of the meeting tonight? What about that?"

"Yeah, trying to heal is a good thing to do." We were quiet for a while.

"Or we could talk about why you never tell me where you're at," I huffed suddenly. Aaron returned an angry look, but I didn't give him a chance to speak. "We could talk about the fact that you never bring up Zachary anymore. Or that you haven't touched my stomach once since I told you I'm pregnant."

"What do you want me to say?"

"You're like a parked car, and I'm trying to tow you along!" I fumed, my jaw locked tight. "Yes, you support me—which I appreciate—but you never open up. You go to work and come home and talk all night about your stupid job. It felt like you abandoned me when I needed you the most, and now you think everything is okay between us. I'm terrified about this pregnancy, but you don't even care!" I did not, at that time, understand the deep undertow of male grief.

"How can we make our marriage better if you always see the negative?" Aaron hissed back at me.

"I'm trying here."

"Me too. But if we are going to get through this you have to forgive me. You have to trust me again. I've learned; I won't leave you next time."

"Next time?"

"I didn't mean it that way."

Week 11: Painting

I watched Hannah work in the art studio in our basement for months while my fingers itched for my paint-encrusted brushes, for blank canvas, paper, pens, and unnumbered hours spent in trancelike meditation of material, texture, line weight, flow, and color. I missed the magic of the first brushstroke, the ugly underpainting, experimentation, and the *happy accident*. I wished to work late into the night, the shifting shadows the only revelers in time's eclipse as I lost myself and found myself and lost myself again and again in the work.

When we moved into our new house six months after Zachary died, Aaron and I fixed the basement and set it up as a studio. It was a bright, south-facing space, a walkout with one wall of large windows that funneled the sunshine. We set up my tall wooden easel in a nook by the windows, a space I shared with a blue tub of splintery building blocks, an A-frame easel for Hannah, and a plastic kid's drafting table I'd found at a garage sale for five dollars.

I sewed together canvas and plastic-lined painter's drop cloths and spread them across the floor to catch careless drips. Aaron built a long rectangular table out of three smaller tables for Hannah and me to share. I covered it with a piece of white waterproof fabric intended for the seat cushions of motorboats. Random storage units surrounded our table and easels in which I tidied my supplies into well-organized white boxes, all clearly labeled. I did everything but make art.

After setting up the studio I intended to paint right away, but my Year of Distraction demanded other priorities. I found my commercial photography business the ideal escape to drown in without it seeming suspicious. Art was dangerous. Creativity set wild in me painful secrets best suffocated beneath the surface. If I surrendered myself unguarded to its processes, I might have acknowledged the sharp regret that I did not die in Zachary's place, and the even-more-terrifying reality in that, spiritually speaking, I had.

In putting the hectic pace of my Year of Distraction behind me, I gradually began to putter in the studio, creativity stirring, yet I was tentative and did not know where to start. In the meantime, Hannah used the space well. I gave her plastic yogurt lids where I squirted blobs of washable gouache and then let her be free, within reason. Hannah usually painted on a long rectangular piece of paper I tore from a roll on her easel. She stood on a chair and mixed her paint into a puddle of swamp-water brown, making a few graphic strokes before painting her nails, then the palms of her hands, and eventually the tops of her feet in a clever deception that looked like shoes.

My brushes, on the other hand, sat dry and bristling until one afternoon when I dunked a select few into an old peanut butter container filled with water. Mixing my colors was seductive. They slipped around on my palette and blurred into one another. The actions of my hands, the mixing, stirring, color-pairing, were automatic from years of practice and instinctually pleasurable. Hannah clamored for my attention, hanging on me and pulling my spotted paint apron off my hips. I set her up with paints and paper of her own at the table beside me.

Back before my canvas, I worked intuitively. I chose translucent gold, copper, and titanium-white acrylics and wedged open a can of the tea-biscuit tan we had used to paint the main floor of our house. A gloss and self-leveling gel allowed the hues to spread in wave-like stripes with each brushstroke across the three-foot-by-three-foot primed canvas. The marks stretched like the horizon with an area of warm sunbeam-gold clumped gracefully in small mounds. Turning the canvas ninety degrees, I let the copper drip downward, peachy undertones and flecks of gold trailing behind. The copper created perfect circles as it fell onto the floor at my feet.

My nerves gradually thinned themselves like spilling paint, relieved from the tension of containment, like my sorrows, however briefly allowed to flow. I changed brushes from a fine tip to a bulbous commercial brush I had owned for ten years, which was now stained with deep, crunchy rust on the silver buckle holding its bristles. Changing plans thoughtlessly, I used a paint roller for a time before returning to detail with a medium-spread white bristle.

"Mary Had a Little Lamb" began on our children's playlist, and I hummed along with Hannah as she sang. Barney was up next with the cleanup song. Then "Yankee Doodle." I painted without a plan, without a concept or direction; I didn't need one—hadn't ever needed one, really. My gestures became a rhythm, which became a dance, my feet shuffling and smearing the drips beneath my toes as I worked.

Eventually Hannah needed attention. She was cold, having tossed her outfit an hour before, and was only in her diaper and painted wardrobe. Her chest was covered with greenish-blue squiggles. The fronts of her legs right down to her toes were also adorned in cryptic patterns. The paint was dry and flaky and pulled at her skin. I carried her to the bath, where the water became a swirl of color that slipped down the drain without fuss.

"Hi, Hannah! Hi, Mommy!" Aaron said when he arrived home from work.

"Read to me!" Hannah thrust a book into his hands before he had a chance to remove his winter jacket. They sat on the stairs while Aaron's deep voice humorously animated a few stories in a *Fancy Nancy* anthology. I slipped into the studio and stood a few paces back from my painting, which was drying in the corner. I watched it as if it were slowly slinking along like the clouds, and in some ways it was. Its edges became the border of my vision, and the colors vibrated.

Outside the studio windows the sapphire sky had slipped into caramel; cloudless, silent, and smooth. It told no story of time. The sky was ageless, but I was not. One year was spent, but I looked older by two. In my painting I had added layer upon layer of pigment, some thick, others a wash. The canvas was rich and labored over—in some places begrudgingly, in others with textured grace.

Week 12: The Elephant

It was strange, but I no longer expected to encounter God in church, or at Mourning Together. Yet that was where I found Aaron and myself, since I had committed us to attend the final session. Tania had phoned the week before, and I had answered quickly without checking the caller ID. "We're thinkin' 'bout you," she said sweetly. "The group missed you again last night." I had fumbled through a response, blaming busyness and Hannah's cold. Tania told me only one meeting remained, and I promised our attendance.

The subject of the final session was heaven, and the discussion was evangelically Christian in nature: *A person can't get past the golden gates without Jesus; salvation is a gift of grace not earned by good works; heaven is wonderful—a place without pain or sadness— and our loved ones, if they were also Christian, will meet us there.* All of a sudden Mike, the widower, spoke up and startled us all.

"I'm not a Christian per se," he began. "My beliefs are broader than that, but I do believe my wife, Lane, is in heaven." Bruce and Tania shifted in their chairs and glanced quickly at one other, but Mike paid no heed to their discomfort. His voice was level, deeper than I remembered from the first week, and confident, yet he seemed younger than his weary expression portrayed.

"We didn't go to church. Lane and I didn't accept Jesus into our hearts," Mike continued. The expression on Tania's face, one of pitying disapproval, made me want to crawl across the table and slap her.

"Well, maybe Lane accepted Jesus before she died and never told anyone," Bruce suggested. "We can always hope."

Mike ignored Bruce's comment. "I still vividly remember my last moments with Lane. She lay in the hospital bed. I sat beside her. She had cancer and had shaved her head six months before, but small patches of blonde were growing back. I rubbed her head gently, and she pushed me away. 'I'm not a rabbit's foot,' she said. 'You can't rub me for good luck.' She could always make me laugh."

Mike looked at the table where he leaned forward, his hands folded. "Lane knew it was the end. Then, suddenly, we both felt a strange, almost spiritual vibration enter the hospital room. It stayed there. It took my breath away actually. I knew without doubt that it was a momentary brush with something bigger— then Lane died."

The library was silent. We all still sat in the hospital room Mike described. Still with Lane. Still breathless in the presence of the unexplainable, and still with the God Mike knew—the one I wished to know. Bruce's lower lip trembled slightly. "We should not rush to judgment," he said finally. "We do not know other people's hearts."

"I'm searching, you know?" It was Aaron's voice. "My friend Jake told Alexis Marie and me about an analogy of God as an elephant." Martha snorted. "We humans are blind, and each one of us touches a different part of the elephant."

"Yeah, that's right," I said, remembering. "One person may feel the tusk and know God to be strong but cold and distant. Someone else may touch the skin and experience God as rough and callous yet all-encompassing. Another person may sense the elephant's breath and believe that God is warm and loving."

"But it's all the same elephant," Tania chirped.

"Exactly."

With effort I struggled to mask my excitement as the last session of Mourning Together neared its end. Eliza, Mike, Rita, and I seemed to flip our workbooks shut simultaneously. The tiny library vibrated with energy.

My notes on heaven were sparse and danced between almost illegible scratches and doodles of flowers and geometric shapes. Jesus's heaven was familiar to me. As a youth I had read the Bible cover to cover—twice—and after high school I had studied theology for a year before dropping out to attend art school. Heaven, a year after Zachary's death, seemed as obscure a subject as something viewed through a filthy camera lens. No matter the technical adjustments, the shift in depth of field or shutter speed, details were lost and clarity made irrelevant—but maybe that was the point. For me, in that moment, heaven didn't matter.

Along with my workbook, I also closed my search for God that night—not completely, but in many ways I surrendered to the realization that I had done my part. In my Year of Distraction, I had discussed faith with a Muslim leader who sat beside me on a three-and-a-half-hour flight from Edmonton to Toronto. He shared his beliefs in a graceful and kind manner as I lamented my arduous pursuit of a savior. In the end he said, "I think you have done all you can do. Now it's God's turn." His words resonated at the time, but they again chimed in my ears as I sat inside that Presbyterian church. I wished to be free of structured religion, to know spirituality in an intimately personal manner—and to be found, if there was indeed someone searching at all.

We passed photographs of our loved ones around our misshapen table one last time. Mike spoke of Lane's practical jokes and about the time she literally scared the pee out of him. Rita bragged that her daughter was once the best cyclist in Alberta and that she would bike twenty-five kilometers to Rita's house for dinner every Sunday night. Her food was that good, Rita said. Martha's husband had been a particular man with a peculiar pet peeve. He hated the skins on food, she told us. Martha spent fifty-four years peeling his apples, his potatoes, his cucumbers. Even tomatoes and peppers; she laughed, and her face flickered with remembrance.

Eliza's husband had played professional baseball in Arizona. He gave up the game at thirty-one. They had hoped to have children and teach them to play ball. Bruce's father had hated leftovers. Tania's mother had made quilts. When Tania and her sister packed up their mother's apartment, they had found over two hundred ornately patterned quilts hanging on the walls, stuffed under the beds, and lining the backs of the couches.

Our group leaned in to hear the tangible memories of lives fully inhabited within time and space—but what were Aaron and I to say about our son? His experience of the world was small, although no less affectionate. I could have shared the vivid maternal imaginings I conjured for Zachary's life. He would have been an active kid. He moved around in the womb as if he knew that that was his only chance to stretch, kick, and dance. His weak heart said *Just one more beat, just one more*, for months, until the end, until birth. He had held on so the slippery coolness of air could goosebump his skin just once, so he could listen to the full volume of his father's voice, so just one time he could snuggle to his mother's breast and feel her heart beating from the outside in instead of from the inside out. He was a determined little boy.

"We were so excited to have Zachary be a part of our family," I choked out when it was our turn.

"Oh, my dears," said Tania, batting her eyes and pouting her lips in sympathy. "But at least you have another chance with your next baby." Her gaze dropped from my face to my abdomen as she spoke with such certainty. I smiled, though weakly.

What is certain in life? The cat-and-mouse play of the sun and moon, the patterned ebb and flow of daily tides, or the landscape's subtle shift to radiance each day and faded glory in the night? So it seems, till the tides breach tsunamis and acid rain falls from the sky, burning the skin

of the earth and the work of human hands. Solid ground beneath our feet rumbles and gives way to labor pains at its appointed time, yet without warning. Lives return to the mud and streams. No one can predict it. What is certain? Only death.

I once believed in certainties, in the certainty of certainty, its character trustworthy, reliable to a fault. I once believed in absolute right, absolute wrong, of nature's constant, of God's perfection. My naivety and trust that *everything will be okay* did not survive Zachary; it passed forever along with my son. Certainty followed my child to the grave.

As per my wish, Aaron had begun forming a vocabulary for his feelings and started musing about plans for the coming summer. He proposed we spend lazy afternoons in the yard where Baby and I could sprawl beneath our striped beach umbrella as he and Hannah kicked a ball from fence to fence. Aaron eagerly anticipated walks around the pond with the stroller, camping trips to the Rockies in a few years, and he already brooded over the early months of sleeplessness that were sure to be. He also asked me if I was going to breastfeed and how soon after the birth we should visit our out-of-town family. I grew uncomfortable in these conversations, unsettled by even the tentative formation of plans.

"How can we know?" I said.

"We just have to," Aaron responded, and I could sense my question saddened him greatly.

"It *will* be nice to have the summer together," I managed quickly as I tried to keep him from drifting from me like smoke. With that, the corners of his mouth twitched upward, and I could see in the glaze across his eyes that he was ruminating, even just briefly, on all that I could not see.

Our discussions haunted me.

Will our words betray us?

Tania and Bruce passed around tea lights in sculpted glass holders, and we each brought our little candle to life. "Zachary." Aaron held my hand tightly as he spoke. "I love you. I wish I could have had more time with you." Everyone said "Goodbye" and "I miss you" and "You'll never be forgotten" around the circle.

The mood shifted once we completed the round. Joe rose to refresh his coffee, and Eliza wrapped her knitted scarf around her neck. No one rushed to leave; everyone lingered in small conversations as well wishes for the future were exchanged.

"Oh, Alexis Marie, Aaron," Tania interrupted. "Last week the group filled out evaluations of the program. Since you weren't here, can you do it now?" She passed the paper to Aaron, who was standing with Joe at the snack table. Aaron passed it to me, obviously disinterested as he resumed his conversation.

What should I write? I drummed the table with my nibbled-short fingernails. *The snacks were a highlight, I can write that down.* Each week Bruce and Tania had brought one group member's favorite snack, which we had listed during our first meeting.

I laid the questionnaire on the table and dug into my purse for a pen, when all of a sudden there was a bright light in front of me. My first thoughts were jumbled in confusion. "Fire!" I screamed when the flame's heat warmed my cheek. Instinctively, I jumped to my feet and grabbed the un-burnt corner of the blazing paper before shuffling awkwardly to Aaron, not sure what to do as the flame ate its way toward my fingertips. Aaron took the paper and swiftly dunked it in the jug of water beside the snacks.

All eyes stared at me blankly. "What . . . what was that?" I stammered.

"You put the questionnaire on top of Zachary's tea light," Aaron whispered.

"Tell me what you really think," Tania said, half joking.

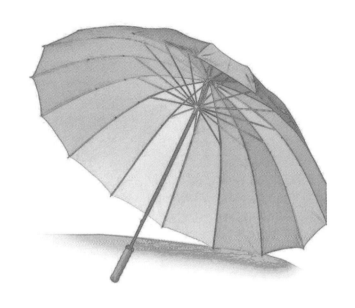

PART 2

SECOND TRIMESTER

Week 13: See Zachy

There were Zacharys everywhere. My senses were
heightened, my ears pricked in interest like a horse hearing things
from great distances beyond its periphery. The sound of even the
softest-spoken *Zachary* had me spooked, ready for flight.

There was a Zachary in Hannah's gymnastics class. The coach
read the roll call of aspiring toddlers each week before warm-up:
"Matthew, Hudson, Hannah, Zachary . . ." Each time, I was startled
at the sound of his name and saddened by the eager little boy who
raised his hand as he sat with his mother on the foamy blue floor.
Her Zachary was present.

There was also a Zachary on the three-and-a-half-hour flight
Hannah and I took to Phoenix, Arizona, to visit my parents at
their vacation home. My girl, full of two-year-old energy, bounced
from my lap to her seat by the window and back again as if she
were still in gymnastics, contained but for her screams of delight.
A mom and her two kids sat in the row behind us. Her son was,
of course, named Zachary, and, as any caring mother would, she
used her son's name often and lovingly throughout the flight.

"Do you want a snack, Zachary?"

"Zachary, are you cold? Do you want my blanket?"

"Almost there, Zach!"

He looked to be nearly eight and wore a baggy lime-green T-
shirt. He was well behaved and ate from a Spiderman lunch box
his mother gave him. He played a Game Boy on his lap. I grew
motion-sick.

As the passengers waited to deplane, Hannah stood on her seat, peeking with curiosity at the people behind us. The boy named Zachary saw Hannah and hid behind his inflight magazine, popping his head around its spine to peek-a-boo at her. Hannah screamed with laughter when she caught on to the game.

As the first row began to file out the cabin door, everyone else shuffled in readiness and impatience. In those last moments on the plane I had the illogical urge to turn to the mother who had sat behind Hannah and say, "I lost my son, Zachary. About a year ago." The strange thing was that I simply wanted her to know.

Hannah did not adjust well to the time change from Edmonton to Phoenix. She slept fitfully, and the nights were drawn out like a necklace, beaded with successive scream-filled wakings before she rose for the day at dawn. The room I slept in was attached to Hannah's by a Jack and Jill bathroom. I brushed my teeth and washed my face in near silence, but inevitably she'd start screaming an hour after I had fallen asleep.

It was almost 5:00 a.m. Hannah and I were sitting on the leather sofa after a jarring night terror, and together we slipped into a cozy slouch. Hannah, more alert than I, plunked a *Dora the Explorer* book on my lap. It was about becoming a big sister; Dora was on an adventure to get home and see her mommy's new baby.

"Hannah, Mommy's having a baby, too," I said, half asleep.

"Baby?"

"Yes, you are going to be a sister."

"See baby." She furrowed her brow, looking around the room.

"Your little brother or sister is in here," I said, pointing to my belly.

"Brother," she said, and the word startled me. *What if I have another boy? Will events repeat themselves?* Hannah looked at me ardently. "See Zachy," she said. Hannah had attended Zachary's memorial, she had played with the teddy bears we collected and donated to the hospital in her brother's name, and she had surely heard me weep in the nursery across the hall from her room—and she'd listened as Aaron and I argued during dinner. She knew. I was having a baby, but Hannah and I were both still searching for the child that came before.

"Hannah hold Zachy," she continued.

"Oh, Hannah, that would be nice, wouldn't it?"

"Zachy hold it Hannah's hands." She raised her palms as if cradling a tiny bird and rocked them quickly back and forth.

My emotion constricted my throat, my voice an octave higher, and I couldn't help but cry, "Mommy misses Zachy *so much.*"

Hannah was fed up with talk. "See Zachy," she whined with a pout. "*Zachy* hold it Hannah!" she yelled.

"Zachy is not here." I rubbed her face, brushing her long bangs away from her eyes. "But if he was, would you . . . tickle him?" I wedged my fingertips into her armpits and tickled around her stomach; Hannah giggled and flopped back on the couch. I kissed her cheeks and neck. Her neck was ticklish, just like mine.

"Hannah tickle Zachy belly," she said and wiggled her fingers in the air in front of her nose.

"Would you . . . tickle his toes, too?"

"No," she looked at me sternly.

"Oh, okay. No toes. Would you—" I thought for a moment. "Would you say *Love you* to Zachy?"

"Yeah!"

"Would you sing 'Bah Bah Black Sheep' to Zachy?" I started singing the song, but I didn't get far before Hannah began to wail for her brother.

"Za-keeeey!" Large orb-like tears filled her eyes and jumped from her cheeks to speckle her pajamas. *Oh, what have I done?* Hannah's cries woke up Mom, who ran out of her room in her nightgown as if the fire alarm were blaring, her bare feet slapping the tile floor, her eyes dilated, straining to focus. She hobbled over and let Hannah climb into her arms.

Am I scarring my child?

"Go back to bed," Mom said over Hannah's back, my girl wrapped around her grandmother's chest like a shell. Exhausted, I obeyed.

Lying on the mattress, my mind was bogged down by wanderings. I twisted the blankets into guilty knots as I searched for the sweet spot of sleep. Mothering after Zachary's death was exacting, both a blossoming joy and a root of resentment. They coexisted equally, which was no surprise. Every part of my *new normal* was spliced in duality. Longings I feared to acknowledge lived darkly inside of me, one of which was the desire to escape. I imagined fleeing to a foreign city and starting over alone. Ignoring practicalities, I saw myself painting, my clothes stained in color, surrounded by eight-foot-tall canvases on every wall. There I could be singular in attention to feeding my sorrows.

When we moved out of the house that was home to Zachary's nursery, the neighbor on the corner stopped by as we hauled boxes to the moving truck. She told me she had a stillborn child, her first, and all she did was lie on the couch—for a year. She envied that I had Hannah. I hated myself for envying her couch, her year.

Inwardly, I defended my unrelenting love for my girl to the irrational grieving woman who lived in my shadows. In bed in my parents' home, I imagined dissecting my inner self into many smaller selves. One part *Mother.* The second part *Artist.* Another part *Mourner.* I thought about dividing my identity again and again into disparate pieces too small to contain fear or worry, until I eventually fell asleep.

Week 14: X-Mas

The swirl of snow and ice met Hannah and me at the airport as we returned to Edmonton from Arizona. Aaron drove us home, and even in the black of night the streets dazzled with blue icicle lights and tall pines that glowed red, yellow, and green from strings of LEDs buried beneath their snowy branches. Nativity scenes lit by halogens remained awake most of the night, and ten-foot tall inflatable snowmen cast soft shadows across the wind-carved snow.

A few days before Christmas, Aaron accompanied me to a prenatal appointment with Dr. Stilles, where the baby's heartbeat was the expected 150 BPM. The appointment was routine, nothing out of the ordinary, and I did not speak of my worries.

"Any plans for the holidays?" Dr. Stilles asked, half-listening as he filled out my chart on the computer, the keys *click, click, clicking* noisily.

Aaron and I looked at each other. "Cinnamon buns Christmas morning," Aaron chuckled, his wide smile creasing his handsome, angular face. Since we married in 2007, cinnamon buns had been our tradition. We had even baked them the year before in our kitchen at the Maui hotel, eating breakfast on the balcony overlooking the first cherry-colored light of Christmas day.

Hawaii was our escape two months after Zachary had died. We had decided to leave town last-minute and cut into our savings to travel at one of the most expensive times of the year, when Aaron had time off from school, all with the hope of a week of forgetfulness over the holidays. Despite the fact that our sorrows had stowed away in our luggage and slithered along the beach with us as we took long walks, it was nice to change the visuals of our everyday experience. The colors were different there; blue-greens of both lush landscape and sea, the gold of sun-loved skin, and Hannah's fuchsia ballerina bathing suit with its crinoline skirt that sprinkled sand like pepper into our suitcases.

I had booked a suite with an ocean view, hoping to sit and let the soothing meditation of the waves replace the discordance in my head. When we arrived, though, we found that the room overlooked the resort and faced the other wing of the hotel like a giant U. The sea was visible only if you leaned dangerously over the balcony railing. I wept in the echoing lobby, and the manager, a trim middle-aged man who endured Zachary's story, grew teary-eyed. Aaron was uncomfortable and rocked a sleeping Hannah a few paces away.

We followed the manager to the top floor of the resort, where he opened a broad door with an ornately shaped metal key. "Merry Christmas," he said, putting the key in my hand. The door opened to a private three-bedroom two-thousand-square-foot suite at the tip of one arm of the U. I embraced the manager in gratitude and wept for the second time that day.

Our family of three traded our winter coats and boots for tank tops and sandals. Aaron and I read books while drinking red wine in the shade of tall palms, and Hannah built lopsided sandcastles, buried Aaron's feet, and screamed at the waves disapprovingly. It was her first time at the ocean. Through Hannah's squeals and Aaron's *Be careful*s to our girl, I sat and listened at the water's edge. I quickly realized that my fears whispered even in the *swoosh* and *splash* and *trickle* of the briny surf. Even five thousand kilometers proved not far enough to silence the pain.

"Are you okay?" Aaron whispered, interrupting my memory of the year before. "You're so quiet," he observed as we left our prenatal appointment with Dr. Stilles and got into our car.

"I don't know. Am I supposed to be okay?" I slammed the door. Aaron studied me with wide eyes but said nothing. He flicked the radio on and a Christian carol extolling baby Jesus confronted me. I grimaced as I braided and unbraided my long blonde hair. One of our well-meaning friends had told us, "God understands what you are feeling because he too has lost a son."

I changed the station.

"I don't want to read the birth story on Christmas day," I snapped. That had been a tradition in Aaron's family growing up, one he had once, early in our marriage, told me he wished to continue with our children.

Aaron paused. "That's fine with me." He was wearing his sunglasses and I couldn't see his eyes.

"Do you remember at our last Mourning Together meeting, remember how Martha said to me, 'You were meant to lose a baby'?"

"Yep. She's insensitive. Ridiculous old bat—"

"Still, I can't get her words out of my head, even at Christmas, even after hearing Baby Number Three's heartbeat just now."

"Try to think positive." Aaron tapped the steering wheel to the pulse of the music.

"What loving God would want me to lose my child? This wonderful baby Jesus, born in a manger, the lover and savior of mankind?" I huffed loudly and continued to play with my hair. "So if I was *meant* to lose Zachary, then what if I'm also *meant* to lose this baby?"

"Our child."

"What?"

"You said *my child*, not *our child*."

"Oh, give me a break. You know what I mean. Fine. Sorry. *Our* child. So what grand work does God have up his sleeve for the death of another one of *our* children?" I shook my head and gritted my teeth. "No. No Christmas carols. No Jesus in a manger. I want Christ out of my Christmas."

"Whatever you need."

"Well, how do you feel about everything?"

"I'm angry too, not like you, but for me . . . I can't help remembering that it was Zachary's original due date on December 20."

"I didn't think you remembered."

"Of course I did."

"Sorry," I said, squeezing Aaron's hand. "You were so quiet."

He nodded slowly. "And me, I spent that whole day in a catatonic state, moving from one task to another, never able to focus. You know, I said to Mom, 'I should be planning a first birthday party right now and complaining that I need to buy both birthday and Christmas presents for Zachary all at once.'"

Aaron turned the corner and was still exhaling as the blinker snapped back into place. "Hey, did you ever find that garland for the fireplace?" He tried to change the subject.

"Yep."

"Where was it?"

"In the third bedroom, among the boxes of clothes and nursery gear meant for Zachary, the boxes labeled *Baby*."

"I'm sorry, hon."

"The doctors said everything was okay with Zach right up until everything was not okay. How does that work? I don't know. How can I ever feel comfortable this go-around?"

"I hear ya." Aaron kept his eyes on the road but ran his strong hand through his dense coffee-colored hair that was flecked with white around his ears. The traffic thickened as we approached the city center.

"I'm going crazy. All I have known for so long is death, and now I'm supposed to be magically chipper?" I looked at myself in the visor mirror. My face was pale and my lips tight and thin. I stretched out my jaw and practiced a smile. The braid was lopsided, and I undid it and pulled all my hair back into a messy ponytail. *What does it matter?*

"I don't expect you to be chipper," Aaron said sadly.

"I appreciate that, hon. I really do." I looked over at Aaron while he drove. "Don't get me wrong, though; I want to be. I want to be carefree and hopeful and *la de da*." I waved my hands around in the air, my fingers flailing.

Aaron chuckled. "Sometimes I see glimpses of that in you."

"You're right, for sure. Like when I heard Baby's heartbeat just now. I felt amazing and didn't want it to stop—then Dr. Stilles turns off the Doppler before the last beat has even passed through my ears and I'm back to . . . back to this nervous, freaked-out person pulling out my motherfucking hair."

"Well, maybe we'll learn more at this next appointment," Aaron suggested. We hadn't told Dr. Stilles, but immediately following our meeting with him we were headed downtown to River Valley Medical Center to have another ultrasound ordered by Dr. Barker. Even though Aaron and I had decided not to see Dr. Barker for prenatal care and had chosen to have minimal testing, I still could not part with the ultrasound appointment. I needed more information; I needed to see my baby and watch the face of the technician for his or her unspoken response.

꙼

The technician wore holiday scrubs that matched her rosy cheeks. "Your baby is seven and a half centimeters long," she said once the exam began in the darkened room. "Baby is moving a lot."

"How does it look? Is everything normal?" My jittery words came out at sonic speed, my eyes locked on every possible tell on the technician's face as if we were playing high-stakes poker.

"Your baby is still very small. Everything we can see at this time looks great."

Overanalyzing her words, I began to worry about everything she could not yet see. "What about the heart? What about the lungs? What about the brain? What about the kidneys?" Those were all the places tumors and cysts were discovered in Zachary.

Aaron explained my spastic behavior to the technician, and she leaned closer to the monitor and sucked her teeth, analyzing. "Baby's tiny hands and feet are in place. The spine, this arching white line right here, appears strong. You can see Baby's jaw and nose bone here, and also two tiny femurs, and the skull. Baby's ankles are crossed."

The ultrasound was like looking at a black cloth with white bones lined up in order. They sat together with such fragility, as if I could shake the blanket and free them into some new arrangement, something that would expose a hidden corner of my fear. My anxious fingers wished to group and regroup them, to hold the fairy-sized skull in my hands, stroke the smooth porous forehead, to know my child that intimately.

We lingered a moment to watch the screen in real time. Baby rolled and adjusted. Then a stretch. So early in my pregnancy, I could not feel these movements, but watching them was my hope's manifestation. Ring by ring, even the fingerprints of my baby were being carved into the pads of its fingers and toes, lifelines I prayed would swell and spread like the aged bands of the Methuselah tree in the White Mountains of California, the oldest and wisest in the world.

Aaron and I listened to our child's heart for the second time that day. It spoke.

I am alive.
I am well.
I am here.

The technician did not pull her wand away quickly, as Dr. Stilles had done. She paused.

I am alive.
I am well.
I am here.
I am alive.
I am well.
I am here.

"Everything looks good!" Aaron repeated the technician's words as we walked down the stairs and out of the building. He didn't look to me for a response; maybe he said it to himself. "Everything looks good," he echoed.

$\wp$

On Christmas morning I was the first one awake. "Was our trip to Hawaii really a year ago?" I asked Aaron as he rubbed sleep from his eyes. "Last year we sweated in shorts, and here we need to turn on the gas fireplace. I'm chilled to the bone."

The smell of baking buns sugared the air, which had grown cozy-warm from the fire. Aaron clanked pans and rattled glasses on the kitchen side of the island after offering to make breakfast. He hummed "Deck the Halls" and shuffled around in his slippers and flannel pajama pants. I kept Hannah entertained, playing with small toys and trinkets from her velvet stocking and treating her to Smarties from a candy-cane container.

To my surprise, only fifteen minutes later, Aaron called, "Everything's ready!"

Hannah pounced into my arms, and we headed to the kitchen table, where Aaron had placed plates of cinnamon buns at our respective seats. The pulpy orange juice was already poured and waiting. Aaron grinned with pride. On Hannah's tangerine plate was one medium-sized bun oozing white frosting, and there were three large buns waiting for Aaron, and three for me.

"So . . . we are having cinnamon bun, cinnamon bun, and cinnamon bun, I see." I slipped my arm around Aaron's waist.

"What do you mean?"

"Did you make anything else?"

"No . . ." Aaron answered with a look on his face that asked how I could ever suggest we needed anything more.

Week 15: Resolutions

The temptation to check myself out in the floor-to-ceiling mirrors that lined the track at the YMCA was too much for me. Every lap I ran, I turned to look. A slight muffin top was developing around my waistline, protruding just enough for the self-conscious child inside me, teased to no end in school, to shift into survival mode. I sucked in my gut and pulled the waistline of my black yoga pants above my belly button to conceal the bulge. Then I ran an extra lap, as if that would make all the difference. *I must have eaten too much over the holidays or slacked at the gym*, I thought to myself. *That must be it. Wait. No!* "You are pregnant, silly," I reminded my reflection.

Pregnant women crossed my path daily, as if their bellies had all popped in unison like clones. They embraced their perfectly egg-shaped midsections through stylish maternity tops while I looked on in horror. I worried for them—and for myself. *What if it's not for keeps?*

People rarely asked any more about Zachary or how Aaron and I were coping, even when we were all together at Christmas. My in-laws had donated to The Arthur Memorial bereavement program; the donation card was in a tiny stocking Aaron's mom had sewn from red felt and faux white fur. My tears were the only conversation. Still, after over a year, people did not know what to say. My pregnancy was a relief for many close to us—an outward sign to them that Aaron and I were in fact moving forward, though internally I still resisted.

"Of course I'm happy!" I defended my motherhood to those who questioned my melancholy. I had an adorable and intelligent daughter and, from what we could tell, a healthy baby due to arrive in six months. *Stop moping. You have so much to be thankful for,* I reprimanded myself. I ate my pain, never letting it escape farther than my breath, and it lived inside, growing sickly in my gut. I was happy but also feeling a hundred other emotions, all of which I encompassed completely. I felt no one understood and that my pregnancy was supposed to blanket all other states of the heart, if not suffocating them to extinction at least concealing them for the sake of propriety.

New Year's came, and in the early morning, when only the clock's clicking arms kept me company, I wrote in my journal by a dim lamp before sunrise. My pen scratched the lined pages, forming three resolutions I had the will but not the plan to execute. Resolutions were risky, and I wrestled with the future, but I knew something had to change.

Make peace with my past.

Search for God; find balance, faith, and peace.

Do some good in the world . . . but what?

Week 16: Anxiety

It was a strain to focus. Numbers on street signs broke free of logical chronology. *Watch the speedometer. Not too fast, not too slow. Mind the lights. Red. Brake. Stop.* My thoughts flashed in and out of the past. Blood. Silence. Tiny hands and feet. *What day is it? What time? Time of death: 9:30 in the morning.* Ashes. My enlarged heart beat violently against my chest. Horns. *What's happening? How long has the light been green?*

Week 17: Painters White

Painters White was a color more akin to muted lilac or diluted mud water than actual white. It was a canvas, a stage before paint, although it was not a primer. It felt like the most unfriendly space for a baby when I first walked into our third bedroom that day, ready to clean.

The week before, nesting was the last thing on my mind. I had somehow arrived safely at Dr. Stilles's clinic and asked for an impromptu Doppler exam. Even after hearing my baby's heartbeat I was still distraught. *What's wrong with me? I must be crazy,* I muttered to myself. In a previous appointment, Dr. Stilles had warned me that the second trimester might be a challenge. In the first twelve weeks I could cling to my nausea, sore breasts, and utter exhaustion as palpable markers of hormonal development. By my sixteenth week, however, all side effects had dissipated, leaving only my slowly expanding waistline and similarly inflating fear. With Baby Number Three, everything hinged on the fact that I could not conceptualize giving birth to a child that lived.

"You may need to see a psychologist," Dr. Stilles had stated matter-of-factly. Slowly, I began to recognize how very poorly I was actually doing. "For anxiety treatment. Cognitive therapy," he continued. In the meantime, he expounded on the mental tactics I could attempt to maintain a positive outlook. The doctor's compassion and encouragement, along with a list of books he recommended on anxiety, proved the impetus I needed.

I entered our third bedroom, which had become the junkyard of moving miscellany, and surveyed the terrain. The blinds flicked open with a thwack of faux wood, letting the cool white light of winter spill in amid an airborne wave of dust. The room felt cold and bleak. Still, I needed to be in that space, I ached for another child, and I was hyper-eager to put myself to work on normal tasks.

Less than a year before, when the snow still lived within the shadows in the early spring, only six months after Zachary's death, Aaron and I had begun to search for a place to heal. While attending an open house, we had noticed the owners of a home across the street throwing their belongings onto the front lawn. A pair of pants blew across a snowdrift. An oak table hit the ground hard and a leg snapped. Inquiring, we learned that the house was being repossessed by the bank after it had been used as collateral on a suspect business deal. When we were allowed inside we found an imperfect property in a perfect location. This, we decided, was to be the place of our fresh start, a home where we could live without the constant reminders of our son's death.

In our old house, the kitchen summoned up the hours I had spent in a lake of my own tears on the linoleum. There I had laid motionless, like a lonesome island, weeping away what strength the daily hospital visits had left me. Then there was the bathroom where I had watched my breasts drip creamy colostrum, the first milk, onto my deflated stomach, onto my toes, my body in denial its baby had died. The front room was another haunted realm. It was there that I had sat on the couch with the lights off and listened to my pastor warn me that termination was murder. My body trembled while the pastor stuttered in discomfort with his own doctrine.

I was the one who had brought up the idea of house-hunting, needing an escape, and Aaron had eagerly agreed. "I just might need it more than you," he said, but he never explained why. The search started a dialogue between us about likes and dislikes, foundations and structures, fixer-uppers or new-builds, and where we wished to plant and root ourselves for the years to come. *At least we are talking*, I thought.

Aaron and I repainted the entire house, which had been nicked, scuffed, and dented during the rapid foreclosure. Every room was repaired and resurrected, except for the third bedroom. *What color do we choose for a space in limbo?* At that point we had not received the news we could have more children. Thus, Painters White was what the room became.

In many ways I convinced myself that I did not need medication or a counselor. I hoped that as I cleaned the nursery my inner mess would tidy itself as well. I packed Aaron's random screwdrivers, loose nails, pliers, and picture-hanging kit into a Dewalt bag. Then I sent him a text: "Don't be mad. All your tools packed up from baby's desk. Put in garage. I'm NESTING!"

My artwork, which had been buried in a corner, I placed purposefully throughout the room, ready to hang. I stacked the suitcases inside themselves like Russian nesting dolls and tucked them away in Hannah's closet. The infant bath found its home in the Jack and Jill tub. I also adorned the bathroom with a large piece of coral I had plucked from the Pacific Ocean as a child, and Aaron's late grandmother's green, yellow, and royal-blue vase filled with pink lilies. Clothes were hung and boxes flattened. After a few hours of sorting and cleaning, the tan carpet appeared.

Hannah was also nesting, and we visited The Home Depot like fowls gathering supplies. As we approached the long wall of swatches displayed in a prism of color, our eyes were charmed after the hours spent with Painters White. Hannah began pulling handfuls of paint samples and chucking them into the cart. "One at a time, please, my girl. Okay, now; if Mommy has a boy, how about Seafoam Spray Green and Sugar Pool Blue?" Hannah studied the colors intently, then nodded her approval. "And for a girl, hmm. Sorbet Pink and Apricot Ice?"

In those moments, I chose to be happy, to practice my own brand of cognitive therapy, as Dr. Stilles had suggested, even though I still did not fully know what that meant. That night, Aaron was startled but impressed when I showed him the breadth of my bird-like arranging. I think he was relieved his wife was doing normal things, not still pacing worn lines or journaling her fears with dark language. This alternative was better.

Week 18: Studying

The books Dr. Stilles recommended arrived on my doorstep in a brown cardboard box, and I immediately began reading about anxiety and post-traumatic stress disorder. It was the first time I viewed my experience within the context and vocabulary of psychological analysis. I learned about self-nurturing skills, realizing I didn't have any, and about the ways a meaningful life can reduce depression. As I contemplated a list of the causes that maintain debilitating beliefs, I nibbled a cuticle anxiously until it stung and bled. Then I scanned the chapters on mindfulness and meditation and realized I had a lot of work to do.

Week 19: Gender

I expected the technician to say, "Girl." The word was already formed in my mind like a stencil ready to be colored in with confirmation. *Girl.* All my motherly intuition pointed in that one beautiful direction. Beautiful because this pregnancy would be different from the last in that one fundamentally defining way, beautiful because then the scathing, scratching fear of déjà vu could unclaw itself from my leg. Yet, the technician held her position with the wand on my rounding abdomen and pointed to the monitor, and the one word from her mouth was not *girl.* It was so dramatically opposite from *girl* that I almost did not understand what she had said.

"Boy. You are having a boy."

"A boy!" Aaron looked down at me, beaming.

"Boy?" I repeated. And repeated again and again. "Boy. A boy. I am having a boy . . . Is he healthy?" I asked eventually, using the masculine pronoun for the first time. "Can you check? Can you double-check, please?"

The technician drifted the wand across my stomach, "Yep, your baby is definitely a boy, and he is in good health. Developmentally right on schedule."

At home that night my anxiety continued to churn. "I already slip up and call the nursery Zachary's room," I told Aaron at dinner as I scooped a bite of noodle casserole onto a yellow plastic spoon and zoomed it like an airplane into Hannah's mouth.

"I'm sure once he's here you won't make that mistake."

"Baby," Hannah said with her mouth full.

"But what if I do?"

Aaron shrugged his broad frame. "You carry on."

"What if I call Baby Number Three by Zachary's name? I don't want it, him, to feel like he's living in the shadow of his dead brother."

"Zachy," Hannah smiled.

"Good girl, Hannah." I stroked her hair and leaned over to tickle her nose with mine.

"I know what you're saying." Aaron rubbed his round chin with his hand. "I don't know what to tell you. It's gonna happen."

"Now, obviously, all the baby girl names we chose won't work. We're back to square one. When the technician said, 'Boy,' all I could think about was the fact I didn't have a name."

With Hannah asleep, Aaron and I lounged in bed on top of messy sheets. We leaned against the fabric headboard with our laptops propped on our knees and searched the Internet, our fingers tapping away to different rhythms. The desire to name my child felt like an apricot pit caught in my throat; the need for relief was urgent. I had eight tabs open with popular baby-name sites.

"What about Isaac?" Aaron suggested.

"I knew an Isaac growing up. He was a bully."

"Okay, what about Daniel?"

"Are you goin' all biblical on me?" I asked, and Aaron smirked, raising his eyebrows.

"Just promise me we are not going to name our kid Apple or Pear or Door-Knob," he snickered.

I punched his arm playfully, and he pretended it hurt. "Of course not," I said. "This is really important to me."

"It's getting late. Can we continue this when I'm home from work tomorrow?"

"I can't. I just can't. I need this boy to have a name. He needs to have his own identity."

Aaron sighed loudly. "Right now? We still have five months . . ."

I glanced at him quickly, but he must have caught the *Please-I-need-this-or-I'm-going-to-go-crazy* glint in my eyes.

"Okay, right now," Aaron said, and he unfolded his laptop once more. We read through thousands of boy names: biblical, historical, modern, cultural—and they all began to string together into one long sentence, the names of all the boys of the world.

To the rhythmic *click, click, click* of Aaron's fingers on the keyboard, my eyelids began to flutter, and the words on the screen blurred. For a moment I was somewhere else.

I am alone in Baby Boy's room, in the nursery. My stomach is ripe and heavy, and I can sense my child inside orbit slowly against my organs. Aaron's deep, kind voice and the giggles of our girl rise to meet me through the floor from the kitchen below, where they scrape a large spoon along our metal mixing bowl, baking. Their echoes are a joy to me. Contentedness and expectation sit firmly on my chest, unmoving, and there is peace in the room.

The window yawns widely above the built-in desk where a green, fleece-covered change pad and nappies wait. The warmth of golden sunlight and the scent of pine needles and blossoming wheat from the nearby forest and farmers' fields are welcomed into the space. The breeze blows the white curtains; their delicate black-ink drawings of trees and leaves and birds come alive with movement. The curtains, still untrimmed, flow from the window top downward over the desk and to the floor, reaching into the room like long arms and legs desiring to plant themselves on the walls. Two of the walls are blue, like the sky on a patient day, and their opposites ground them in minty-green fields that roll away like uncoiled sod toward the horizon. Within the nursery, both the sky and the earth rest comfortably, both within grasp, both of formable materiality like clay; touchable, impressionable.

The crib, meant for Zachary, sits centered on the largest blue wall. Its mattress lived in plastic for two years, but the rocket-ship bedding is new. To the right of the crib stands Aaron's late grand-

mother's side table that I had sanded, until my fingertips blistered, and then restored with a deep, chocolate-colored lacquer. From its place on the side table, my childhood lamp with a shade made of strung amber beads splays a pattern over the wall like a light projector. In one corner is a muted-cobalt dresser, and across from it sits the glider where I held Hannah to my breasts, where I rocked her to sleep.

I rest here in the earthiness of the nursery, in its gentle energy, its connectedness. Standing in the middle of the room, the Spirit of Birth stirs in the warm gale from the window that nearly raises me off the floor. I hear Hannah's laughter and her pattering footsteps, half-speed, as Aaron chases her in the distance of my periphery, and then they are in the nursery, running circles, and I wonder. Maybe they were always with me. All things: the sky, earth, branches and wooden furniture, the fragrances on pinkish wind, and Hannah, Aaron, and me; everything spins and floats, weightless. My lungs fill with the Spirit's breath, and I am ready to push . . .

In the margins betwixt awake and asleep, where consciousness is a thing held in the hand and toyed with, I nudged my dream in a precarious direction. It was a place my alert mind refused to venture. Even the idea of it—of imagining the call to birth progressing to the delivery of Baby Number Three, the stiffening and breathlessness of contractions—forced my sleepy vision to shatter against an impenetrable barricade. I couldn't see that far. Beyond the nesting, arranging, ordering, puttering, and surface decorating, there was nothing.

I had only ever gone into labor at our last home. Imagining it with Baby Number Three transported me back there, among the sacred and the tragic memories. Hannah's birth, Zachary's death; yet that was my labor place. I strained to wrangle my wayward imagination, but everything beyond the suddenly silent and uninhabited nursery was impossible to conjure, completely veiled.

Sitting up in bed, back in the present moment, my wrist

cracked from the position where it had cradled my cheek as I dozed. Beside me, Aaron continued in the search. He suggested a name. Then another. "What about this one?" he pointed to the screen. I shrugged, ambivalent to them all.

Week 20: Horse with Blue Eyes

Pulling out of the garage one morning and turning onto the snowy road toward Mom's house, it was as if I were piloted directly into a cloud. With less than a kilometer behind me, it was without doubt no ordinary winter morning. The new world was buttered with hoarfrost so thick its icicles dripped off branches like tiny rapiers, and everything, from the stark white horizon to the cloaked roadway, glowed in the diffused February light.

"Moon!" Hannah yelled from her car seat in the back, pointing at the misty orb low in the sky.

"That's the sun, Han."

"Moon!" Hannah called again, and I let myself see through her two-year-old eyes. It was in that moment that I relented to my own childlike curiosity. I dropped off Hannah with her grandmother and, instead of heading back to the house to work, traced the back roads of south Edmonton that divided farmers' fields and dense patches of trees, my camera bag sitting on the passenger seat beside me. "Frost chaser," I called myself. I couldn't remember the last time I had felt such unguarded anticipation—not since early in my pregnancy with Zachary, at least. The thought made me shudder.

Hopping out of the car, I struggled to zip up my coat, but it would not stretch past my belly button. Finding a scarf in the backseat, I wrapped it around my neck and waded through a sloping drift to an area of brush that peeked above the snowy surface. I attached my macro lens and photographed frozen seedlings that balanced upon the skeletons of wildflowers and were caught in the slight breeze, rocking their loads back and forth.

As I was about to return to the car, something caught my eye in the field opposite. Squinting, I could barely make out a dozen ghostly figures, like faint ink splatters, dotting the white page of the foggy pasture. Intrigued, I approached the toppling wire-and-wooden-stake fence just past a gully of knee-deep snow. Shivering at the fence, it was all I could do to stand still and wait, my breath wafting around me in delicate plumes.

The ink splatters took on form and moved gracefully toward me. As if dreaming, I imagined hearing their every step, crunching the snow as their hooves trod heavily in their watchful gait. Tall horses emerged into the clarity of the frigid air, the distance between us condensed as they approached, unafraid.

I expected the horses to be tentative, leery of my hooded silhouette and untrusting of the camera around my neck, but they did not slow. As if foregoing the dream, they walked right up to me, pressed their noses to my arms, and blew their breath into my palms. They nuzzled in affectionately, and I stroked the coarse hair on their warm hides.

A patchy white and brown horse approached after its two smaller black companions nibbled at my sleeve before moving on to wrestle in the snow. The patchy horse was taller than the rest, and it looked at me with confidence and understanding in its sky-blue eyes; understanding and sympathy. Zachary had also had blue eyes, or so Aaron had told me. I had been too afraid to look for myself.

My hands stroked up and down the bridge of the horse's nose and broad cheek. We stayed like this for many quiet moments, enjoying each other's warmth. The blue-eyed horse eventually turned toward its frolicking friends and, after looking at me again for one long breath, joined the others as they retraced their steps back through the mist.

As I stood there, I hadn't noticed the breeze that skated upon the frozen earth behind me, not until it tipped the balance of snow resting on the tree branches overhead. I was caught in a flurry of fat snowflakes that whirled lazily around me. I breathed in the sharp, clean air and felt strangely alive. Raising my camera, I held down the shutter in rapid fire, capturing the whirl of white that gave visible form to the hand of the wind.

All of a sudden, a familiar voice broke the silence of my winter trek, though I was alone. Listening to her words, tears froze on my cheeks. "You have lost your child, but *you* are not lost," my own voice whispered—but the words did not make sense. Zach was dead, and I too felt death's cold spreading outward from my core. Like the fog of the morning that seemed to pass right through me, I once more sensed the powerlessness to alter Zachary's fate. Covering my mouth with my frostbitten fingers, my mind filled with images of my baby boys, both the one to come and the one then gone.

"Your child's identity is not your identity. *You are alive.*" My words hung in the air.

For so long I had felt like an apparition, just the shell of a mother in mourning. My mind wandered to Hannah, to Aaron. I had been strong for so long but, as I shivered in the last touches of the windblown flurry, I allowed the frozen places of me, the wounds and walls of self-protection, to fissure and crack like ice in springtime.

As my eyes remained fixed on the distant place where the horses had slipped from view, my hands, trembling, dropped from my mouth to the arch of my rounding abdomen. The baby within me kicked lightly, a sensation as faint as the snow melting on my skin. I had wondered for the last twenty weeks, *How am I going to do this? How can I bring a new life into the world while feeling so very distant from it?* Yet, in that moment I knew.

I had not completely forgotten who I was. It was true that a part of me had passed into white like the horses, but I now saw that I would survive, that I must survive—not only for Hannah or

Aaron, or for my next child, but for myself as well. The thaw was coming; I could sense its stirring, its deep earthy groaning. A new season would soon replace my winter of the soul.

After that day, whenever I passed through those back roads, I watched for the horses. Sometimes I caught a glimpse of the mares grazing in the sloping fields. Their shaggy coats danced in the wind as they galloped, unbridled and unbroken. Yet, in all the years since that one quiet day, I never again have seen the horse with blue eyes.

Week 21: The Name

Sports were the predominant theme of boy's infant and toddler clothing. Sports and animals. The ultimate was an animal playing football or baseball. Already I had an impressive collection of sleepers, onesies, T-shirts, and corduroy pants for Baby Boy. My cousin contributed a heaping bag of hand-me-downs, and Mom purchased gifts stateside. Then there were the adorable outfits from Costco that beckoned me every time I shopped for groceries.

After Hannah was born, I thought the other gender's apparel could never match the cuteness of pink polka-dot dresses, flowery tights, and sparkling headbands, but in fact I grew fond of trucks and camo-green. My apprehension over Baby Boy's gender was easing as well. Superstitiously, I took these shifts as an omen.

After Zachary died, I was too economical to give away the clothes I had amassed for him. True, they were in perfect condition, but the motivation was deeper and more elusive than even I could understand. All I knew was that I could not part with the clothes, while at the same time I could not bear to look at them.

Eventually I hung every sleeper, shirt, and pair of pants on mini-hangers in the nursery closet. *I'll deal with them later*, I told myself. The price tags, though, remained hinged to collar labels and sleeves, as they held a peculiar power over me. The tags were a line of commitment I could not cross.

I sat on the cool tile floor of our Jack and Jill bathroom one morning, encouraging Hannah to use the potty. She perched comfortably on the padded child's seat as I worked my way through her stack of books. "Mommy, read it," she said, and she passed me a worn anthology of children's stories I had found at a garage sale the past summer.

"All right, Hannah," I said in my firm but loving mommy voice. "We'll read this one last story, and then you are getting off the potty. Deal?"

"Deal!"

Randomly, I let the anthology fall open and flipped to the story's beginning. It was about two curious yet well-mannered bunny rabbits on a treasure hunt in a park. They found a toy boat, a locket, and a ring and shared their treasures with their friends.

The opening page introduced the bunnies. All of a sudden, the name of the second rabbit grew bold before my eyes. It was as if I were hunting for a treasure myself, scanning words and letters jumbled in a monumental puzzle; the search for my baby's name. Then, four seemingly random letters fused together, and I saw it, what I had been struggling to find for weeks. *The* name.

Eden.

It was as simple as that.

Eden.

I said the name aloud. Then I said it again. And again. I asked Hannah to say it. "Eden," she said clearly. *Eden.*

On the bathroom floor, I shivered violently in what I can only describe as a mashup between déjà vu and enlightenment. The future I had strained for so long to imagine was all of a sudden aglow and crisp before me. It moved, flickering like reel film. In it I saw my son, my *Eden.* He was a child around two years old. His ashen hair blew in the breath of autumn as he ran through unkempt grass and brittle leaves, his jacket unzipped and flapping. *Eden's* face reflected the peachy late afternoon sun and wore a smile of unabashed delight.

Then *Eden* was in school with a notebook he doodled in with a yellow HB pencil. Forward in time, he and Hannah were teenagers in the basement where I was attempting to take their picture in front of one of my backdrops. They pestered each other and refused to sit still; "Come on, Mom! What's taking so long?"

The pride in those prospective tomorrows pinned my back against the bathroom wall—but I was not in the bathroom. *Eden* was an adult. It was his wedding day. I could see him and his friends goofing off in their suits and shiny black shoes. He was so tall, and I felt warmth through his long arms hugging me, his voice vibrating in my ears as he said goodnight. The light of the vision, which illuminated years forward, eventually faded as the bathroom walls defined themselves again. Hannah still sat there on the toilet beside me.

"Eden!" I yelled joyfully. "Eden!" Hannah joined in, screaming and repeating the name in her high-pitched squeal. We laughed until we were winded and our voices rang against the walls and tile floor like a wind chime, the sound bouncing off itself into new directions. Giggling, arms raised, we hollered and flailed and stomped our feet.

Eden. That was it. *Eden*. I quickly found my phone and Googled the name.

Of the associations that came to mind, the Garden of Eden was the first, then Mount Eden in Auckland, New Zealand. Mount Eden was a majestic volcanic mound that rose up out of the city core with a herd of roaming cows grazing on the cusp of the deep, grassy crater. Aaron and I had visited Mount Eden many times when we lived in Auckland, watching the sun set across the 360-degree view, the Sky Tower—the tallest building in the Southern Hemisphere—silhouetted against the evolving color of the evening sky.

I found the answer I was looking for.

Eden meant *delight*.

I called Aaron at work. "I like it," he said. "I really like it," and I knew without a doubt that Eden would be our son's name.

The next morning, awakened by Hannah's soft yet insistent voice, I picked up my girl and carried her into the nursery. We sat on the floor and, one by one, I removed each price tag. I gave them to Hannah, who held the tags to her ear like a telephone and talked to the printed pictures of grinning babies.

Tenderly, I ran my hand over a cotton grey-and-blue-striped onesie with a superhero puppy flying across the left panel. *Eden will wear this.* Grinning, I thumbed a forest-green and mustard-yellow football jumper. A raccoon and the words *Daddy's #1 Draft Pick* were stitched across the chest. Then there was a red-and-maroon-striped newborn onesie with a silver robot walking across the front. *I'm Nuts for Mommy*, it said, above a colorful collection of screws and bolts.

"Maybe we'll take Baby Boy home from the hospital in this one," I said to Hannah, and she nodded.

Week 22: Magnetism

"You can't live in fear." Aaron looked at me slyly, a smirk across his wind-burnt face as he towed Hannah, who relaxed on the old wooden sled, on a ride to the hill. The cold air pricked our skin, but Hannah relished the nippy chill, even scooping handfuls of snow with her mitten and filling her mouth. She was determined that wintery Saturday mornings were best spent outdoors.

"Yeah, yeah." I laughed off Aaron's new catchphrase. Whenever I started worrying, he would pop into my thoughts and say, *You can't live in fear.* Every time. "There are so many what-ifs," I replied. "I wish I could be one of those Zen moms that live in the here and now, you know, present in the moment. Then maybe I wouldn't worry so much."

Aaron flared his nostrils. "I don't think those moms exist. And even if they did, you'd still worry."

"Gee, thanks!" I rolled my eyes, which matched the color of the shadows on the icy-blue snowbanks. Everything was going well with the pregnancy, but the unknown still terrified me. I found myself diluting my worry for others' sake and out of fear of appearing crazy. The last person I wanted to become was the clingy, paranoid mother scared of all the ways her children could die, frightened of every natural stage of letting go. I did not want to mourn Hannah or Baby Number Three's first day of school or their first sleepovers.

"Just try not to get ahead of yourself."

"If only you knew."

"Just look at you. When you were younger you did all kinds of risky things—and you're fine."

"Like what?" I snapped.

"Um, gee, let me think," retorted Aaron, mimicking my sassy tone. "What about that time you slapped a girl in the bathroom during the Catholic school dance?" I nodded. *Yes, there was that.* "Or what about all the concussions your mom told me about? Let me count." Aaron pulled off his glove and straightened a finger with every instance. "There was that one time sledding, correct?"

"Uh-huh," I said quietly, and we both looked back at Hannah, sitting merrily in her little toboggan.

Aaron continued. "Then when you played shinny hockey without a helmet. What else? Hmm. Oh yeah, that ATVing accident in college. There are more, aren't there?"

"I think you've made your point."

"I'll never forget that camping trip we took with friends back in 2003."

"The summer we started dating."

"We were in Jasper at Horseshoe Lake. All us guys were arguing about who should cliff-dive first. And all the girls were waiting for one of us to be the macho man. Remember that?"

"I do."

"And, then, swoosh." Aaron gestured with his hand. "Without saying a word, you ran past us all in your little bikini and jumped off the cliff into the lake. That was pretty cool."

"You're forgetting the part where I tried to plug my nose and ended up punching myself in the face." Aaron cracked up, leaving a trail of his breath in the air behind us.

"But you were fine."

"Yeah, but I don't want Hannah cliff-jumping. Or Eden. Just thinking about it freaks me out."

"Eden!" Hannah overheard and yelled her brother's name.

"Shhhh, Hannah! That's a secret!" whispered Aaron, momentarily stopping in the ankle-deep snow to give Hannah a stern look. He turned back to me. "It's all these adventures you've had that have given you such great memories." We continued our trudge to the park.

"But what if something bad happens to another one of our kids?" I choked. "I don't know what I'd do. I don't think I could handle it."

"You could."

Aaron's confidence infuriated me. *Why can't he understand?* We had the same experience, yet the world moved on at a different pace for each of us. *Does he ever wonder if Eden will survive?* All of a sudden I felt very alone.

"Ready, Mommy?" Aaron asked as we reached the top of the hill. Hannah clapped her mittens and bounced in the sled.

"I'm actually feeling a little tired from the walk," I exaggerated, rubbing my belly. "Mind if I sit here for a couple minutes?" I pointed to the bench at the apex of the slope.

I could hear Hannah's happy shrieks on the way down followed by her continuous giggles as Aaron pulled her back up. The hill was busy despite the cold, and everyone kept moving for warmth, which meant I was alone on the bench with my wandering mind. I thought back to the camping trip in Jasper in 2003. I was nineteen at the time. After cliff-diving, I had come out of the water with my nose bleeding from the self-inflicted blow. Aaron had not comforted me; it was another friend who wiped my face with his towel, sitting with me until the bleeding stopped.

Aaron apologized for it later, and I forgave him quickly in the intoxication of young love. After our friends went to sleep in their tents, Aaron and I snuck to my car to dampen our lips with each other's tongue. Heat perspired on the inside of the vehicle's windows.

Aaron was athletic and strong, with kind features and a large grin. He was two years older and a foot taller. We spent four years together at the University of Alberta, he in athletics and me in fine art. We were an unlikely pair. I played volleyball and slow-pitch with him, and he would read, watch movies, and discuss life with me while I painted in my studio at school or in the basement at home.

It was not only our interests that were distinct, but our upbringings and families as well. Aaron was raised in a conservative Christian home; his father's way was the only way, and no one swore or gambled or drank. I, on the other hand, grew up with a working mother and my stepdad, Ken, who, to make his point, would say things like, "Does Dolly Parton sleep on her back?" My family appreciated a good drink, and we were loud both in our arguments and in our laugher. It never occurred to me at the time how different Aaron and I were; the chemistry and depth of our relationship made all things seem manageable, even beneficial.

As I sat on the bench at the top of the snowy hill, I began to realize that the nine years Aaron and I had spent together, which had entwined our souls into an inseparable knot, still had no bearing on the way we grieved—or healed. Aaron was the type of person who always saw the good in people, in life, and in me. For as long as I had known him, I wished to be like Aaron in that way. Yet, our reaction to my third pregnancy said everything.

Aaron and I maintained our decade-long routines as if it were someone else's baby that had died, but the foundation of our marriage had shifted, and tiny cracks were visible. After a while, I stopped bringing up the abandonment I felt when Aaron swiftly returned to work after our loss, when I was still reading and re-reading the sympathy cards aloud in our lonely home. There never seemed to be an escape from that pain of absence, although silence masqueraded as relief, at least for Aaron.

At twenty-two weeks, I remained the only one who could sense Eden's movements. He was just shy of a foot in length and weighed about the same as a block of butter. He loved to stir in the evenings. Aaron and I would lie together on the couch, my legs across his lap, and watch TV, or read in bed and talk until we fell asleep. It was then that Eden would test the limits of my womb in what felt like, at first, faint butterfly wings against my skin. Later, the movements resembled patterned knocks. It was our private language;

one knock meant *Hi, Mom!* Two was, *I'm having fun!* Three said: *Can't wait to meet you!* Midway through my pregnancy, it was not Aaron's reminders to not live in fear but Eden's presence that sustained me.

Week 23: The Business of Happiness

"What are you up to?" Aaron asked one evening. I was hunched over my desk revising my artist's statement. The sun was already asleep beneath the fold of the horizon, and the only light in the office glowed from my monitor. Aaron flicked on the light in the ceiling fan.

In my periphery I could see his tall silhouette lean on the office doorframe as he watched me. "I'm preparing a submission for a few galleries," I mumbled. It must have been close to eleven.

"For the large landscape paintings you've been working on?" I shook my head no. "For the abstract gold series, then?"

"Nope. My new marble photographs."

"Ah. Well, are you coming to bed soon? It's late." When I failed to respond quickly, fumbling over a line of revision, Aaron pressed his point. "You need to take care of yourself."

"I *am* taking care of myself!" I snapped back over my shoulder. "*This* makes me happy."

Aaron responded in turn to the annoyance in my voice. His eyes grew wide, and he stepped back from the doorway into the shadow of the hall. "You look more stressed than happy to me," he mumbled as he closed the office door behind him.

"Whatever."

Aaron heard me through the door. As a teacher he despised that word, and I knew it. "What did you say?" he asked as he briskly swung open the door. I ignored him. "I'm very happy you are enjoying yourself, but I thought you were supposed to be slowing down. Remember your Year of Distraction? The burnout?"

"I need this. Can't you understand that?"

"Where's the balance?" he fumed. I did not answer. "Fine," he said, and he stomped to bed.

Later that week, Hannah and I plowed through the snowy streets of downtown Edmonton for a press conference at City Hall. One of my art patrons, a businesswoman who had purchased many of my paintings over the years, had nominated me for a local art award. Hannah and I stamped our boots at the entry to the marble foyer leading to the indoor amphitheater. The announcement of nominees was already underway.

Pulling a tangerine lollipop from its plastic sheath, I bribed Hannah to stay quiet in the stroller. "Okay, Mommy," she mumbled and reclined. Together we ventured only a short distance into the large hall and found a spot where I could stand with the stroller beside the bubbling coffee machine. The long list of nominees in my category made me wonder why I had wasted ten dollars on parking. "Everyone is a winner!" each corporate sponsor admonished. I rolled my eyes, cursing my twenty-eight years' worth of bad luck.

The only time I had ever won anything was in grade five. During the assembly following the school's Thanksgiving Turkey Trot, my raffle number was called. The trouble was that I'd torn my ticket to pieces; by the age of ten I was already acutely aware of my unlucky streak. Timidly, I dragged my feet to the front of the gymnasium, passed the principal the shredded red ticket, and collected my prize. A seven-pound frozen turkey.

Five minutes into the press conference, all that remained of the lollypop was a wilting stick. Hannah, squirming and whining, began vehemently spitting pieces of paper from her mouth. I whispered in her ear, "Please, Hannah. Please be quiet," taking the damp stick from her gooey fingers and wiping her mouth. She refused to sit still. People turned. Press reporters cast sour glances in our direction as they held their recording devices midair. Anger flared in my throat. When it was clear we couldn't avoid a scene, I turned the stroller harshly and left.

On the drive home I longed to yell but bawled instead. Hannah was a child; she was not to blame. "What matter, Mommy?" she asked with tenderness.

"I'm just a little," I sniffled, "a little sad—but I love you so much, my girl. So much. You make Mommy very proud and happy. And you know what you are to me, right?"

"What?"

"Hannah, you are my sun, my moon, my shining stars."

"I know, I know," she giggled.

It was the truth. Hannah was my joy, my solace and treasure, yet the life I wanted, the one I had planned for with Aaron, Hannah, and Zachary, was gone. In my struggle to reconstruct a new kind of happiness, every detail of what was real and what really mattered seemed askew. As an artist, I was alive and powerful: a flowing, graceful, authentic, and free spirit, untroubled and at peace, particularly in the most private acts of creativity. On the other hand, as a mother I felt inept. Each day was a gnarling struggle to be on time, guard my patience, gauge the correct number of apologies for raising my voice, to wedge my passions into particled quadrants of time: an hour while Hannah napped, two before I went to bed, and maybe an afternoon or morning on the weekends if I wasn't dog-tired. I needed a win, I felt, even in just one area, to somehow balance all the loss. In my heart, though, I knew no number of awards would make a difference.

"You're not going to work on your submissions tonight?" Aaron asked civilly on the eve of the press conference, noticing my avoidance of the office.

"Not tonight." We headed upstairs to our bedroom together,

Hannah's nightlight shining on our feet from beneath her door.

Aaron started pulling clothes from his dresser for the next day of work while I slipped into my nightgown and brushed my teeth. "Maybe we should figure out when we are going to tone down the ambition," Aaron said while folding a shirt. He did not look up.

"What does *that* mean?" I walked out of the bathroom, frothy toothbrush in hand.

"You know, you've been pushing yourself really hard lately."

"Because I love it," I said, wiping white paste from the corners of my mouth. "What, you just want me to put it all aside, sit around, be a good old housewife?"

"I'm not trying to be a male chauvinist pig."

"Are you sure? Because you're doing a fucking good job of it!"

"Give me a break, Alexis Marie. I can't say anything without you blowing up at me." Aaron threw his pants across the room and his belt buckle nicked the wall, leaving a tiny dent.

"I'm fucking pregnant! What do you expect? I'm a huge fucking ball of fucking hormones!"

"Stop swearing!" Aaron threw his shirt to the floor.

"Stop throwing things!"

We huffed and fumed in silence for some time, circling around each other while getting ready for bed, never once touching as we passed the other at the closet or in the bathroom. Climbing into bed, our tempers spent in the huff, we lay beside each other, stiff as parallel floorboards until I finally relented—a little.

"I do feel very tired. Slowing down would be good, for both Baby and me, I'm sure."

"I don't always say things the right way. I'm sorry. But you don't wanna be working like crazy and all tired when Eden arrives. I'm just worried about you, okay? I remember how the year after Zachary wore you thin." I placed my hand on my stomach where Eden was readjusting and Aaron did the same, briefly, before quickly sliding his hand to my chest beneath my left collarbone. "I'm still worried about your heart."

"Sorry for swearing and losing my cool."

"Thanks."

"You have to understand, though, Aaron: I need my art. I need to be able to express myself. It is the one thing in all the lostness of my life that I can control. I couldn't stop Zach from dying, my heart may explode at any moment, who knows, and it's out of my power whether something bad will happen to Eden—but in my art, I decide."

"I never thought about it like that."

"You're right, though. My Year of Distraction was brutal—for all of us. I see that. I can probably tone down the submissions, the business side of things. I can do that, but I still need to create. I feel that urge now more than ever. And it kills me to compartmentalize. I can't switch back and forth between artist and mother—it's not one or the other in me. They are both who I am." I was slowly coming to acknowledge the shifting season of my body, and it was a time I wished to enjoy, despite my equal if not greater fear of it. "I can't just twiddle my thumbs until June 25. I'll go crazy."

"I love you so much, and I believe in you as an artist, I really do. It just kills me to see you stressed and tired. I think I didn't appreciate before how art is an escape for you, a distraction—but a good distraction. Like my work is for me. I love what I do. Maybe that's why I went back so quick: I needed it. It's my job to provide for you and Hannah, and to protect you. That's why I say the stupid things I do. I love you." We filled the gap between us in the bed. I leaned in, resting my cheek on Aaron's chest, and his strong arms blanketed my shoulders, his heart thumping in my ear.

"I love you, Aaron."

"Do you?"

"I do—but just for the record, you're not a jerk who's trying to crush my dreams, right?" I heckled, squinting my eyes up at him playfully.

"Well, maybe just a little," he jeered, the heat of our snuggled bodies also warming our conversation. "No! Not one bit. At the end of the day, you know best," Aaron continued seriously. "But maybe I know second best."

"Maybe. Maybe second best."

Week 24: Abstractions

Dr. Haverson met me in the wallpapered reception area and shook my hand. Her cheeks were rose-colored, and her hair was grey and chopped short. She smiled with her eyes and waved me to follow her into to a small office. I instantly liked the forest-green wing chair in the corner, meant for me, I could tell, and the quaintness of the space lit by one long window that reached from wall to wall. Formalities of paperwork aside, we began to talk.

"Thank you for fitting me in so quickly," I began.

"Your mother sounded very concerned on the phone."

Only a few days before, everything had climaxed. Hannah was cemented in a long stretch of night terrors where she would scream like a banshee, kicking and fighting Aaron and me in her sleep. The days and nights conjoined themselves into one ceaseless loop. While Aaron was at work, I nearly taped my eyelids open so I could play with Hannah and her matchbox cars; build wooden puzzles, which were always annoyingly short on pieces; and hobble to the park, where I dozed on the slide in the sun until some kid kicked me in the ass. When not pining for rest, I was ardently craving focused time in the studio, to be lost in the soulful state of making art. The symptoms of withdrawal were apparent; I was easily aggravated, sad, unmotivated, and depressed.

The day before my first meeting with Dr. Haverson, I could hardly keep my eyes open, yet Hannah giggled and jumped on the couch where I had just flopped like a sack of potatoes. I looked up at my cheery girl and begged, "Can you please give me five minutes to rest? Just five minutes? Then Mommy will wake up, deal? Then we'll play, I promise." The words mixed on my tongue in an exhausted slur as I drifted off, but Hannah was determined.

BAM!

Stabbing, burning tenderness erupted across my left eye and crescendoed in a scream of pain that woke me instantly. Hannah wanted my attention—and she got it—head-butting my face, where my glasses contorted and jammed deep into my eye socket. I shot up from the couch seeing grey as flaming arrows arced backward into my brain. Reaching out to find the coffee table by touch, I slipped to the floor and rocked back and forth. My watering eye failed to focus. Hannah crawled up beside me, delicately collecting the tears from my cheeks and rubbing my leg with her short, pudgy fingers. Pulling her onto my lap, we cuddled while my chest pulsed sorely in and out as I restrained myself from weeping and beating the floor. My love for Hannah was all-encompassing; I would do anything for her, yet I had nothing left to give anyone.

I am so fucking lost in my own life. The thought dripped with bitterness. My insides were grated by the sharp guilt I hoped would numb me to the disconnectedness. My life was perfect, beautiful, blessed. *What's wrong with me?* In trying to survive my pregnancy, the quest for my own happiness seemed to conflict with everyone else's needs; who I wanted to be raged against who I was. *Calm down! Calm down,* my own words ricocheted within my skull.

Dr. Stilles had warned me that stress could release cortisol, which in turn might harm my baby. Breathing deeply, I struggled but failed to extinguish the combusting emotions and fretfully imagined my sorrows, little by little, sucking away the health of my unborn child. My tortured breaths came faster and faster. I spiraled downward.

"Alexis Marie. Alexis Marie?" Dr. Haverson interrupted my thoughts.

"I had a panic attack yesterday. At home. With my daughter. I called Mom, and she came over. She asked me what she could do, but all I could respond with was a blank stare. I couldn't stop my head, my hands, my one leg, from shaking. Then Aaron arrived home."

"Aaron?"

"My husband. I was crying, but the shaking had stopped by then. I was still. Frozen; I couldn't move. I just stared. At one spot. Thankfully, Hannah played around me, oblivious. I was numb. I felt lost, you know? It was thick, like a rope around my neck. I was suffocating. Mom and Aaron kept asking, 'What can we do?' Over and over. 'What can we do? What can we do?' But everything I said infuriated them."

"Why?"

"Because they are practical, logical thinkers."

"And how do you think?"

"In abstraction. In metaphor, simile, figures of speech, symbols . . . They couldn't understand what I was saying. I was like a puzzle they were trying to solve. They couldn't make sense of me. And I was just so scared they would say, *You have such a good life; you don't work; you get to play with Hannah all day. You are so selfish for wanting more. Why is this not enough for you?*"

"Why would they think those things?"

"I don't know." I paused. "Probably because that's what I think about myself."

"What is the root of your sadness, Alexis Marie?"

"My . . . my baby . . . died," I managed to choke while clutching the neck of my blouse. I told Dr. Haverson the details of Zachary's life and death, I spoke about my upbringing and my fixation on perfectionism and tendency to overthink, and about the tug-of-war between motherhood and my art. My words took form, growing like thorny vines that cloaked the room from floor to ceiling.

"When Zachary died I felt like the ultimate failure as a mother. And every day with Hannah . . . I love her so much and try so hard, but it's like I'm never enough. For anyone." My lower eyelids cupped swells of tears. I blinked them back. Dr. Haverson passed me a familiar tissue box, the kind the hospital stocked, the kind I'd torn through with my tears as Aaron and I were counseled on funeral homes and burial options.

"I don't cry about Zachary anymore," I said, nodding slowly. "My feelings aren't ragged and oozing like they were before. I'm healing, you know? The white blood cells and time are doing their work." I chuckled faintly, but the psychologist just watched me. "I still do bring up Zachary, all the time, actually, even to strangers. When people ask if the baby in my stomach is my second, I tell them no; I say that this is my third, that my second child passed away—but all that doesn't make me cry anymore."

Yet, in Dr. Haverson's tiny office with maroon carpet and a wooden L-shaped desk that she leaned on thoughtfully as she listened, I found myself crying.

"Maybe this," she gestured to my tears, "is a more genuine reaction to how you are feeling about Zachary, how you are feeling about all aspects of your life."

"Maybe . . . maybe." My breathing was tight and short, until I could no longer hold myself back. I wept.

Dr. Haverson watched me patiently and my breathing eventually slowed. Then she and I stared at each other without speaking. Did I even see her full cheeks and round nose where wire rims bounced up and down when she spoke? Did I see the way she sat there, slouched, legs uncrossed? Or how she tapped the point of her pen on my chart to keep her place? No. She was an outline.

In the style of the vintage 3D View-Master, with its circular reels of photographs featuring places like the Grand Canyon and Mount Rushmore, my memory clicked through my own recent images of significance. They were all places of containment: houses with rooms and nurseries, hospitals and their waiting rooms, exam rooms, counseling rooms, the frame of the ultrasound monitor, the borders of X-rays, and my own hands and heart.

Containment yet vacancy. Emptiness.

The connections between these places, the drives to the hospital like dizzying carousel rides, and the expanding and contracting hallways of my memories—they all drew me forward in one direction. Always to the spot where Zach lay motionless beneath a warming lamp. There the procession of images jammed, and I could not advance.

The doctor interrupted the reel. "Your job is to get free."

The statement was simple, yet wildly abstract. *Get free.* It was the kind of response that resonated with my conceptual nature. Dr. Haverson spoke in a way I understood, and I smiled suddenly, like a foreigner hearing the sound of her native tongue. When I had told Aaron and Mom I felt trapped, they didn't know what to say. "How can we help you if we don't understand what you need?" they had responded. I was a mystery to them. Yet, after all my ramblings, hidden metaphors, and poetic drawl, Dr. Haverson, who had only known me thirty minutes, understood my entrapment and responded with an equally abstract call to action.

Your job is to get free.

She paused, pursed her lips. "Freedom. Authenticity. Give yourself grace. This will be a transformation. Allow yourself to be who you are. You *must* do your art."

Week 25: Lifting the Curtain

When I had been twenty-five weeks pregnant with Zachary, my understanding of the world smashed around me with his diagnosis. Like shattered mirrors, each piece reflected my broken innocence, stretching backward in an eternal repetition. Reaching that time marker with Eden, I once more found myself living in a house of glass.

"Mommy eyes all be-doo?" It took me a moment to understand what Hannah was saying. I tilted the rearview mirror so I could see my girl in her toddler seat strapped to the center of the passenger row. We were running errands, and the sun warmed our skin through the car windows, despite the frozen snowbanks, standing more than two feet tall, that bordered the road. Hannah repeated herself, and I read her lips.

"Mommy's eyes are all better?" I replied. "What happened to Mommy's eyes, Hannah?"

"Mommy eyes cry. Doctor says . . ."

"What does the doctor say, Han?"

"Doctor says, 'No more monkeys jumping on the bed.'" Hannah burst out laughing.

We sang the nursery rhyme, and Hannah kept the tune, remembering most of the words. All the while during our duet, I fretted about the effect of my emotions on my girl. Even from the backseat she had noticed my tears. Hannah attended every prenatal appointment with me. She observed most intimately my daily struggle between grief and freedom.

One of our errands that day was to purchase a newborn-baby doll. Hannah was curious about Eden and often tenderly rubbed her own belly, saying she had a baby of her own tucked inside, just like Mommy. I was hoping to find a doll similar in size and proportion to an actual newborn, a baby that Hannah could practice caring for and sharing with before her actual sibling arrived.

The only dolls we found at Value Village had animal faces and, while Hannah was entranced, their anthropomorphized features unnerved me. At the shop of slightly used clothing and toys just up the road, there were shelves of plastic products: water tables, music stations, Mega Bloks, transformers, doll houses, but no baby dolls.

"No more car seat," Hannah fussed as I tightened her shoulder straps.

"Han, I have one more idea where we can find you a baby."

"Let's go!"

Navigating the maze of Toys"R"Us, we eventually arrived at a ten foot tall display of newborn-baby dolls. Some had thick plastic lashes and weighted eyes that stared at us, unblinking, from their boxes where they stood, strapped and inert. Other dolls reclined in their packaging, their little bodies flanked by pink accessories. Every baby wore pink. I was undecided if the display was a bereaved parent's dream or nightmare.

Back in the parking lot, I gently removed the newborn from its twist-tied and cardboard constraints, passing it into Hannah's eager hands. "Hannah hold baby, hi baby," she said. We also bought a bottle that made three distinct sounds when the nipple was compressed.

Looking at the time on the dashboard, my palms began to sweat. "Let's go, Hannah. It's time to go."

"Home?"

"Not yet, sweetie. One more stop." Hannah began to whine, but I told her we were headed to watch baby Eden on TV. In the rearview mirror I could see Hannah look down at her newborn excitedly. You would have thought we were headed to Disneyland. At the opposite extreme, the ultrasound ordered by Dr. Stilles terrified me. *What will they find?*

Hannah played with the baby doll in the airy waiting room of River Valley Medical, where large angled windows rose like skylights above the bench we sat on. Hannah inserted the bottle between her baby's plastic lips and mechanical-sounding wails escaped. Then a suckling noise. Then a burp. Hannah sat up straight with pride as she mothered her doll, which she eagerly showed to her daddy when Aaron arrived.

I had insisted Aaron and Hannah accompany me at every stage of the appointment; I was petrified I might receive bad news alone, as I had from Dr. Stilles about Zachary's heart. I needed Hannah to be grumpy from her lack of an afternoon nap. I needed the distraction of caring for her, of offering a sippy cup, Ritz Crackers, and, eventually, my iPhone with *Max and Ruby* reruns. I needed Aaron to hold my body from quivering off the tabletop and to transcribe the appointment in my notebook so I didn't forget a word. Living people. Touchable relationships. I needed their noise and breath and shuffling feet in the building that had come to represent for me the beginning of the end at twenty-five weeks.

The technician brushed the wand across my stomach like an artist at her canvas, measuring, calculating, recording data into her computer. Aaron pulled the only other chair in the room up beside the exam table so Hannah could perch there and lean on me while she watched her show. Ruby bossed around her little brother, Max, as she did in every episode, and I wondered if Hannah would do the same to Eden.

"Mommy, hiccups!" Hannah said with a giggle. She looked from me to her daddy and waited for the evidence. When she hiccupped again, Hannah's shoulders popped up like a shrug, and Aaron let shock spread across his face. He tussled her hair playfully.

The technician, having completed her measurements, began,

"All the gross anatomy looks good." She approved the greyscale images on the monitor with a nod, aware of our history from my thick chart on her table. Turning toward Hannah, the woman said, "Your brother has hiccups, just like you!" Baby was moving, all right, but I didn't realize it was with the same rhythmic jolts as his sister.

"They are in sync," Aaron chuckled.

"Your baby is waving to you," the technician continued. Hannah's jaw fell open in amazement briefly before she turned back to her show. "That is a good sign, because we often see clenched fists in babies with abnormalities." I twisted my neck to look at the screen; Eden's hands were open, and we could count the little white bones in his fingers.

The technician directed our gaze toward Eden's eyes. "See." She pointed to the screen with one hand while holding the wand steady with the other. "His eyes are moving. They are actually closed, but we can see the lenses refracting light." Eden's heart rate was 167 beats per minute, and from the technician's measurements we learned he weighed one pound and nine ounces. He was lying facedown in utero and still had no hair on his head.

As the technician stood to take her images to the doctor, in a matter-of-fact tone she said, "The radiologist on today is very thorough. Don't be alarmed if she comes in and wants to do some scanning herself. She likes scanning."

Aaron and I waited, holding each other's hands, sweaty and tight. We strained to extend our hearing beyond the room to no avail. "If the radiologist comes in, that's a very bad sign," I whispered to Aaron.

"Everything's fine," he said, trying to comfort me, but we had been in that exact exam room before, in that exact situation—waiting for news. When the door handle turned, I expected to see the doctor, but instead the technician walked in. "The radiologist says she has no concerns with what she saw; she is not coming in to scan."

"Oh, thank God!" I exhaled loudly.

"But—she does recommend you get an echocardiogram of the baby's heart."

"What?" My nerves, after less than a fraction of a second at rest, flared back into heightened awareness.

"She recommends it not because of anything she saw, but just because of your history. It can give you two some peace of mind while providing us a more complete study." I looked at Aaron with panic, then back at the technician with suspicion. *This doesn't make sense; why are they ordering a fetal echo without cause?*

"And for that I have to go to the perinatal clinic at The Arthur Memorial Hospital?" I asked, already knowing the answer, instantly recalling the peachy-color of the clinic's walls, the cheap poster art that hung there, and the circular cell-like hallways lined with doors to darkened exam rooms. *What if we bump into the doctor who pressured us to terminate Zachary's life? What if we see Alice Smyth?* Alice was the counselor who had talked Aaron and me through our options, every day, at every appointment. Already I dreaded the echo.

A few days later, before five in the morning, I woke and rolled out of bed for the ritual emptying of my bladder. I must have slept most of the night on my left side, because when I returned to bed and lay on my right, Eden dislodged from the nook he had been cuddled in. He seemed to wake and stretch from my lungs to my pubic bone, becoming a busy boy. I couldn't recall how long I flirted with sleep.

As I drifted in and out, I entered into the forbidden dialogue with my subconscious. Only a month before, my drowsy brain had erected barricades to the taboo subject of Eden's delivery. Yet, in those sleepy moments, as Eden played my ribcage like a xylophone, something changed.

First, I began to make a mental list of everything I needed to pack. *Which camera should we bring to the hospital? The Sony or the Nikon? What bra will I wear? I don't want to forget my journal—*

or my housecoat. I pictured labor with Eden unfolding exactly as it had with Hannah . . .

꩜

I am in the hospital, and it is November 2009 at Hannah's birth— but also June 2012 on Eden's due date. The warm yet itchy numbness of the epidural slips over the lower half of my body, and I welcome its relief. The time melts surreally, like Dali's clocks, and I am beside myself while also fully, soulfully, enfolded in the moment. Hannah's heart rate drops suddenly. Eden's heart rate follows.

"We need to get this baby out, now!" the on-call obstetrician commands, but not to me; the nurses begin to flutter around my bed. The obstetrician pulls a doctor's covering over his striped dress shirt. He is older, pure white on top with an obvious appetite for heroism. With precision born of acute muscular repetition, he swiftly brings Hannah, brings Eden, into the world, wielding the forceps as skill-fully as dining utensils. Hannah has not one mark upon her head. Eden is perfect.

"I did such a great job, you should name your baby after me!" The obstetrician puffs his chest and laughs through Chiclet-sized dentures. "And name the placenta after the nurse!"

Hannah lies upon my chest, slimy with vernix and blood. Eden nestles into my breast. The crimson stain on my hospital gown is holy. Baby's new skin is wrinkly and furrowed. Hannah cries. Eden wails. The nurse takes my child and records weight and length. She wraps the curled body in a receiving blanket and places my baby in my arms. I have been stitched, but I remember it only vaguely.

Hannah and I, Eden and I, are wheeled to the private room Aaron requested; a queen bed with real linens and a large photograph of the ocean greet us. Hannah sleeps in a basinet at my bedside, and I can see Eden from where I lie in the bed. I get up frequently in the night to nurse and change the meconium-filled diapers and rock Baby back to sleep. Aaron rests through the night, as if he were the one who gave birth. We have visitors in the morning and take photographs of our daughter, of our son. Then we head home to learn a new way of living.

Week 26: Photographs

One Saturday morning, while Aaron played with Hannah in the backyard, I called Baby Before Birth and booked a 3D ultrasound for Eden. If it had been a normal pregnancy, the planner in me would have made the call as soon as I found out I was pregnant. The portrait studio, as they called themselves, was always busy and booked months in advance. When I phoned, the receptionist told me I was just in time; any further along and Eden's pictures may have resembled a child with his face squished against a window.

Baby Before Birth had been the first to detect Zachary's cardiac abnormality—which, since they were not doctors, they could not alert us to at the time. The appointment for Zachary had taken place in early September of 2010 and progressed much the same as Hannah's the year before. Both sides of our family had squeezed into the tiny exam room, where my dad volunteered to sit on a windowsill as we were short on chairs. As a group, we admired Zachary's orange-toned 3D form in real time and counted his toes aloud for Hannah. She was momentarily enthralled before squirming out of Aaron's hands to crawl on the floor, distracting the grandmothers who vied for her sacred attention.

The technician knew something was amiss, yet he granted us our time of happiness and dysfunction without saying a word, sending me home with a DVD of pictures I planned to scrapbook. Those photographs did eventually fill the pages of one lonely volume, but not until we learned the truth of that appointment. After Zachary died, it was all I could do to paste the monotone images onto baby-blue paper and cradle them within plastic sleeves.

There was a time I vowed to never again utter the words Baby Before Birth, let alone step again into its reflective downtown building made of azure-toned glass and steel. The memories of that place were distorted; they had all the qualities of an old, eerie film, something scratched and desaturated. The accompanying score was like a violin solo of wind through the branches of the two skeletal maples that flanked its entrance. When I imagined walking through its doors, I saw the plaster walls crackling inward beneath flickering fluorescent lights. My clicking shoes slipped across the deathly cold marble floor while doors creaked and laughed wickedly as I passed.

A part of me still subscribed to the notion that if I did everything the same as last time I would reap the same result. Yet, it would pain me if Eden, born healthy, lived to wonder at the absence of photographs recording his features as he grew, or at the void of scrapbooks and photo albums with his name scrawled in Sharpie on their spines. When I was pregnant with Hannah and Zachary, Aaron took a picture of me in profile in steady increments. By writing my gestational week on a sheet of paper, which I then held up in the photos, we documented the expanding girth of my stomach and our approaching due date. With each image I grew fatter and happier.

Aaron and I had yet to take even one photograph of me in my pregnancy with Eden. A photo was a record of anticipation. After week twenty-six there would be week twenty-seven, twenty-eight, twenty-nine, thirty, and onward—if we were lucky. I tried to force my mind into expecting this progression, but like a child with her chin pinched so she would look at her scolding mother, the girl's eyes darting obstinately back and forth, I could not bring myself to look into the face of my future.

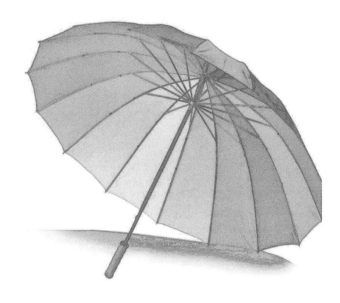

PART 3

THIRD TRIMESTER

Week 27: Snow in the Desert

Spring in Edmonton unveiled itself in gradual ways. The air grew warm and sweet-smelling at the same time as the waist-high snowbanks began their leisurely thaw. The melting revealed grime-caked gutters that lined the roadways like dirty fingernails in a messy collection of gravel spewed from city trucks all winter long. The frigid season had spanned nearly five months, and, as a result, Hannah and I were eager to fly south to Arizona for a visit.

Our itinerary allowed for a week with my parents before Mom and Ken flew back to Edmonton, and Aaron, with our friends Jake and Megan, joined us for spring break. When our plane touched down, Hannah and I found Phoenix already abloom with fuchsia and pearl-colored flowers budding between cacti needles and a desert full of palms and dusty yellow-green shrubbery.

From the moment Hannah and I arrived, my overprotective mother began grooming me for her departure. "There's a restaurant file in the top right drawer of my desk with menus and directions. I have written out some notes for you." There were seven pages in a yellow legal pad. "When do you want to go over it all?" We added two more pages with step-by-step instructions on how to use the spa remote.

"This is the drawer where we store the car keys." Mom pulled open a wooden drawer with a *swoosh* and metallic flash. "Oh, and the mail key. Can you get the mail a few times? Remember, the mail key is on the red curly swimming chain. Box #35." Her blessing of hospitality came with a list of chores.

Mom taught me tricks to remember everything. "You won't forget our mailbox number because the house address is 3225. Take the first and last number and you've got it." She had invented riddles to recall the computer password and organized her house with the logic of "If I were to look for something, where would it be?"

Mom wore her blonde hair in an ear-length bob; atop her nose sat chunky red frames. Everywhere we went people commented that we looked alike, although my hair was long and my glasses were black. Their words were a compliment I was eager to receive, as Mom was very beautiful. When Hannah grew out of her baby rolls, she would share our prominent cheekbones and feminine jawlines.

Mom was a brilliant woman, business-savvy and astute in more areas than I could count. She had always been my hero and perfectly encompassed many extremes at once, from skillful chef to master financial analyst. She was resolute in her independence yet swift to push everything aside in order to spend time with me or Hannah, whom she adored. To any question I asked, Mom knew the answer or was quick to research and call me with a lengthy response. Yet Mom frequently lost her keys, her greatest foible, calling me weekly to tell the horrific story of their latest disappearance.

"Remember to put the car keys and mailbox key back in this drawer when you're done," Mom instructed, sliding it shut with a clamor before we moved onto the next item on her list.

I was used to these collections of tasks, to Mom's directions and running commentary on the mundane functioning of things. I knew when to pay attention. Being a list person myself, and terribly forgetful, I was secretly thankful for every handwritten page of the Phoenix visitor manual Mom had compiled and her GPS-like directions to the grocery store, Target, and the airport, complete with instructions on how to get home either way on the I-10.

Yet, as we set off early one morning to visit the red-rock mountains of Sedona, an hour-and-a-half-long drive, I grew impatient with the conversation. The road trip was fairly direct from Phoenix, and that was also how I was feeling that morning. Direct.

"Mom, can we talk about deep stuff for a while?" We turned left onto Carefree Highway and headed west. Mom snapped out of her monologue of instructions, jarred back into the present, and glanced over at me in the passenger seat with a nod. Mom tried hard to be supportive in the way I needed, and for the first time since Hannah and I arrived, we had a real conversation.

"I got a Facebook message yesterday from this girl I know . . ." I pulled out my phone and read the message to Mom:

> Hey Alexis Marie,
> I have a personal question. One of my girlfriends had a stillbirth at thirty-eight weeks not that long ago. I want to comfort her but I don't know how. What helped you and Aaron when you lost Zachary? Do you have any advice? I thought about taking my friend for coffee or going for a walk to try to get her mind off things. Any suggestions would be great. Thanks.

"And, what did you write back?"

"So, I started by suggesting she avoid saying things like *Everything will be okay*, or *At least you can have more children*, or, even, *God has a plan*. When she asks her friend how she is doing, she should try really hard to just listen and not compare hardships. I explained that her friend had not only lost her baby but her future as well—and that marriage can get complicated . . ." My voice trailed off. "I threw out the ideas of scrapbooking and writing in a journal. Those things were helpful for me. And, I told her that her friend probably wants to talk about her baby, not have her mind taken off of it."

"Those are good suggestions."

"But I still can't shake the question of what helped Aaron and me. How *did* I get through it?" I paused. "Nothing I wrote really gives a straight answer." I strained my mind backward, but the memories were no longer crisp, time wilting the edges of my recollections and replacing details with impressions and emotions instead. "It doesn't feel like Zachary passed away yesterday, maybe a month and a half ago—but definitely not a year and a half ago. It's weird how I can't remember how I survived it all . . ." I stared out the window.

Driving along Carefree Highway, we passed a dusty field where hot air balloons with Native American Aztec patterns of orange and red and blue were beginning to rise over the foothills of Black Mountain. "Air boon! Air boon!" Hannah screamed, pointing. I opened our windows and took a photograph, the air rushing in fast and fresh, rich, smelling of dirt, horses, and history.

Mom was quiet for a few minutes and turned north onto I-17 before she spoke. "Your dad and I went to school with this woman, Roxanne," she began. "Roxanne got married and moved away from the Okanagan. A few years later your dad got transferred to Vancouver, where Roxanne lived, and we somehow heard that her husband had died. I think it was cancer or something. Leukemia.

"We wanted to visit her. The three of us went for dinner, and during the meal we didn't talk about her husband. We drove her home, and she invited us in for drinks. That's when your dad said something like, 'I'm so sorry your husband died; it must be so hard for you.' Roxanne cried. She said, 'Yes, it is hard. People come and visit and pretend it never happened; they don't even acknowledge that he existed. They think that makes it easier for me. I loved him so much, he was the most important person in my life, and now he's gone and all I want to do is talk about him.'

"Your dad and I were just as ignorant as everyone else," Mom reflected. "We sort of stumbled into the conversation. Your dad and I were not sure what to say; we were scared of saying the wrong thing. We asked what had happened, and she was so happy to talk. They were still newlyweds. He had renovated their house. She showed us around. She was so proud of the work he had done."

"Thanks, Mom," I said. "Thanks for telling me that."

"See those cacti?" Mom asked. "The tall ones with arms bent

at the elbow, reaching up to the sun? They are Saguaro. There's a point on this drive where the Saguaros stop. They just stop, and the terrain becomes totally different." Mom was back to her commentary. She knew the drive well, and I sat back in thought and watched her words come true as the miles passed beneath us.

All of a sudden, as we neared Sedona, there was snow. *Snow?* It was the desert at the end of March, yet there it was, just outside my window. The snow filled the gaps between shrubs like grout along Arizona State 179 North to Route 89A, and as we approached the massive, jagged red-rock bluffs of Cathedral Mountain I noticed its base was blanketed as well. The cliffs were capped in white, standing a proud fifteen hundred meters tall.

My mouth hung agape like a cartoon character's as I gawked; I had just left snowy Edmonton and hadn't even packed a jacket. *How can this be?* Mom was also startled and had no answer. Hannah, who had woken quietly, paid no attention to the snow and instead pointed excitedly at a pack of motorbikes that roared past us like a swarm of bees.

We pulled into a lookout point where we could just make out the Chapel of the Holy Cross built atop a low mountain arm off in the distance. I leapt from the vehicle and grabbed my Nikon while Mom unbuckled Hannah from her car seat. I raced to the wood-and-stone-column fence at a small information hut and was greeted by its roofline of ice crystals that dripped sun-glossed dew into puddles on the pavement. Carefully I maneuvered my belly and swollen feet over the fence and landed ankle-deep in the snow of a wide embankment. Green poked through the glistening white, revealing the resilient desert foliage.

"Where are you going?" Mom yelled at me.

"Closer," I replied, my back to them. The truth was I didn't know where I was headed; the trails that led to the base of the mountain were closed. "Snow in the desert!" I yelled in response, as if that were the answer.

Hannah cried out, "Mommy, ca-wee!" When I turned, her bottom lip was in a full downward curl as she watched me longingly and squirmed in Mom's arms. Too enthralled with the landscape for a long debate, I backtracked through the snow in my slip-on flats. Quickly, I sat Hannah on my hip, so she was straddling my baby bump, and began to crunch through the snow once more before Mom had the chance to protest. Hannah instantly laughed, her pout forgotten, and I used my free hand to scoop up some clean snow, crushing it into a ball I gave her to nibble.

Hannah and I ran and played in the snow. I photographed the paradox around us and the mountain that reached to the sky as if it had recently fallen from it, ruddy and newborn itself, an evolving formation of earth and clay. The day was sunny, and Hannah refused her coat. Mom mirrored our movements on the opposite side of the fence, her shoes as impractical as mine. The columned barricade turned to an economical wire as we curled our way around the parking lot.

Snow in the desert.

The dualities within me were painted in white across the fire-colored rock. I again thought of the earth's axis—*Am I burning or am I frozen?* I had pondered that question the day I hosted Theresa's baby shower, back before I learned I was already carrying Eden. The paradox of snow on lava rock was a tender indication that I could in fact encompass many extremes simultaneously. Both life and death could live within my soul. It was possible to be mother and artist, through and through, within one identity. And the anomaly of Zachary's genetics, and my enlarged heart, were both a misfortune and a blessing—though I could not yet have known why.

Week 28: Sex

"Ready to have a whale on top of ya?" I climbed onto the guest bed in Phoenix and straddled Aaron, who nodded hungrily. He was aroused at the sight of my skin and plump, heavy breasts; in his eyes, I was his perpetually pregnant wife with sexy feminine curves. I, on the other hand, felt like a blob that hadn't seen her pubic hair in months and had a pointy weapon for a belly button. I couldn't remember the last time we had made love.

In the first trimester, I had grown nauseous just thinking about bouncing around in bed. In the second, according to Dr. Stilles's gruff female resident, I was pregnant, which was meant to be answer enough. "Biologically, we have sex to make babies." She spat her words out through lemon-colored teeth. My desire for intimacy had shriveled in the second trimester, and Aaron had suggested I inquire about it at my next prenatal appointment. I could tell the resident was thinking something like, *Your husband is just horny; stop wasting my time.*

Then she read my chart. "Plus, you have been through a lot." The sharp edge to her voice dulled as she squeezed my hand tightly with her large palm and long fingers. "You have a lot you are worrying about right now."

Aaron and I had practiced safe sex, if not voluntary celibacy, during the nine months of our genetic testing, terrified of accidentally becoming pregnant before the verdict. After the genetics counselor pronounced us normal, we began making love like newlyweds on their honeymoon, multiple times a night and while

Hannah napped, but it was never frivolous. I knew, with the tensile certainty of steel, that I needed to mother another child. I could not rationalize or explain the urge, except to acknowledge its barking demand in my sleeping and waking dreams, in every conversation, in all that caught my eye, right through to my very biology, which manifested as a head-to-toe physical ache.

I was a sex machine. "Let's do it again."

"Give me a few minutes," Aaron responded as he lay back on his pillow, his chest rising and falling heavily.

"Was that enough of a break?" I asked literally three minutes later. "Are you ready?"

After a couple weeks, Aaron was weary and disenchanted with the process. He wanted the magic: passion, sexy lingerie, connectedness, foreplay, intimacy. I wanted the baby.

Those were sweet times in retrospect, moments I wished I had allowed our affection to help heal my heart. Maybe if I had, if I'd opened myself to that possibility, I would not have continued to struggle with feelings of disconnectedness between us. Or perhaps there was no quantity of time or words or sex that could make me forget.

꙳

Aaron, Hannah, and I had visited Mom and Ken in Arizona for New Year's about two months after Zachary died. Hannah and I were scheduled to stay a week, while Aaron had to be back to the school on Monday. Again I had said to him, "Stay with me. I need you."

"I can't. I have to get back to work. I am trying to take care of our family."

"Your family is here! I need you. Please don't leave me again," I begged shamelessly. I had even talked to my parents about it. "I need my husband."

"We are here for you, whatever you need," they told me. Later, I overheard Mom and Ken reminding Aaron we had a mortgage. They did not understand.

I had been direct and specific; I needed my husband, but judging by the looks on their faces I could have had a brain injury that caused my speech to jumble beyond my lips. No matter my words or thousands of tears, Aaron and my parents could not make sense of what to do with me. I was a person without appendages. I had no hands to free myself and no feet to get anywhere, anyway; no tongue to cry for help; no eyes or ears or a nose. I was completely senseless in my anguish.

Aaron was not going to change his flight. That was clear. I went into the garage to escape the logical conversations that left nothing for my irrational yet fragile longing for companionship. Tension rippled through me in spasms, and my nostrils flared like those of a bull taunted with red. I hit my skull hard, beat myself again and again. There was no outlet for the anger, for the wildness of my isolation, but my own body. I scavenged for something to break, or to break me.

Suicide was not my intention. *What will death accomplish?* I thought. *Alleviate my pain, yes, but also amplify it for everyone in my life whom I care for.* My love for Hannah was greater than my despair, and I would never leave her motherless; I simply wanted to hurt myself. *Then they will see how serious I am. Look! Listen to me, please! The blood will show them,* I had reasoned. Physical pain had become a paper cut in comparison to the state of my aching heart.

Rubbing the soles of my feet on the gritty pavement of the garage, I had hoped to shred away my skin. *BANG*—my hands whaled upon the white pressed-board storage cabinets. Then I ripped open the flimsy doors to see what was inside. The first revealed a jumble of red and blue bungee cords, half-empty paint cans, and masking tape. *No. That won't work.* I slammed the door closed. The force with which I opened the second set of doors created a tsunami of air that blew the hair away from my face. That cabinet contained spa equipment, tubes and filters and fabric shopping bags. I wailed, frustrated. Someone was coming. The garage door opened with a chime from the alarm system.

"Alexis Marie? What are you doing?" Aaron's voice reached from the far side of my parents' vehicle. I raced to the third and final cabinet. There was a collection of golf balls my parents had found on the course, some throw-aways mixed with a handful of Titleist pro V1s and Bridgestones. I found the tees; grabbed a white, splintery one, and began to stab the palm of my hand, boring into myself as if I were hard earth at a tee box.

Aaron grabbed me by the wrists. "STOP!" he yelled, but I thrashed and resisted.

"LET ME GO!" I screamed, my rage widening my eyes, pulling my lips back into an animal snarl and growl. *How dare he? He is the one leaving me!* I threw my body against him. He was too strong, too tall, weighing so much more than me; my one-hundred-and-forty-pound frame was powerless in comparison. We were on the ground. I could not move. His restraint was a picture of my inward state. *I am not free.*

I screamed, "Leave me alone! Go away!" My parents came out, Mom carrying Hannah. I did not want my girl seeing me like that, and my glare in Mom's direction communicated so. Mom quickly turned back into the house. I can't remember exactly how I calmed down or how I convinced Aaron to release my wrists. *Did I bite him?*

Ken asked Aaron to cool off in the house.

"I think you have post-traumatic stress disorder; we are going to get you help," Ken said to me once we were alone. "You need to start painting more, doing the things you love. We need to get you exercising and taking care of yourself." He sat beside me on the small six-inch step at the back of the garage and spoke calmly and evenly.

"Can I purchase some canvases for you?" Ken had asked. I nodded. This gift would later become the impetus for my use of art in healing.

Aaron flew back to Edmonton that afternoon as scheduled. I don't recall whether we said goodbye.

Reflecting on that 2011 trip, I found it eerie to be back in Arizona roughly a year later—this time expectant with Eden. If it is true that men and women grieve differently, they must also heal in distinctive ways. I knew I must forgive Aaron for leaving me when I needed him, although I was not sure how to forget.

I had found a strange peace in Arizona, in the middle of the Sonoran Desert and among the sharp barrel cactus. Once, all I could see was the wasteland, and I had wondered why anyone would choose to live in its dust bowl. I had been ignorant of the spirit of survival in the land. Sometime between the winter of 2011 and the spring of 2012, I began to appreciate it all differently. The landscape had remained the same; I was the one who had changed.

The cacti had perfected the endurance of survival. They thrived. *How can I be like them? How can I make my marriage like the Saguaro?* Aaron and I needed to thrive together, as if we were plants intertwined, roots tangled inseparably, birds building their nest between our two tall arms.

Spring break came to an end. Aaron and I made love twice before heading to the airport. He smelled my hair and told me I was beautiful, stretch marks and all. In Terminal 4 at Sky Harbor International Airport, I kissed him goodbye. The day before, I had decided I was not ready to go home; I was going to stay, just Hannah and me. Aaron had to return to work Monday morning—but this time I did not mind.

Week 29: Laura

I sensed urgency in my friend's words. "Laura wants to talk to someone who knows her pain," she had written in another message about her friend, a woman I did not know, who had given birth to a stillborn child at thirty-eight weeks. While I was still in Arizona, I called Laura, and we arranged to meet for coffee at Starbucks once I returned home.

The trip from Phoenix to Edmonton had been a challenge, but not because of our overweight bag or Hannah on the late-night flight. It was the coming home to my worry, the return to myself and my routine that was agonizing. In Arizona, the heat was my prenatal appointment, the bottomless blue sky my therapist, and the restful and simple days my examinations. The cacti, the stoic thorned statues, were my daily inspiration. It was there I found peace.

In Edmonton, the snow waxed across all the places the sunlight could not reach, hanging on in small clumps within the perimeter of shadows or neighboring our front steps or beneath the roofline of the Starbucks where I waited for Laura. I had arrived early. Shifting from foot to foot, I wondered if I'd see a version of my grief-worn self walk through the coffee shop door.

I still did not know what encouragement to offer Laura. *What am I going to say?* For a while I stood nervously, fidgeting, then sat, then visited the washroom. I munched on the skin of my lower lip, then went on to bite my hangnail. *Should I confess that I survived the last eighteen months since Zachary's death by trial and error?*

Laura had lost her daughter two months before our coffee date. At two months I was still pretending to be strong in my Year of Distraction, holding my head high while internally I was unfastening. I did not reach out to others at that time; already Laura was braver than I.

The roads were peppered with gravel and it crept onto the sidewalks and front lawns, onto brown moldy grass and into my shoes. It was a disease. It crunched as cars passed the front window of the Starbucks, crackling noisily as I waited. I stared out the window and wished I were still in Arizona.

A person in a blue coat walked by, catching my eye, and I looked up expectantly. The man passed the door without entering. Rummaging in my purse, not looking for anything in particular, I pulled out my journal and tried to write a poem, but I had no words. *If I can't even form a thought on paper, what am I going to say to Laura?* I debated bolting.

An elderly woman left the coffee shop and smiled at my stomach as she passed through the door. What if Laura, too, noticed I was pregnant? I chewed another fingernail. Our mutual friend had warned me that Laura was extremely sensitive to her friends' pregnancy news since her baby had died. The neck of my sweater, which I chose specifically for the coffee date, drooped with folds of fabric over my chest, but still it did not conceal enough. I had added a scarf with a busy pattern. *Maybe I can distract her*, I had mused, putting on dangly earrings. *Hopefully she will just think I'm fat.*

I had discovered that Laura and I had many connections in common, according to our mutual friend's Facebook page. Most of those people were from the Bible camp I had attended as a youth. Following a link on Laura's page, I learned she was a banker; her professional picture showed a spunky redhead with a wide smile and a Himalayan kitten on her lap.

A figure entered the coffee shop, and I looked up. It was Laura.

"Nice to meet you," I stuttered.

"Likewise, Alexis Marie. Thanks for meeting me here."

"My pleasure. Wait. No, I didn't mean it that way."

"It's okay."

"I read online that you're in banking." Laura nodded and smiled weakly. Her red hair was pulled tight in a messy ponytail, her skin was pale, and she had blackish rings beneath her eyes. "I worked in a bank one summer when I was in university," I rambled, an anxious habit. "Not as a banker, though, obviously; just as an intern. Some of the bankers were pretty crazy."

Immediately I worried I'd offended her, but Laura laughed loudly. "You are so right," she said. We talked about the investment bankers we both knew, the wholesome ones and the scrupulous few, the big players and the woman who was a serial adulteress with each of her muscular, tanned assistants.

At the Starbucks counter Laura and I realized we both disliked coffee and ordered hot chocolates instead. "So, obviously, I looked you up on Facebook," I began. "Oh, man; that sounds creepy, huh?"

"I did the same with you," Laura chuckled.

"Oh, good. Anyway, we know a lot of the same people. Do you go to church?"

"Not anymore, but I did. Growing up." We realized we were once part of the same denomination, although we had not known each other.

"After Zachary died, Christians kept telling me that things happen for a reason, but that only made me angrier. Outside the church I feel freer to accept that there are things in life that cannot be explained."

"I feel the same way, even though I was disillusioned with religion well before Betty died." Laura said her daughter's name with reverence. "My parents are very strict with it all. After Betty was stillborn, my dad told me, 'Satan took Betty.'"

"What? Are you serious?"

"Yep. I haven't spoken with him since. He made me feel like it was something I had done, some sin I was being punished for."

"I'm so sorry to hear that, Laura—although I know what that's like. I had a family member suggest Zachary died because I got pregnant too soon after having Hannah."

"One of my family members said Betty died because I worked too much."

"I'm sure that wasn't the reason."

"The doctor chalked it up to bad luck. What about you?"

"They told us Zachary's genetic abnormality was random. They said it wasn't our fault, that there was nothing we could have done differently."

"Us, too." Laura took a sip of her hot chocolate.

"If you are comfortable, can you tell me about what happened?"

"Sure." Laura took a breath. "The pregnancy was going great. I felt good. Everything was normal. We were almost there, only two weeks to go. Then one night I realized I hadn't felt Baby move in a while. When I thought about it, I couldn't remember the last time I had felt her kick. I thought maybe the last time had been just that morning, but then I realized that it could have been the day before. I wrote it off for a while; as babies get bigger, they move less, right?" I nodded.

"I ate a whole pile of sugar and lay on my side in the position that always made her wiggle. But she didn't move. My husband took me to the hospital and they did an ultrasound and there was no heartbeat. They told me Betty had died, but it didn't make sense. She was supposed to be born soon. They induced me and I delivered her. She was beautiful."

"Did you take any pictures?"

"Yes, a few."

"I'd love to see a photo of Betty sometime, if you're comfortable showing me."

"That would be—wonderful." Laura teared up for the first time that evening. "We never get to show her picture to anyone. Thank you for asking."

"I'm so sorry, Laura." I watched her wipe away her tears and compose herself. "It's okay to cry."

"All I do is cry."

Laura asked me what had happened with Zachary. I shared my story but couldn't avoid mentioning my growing stomach. "I should have told you on the phone. I'm sorry; I don't want to upset you."

"No, no. You're good. It's the baby news from friends who have never lost a child and are so excited right in my face that pisses me off. It's actually an encouragement"—she gestured toward me—"to see couples have healthy children after, well, you know."

"I hope healthy," I said under my breath before asking, "Your friends are rubbing their pregnancies in your face? Why?"

Laura shrugged. "They're oblivious. Or ignorant. It's usually a scenario like this: they take me and my husband out for dinner and ask how we are doing. I think, wow, this friend really cares, and I open up about my feelings. Then the friend says, *Well*, as if the floor is now open, *I've got good news—I'M PREGNANT!* Seriously, what kind of a response are they looking for?"

"No kidding."

"We pretend to be happy. Talk about the due date and morning sickness and all that crap and then try to get outta there as quick as possible." Laura compared her experience to a person confessing her bankruptcy only to be told by her confidantes that they had just won the lottery. "Your pregnancy," Laura said slowly, "is like someone who has first been bankrupt and *then* wins the jackpot. It is totally different."

We talked about our new hospital phobias and Laura's adverse reaction to the stuffed bear given to her by a nurse once Betty was delivered. Laura shared how angry her husband had become and how they'd taken many trips over the last two months to be alone together. She told me she was not suicidal but that a part of her would have been okay if she had died, because then she could be with Betty, who was named after her favorite grandmother.

A Starbucks worker tapped me on the shoulder. "Just to let you ladies know: we are closing now."

Confused, I looked back at Laura. "What time is it?" We had

talked without lull since she had arrived. We stepped out of the shop and onto the dimly lit sidewalk. The air still had the bite of winter rather than the warmth of spring. "Somehow, life does go on," I said, immediately hating my choice of words, and I apologized. "Oh! Jeeze! That sounds so cliché—but I do feel it's true. Somehow, life does go on."

Week 30: Baby Before Birth

Aaron hopped in the shower with me and swirled the steam. I looked at him, admiring the charming details of his face, his genuine smile and kind, almond-shaped eyes. He still possessed boyish good looks.

"It's going to be neat having a mini-you walking around the house," I said, remembering all the baby and childhood photographs of Aaron I'd seen while we dated, and how proud his mother was to share them. When I looked at Aaron, I imagined the face of my boys, both Zachary and Eden, all at once.

"Do you ever feel that way about Hannah and me?"

"Yeah, with some of her expressions and the way she says things. Just like you."

"I'm thirty weeks, you know."

Aaron did not reply right away. "This is as far as we got with Zachary. Everything is going to be different from here on out," he said finally.

"I hope you're right."

Aaron and I dressed and hustled Hannah out the door to meet our parents at the Tin Palace for lunch before our appointment at Baby Before Birth. The morning was bleak, a white sky with a thin veil of snow across the ground. The rain from earlier in the week had frozen, clumped into slush on the edges of the roads and frosted tree branches and buildings. Snowflakes warmed to dew on our hair as we entered the restaurant beneath a large wooden parrot. I spotted Mom at a circular table with all of Hannah's grandfathers:

my dad and Ken, as well as Aaron's father. Before I even reached Mom, my eyes blossomed with tears.

"I'm nervous," I whispered. Mom squeezed my hand under the table while the tension throughout my body pulled my shoulders toward my ears. I sat on the edge of my seat, barely tasting the chicken sandwich that appeared and disappeared without my having any consciousness of it. I would never forget Dr. Stilles's words. A year and a half before, he had said, "Baby Before Birth called . . ."

"What if something is wrong this time, like it was with Zachary, and we go through the whole appointment not knowing?"

"Everything's going to be okay."

"I hate it when you say that, Mom. Don't say that to me. You don't know. If something is wrong . . . I can't handle it." Anxiety began to fill my insides and sat like a ten-course feast in my stomach. Everything annoyed me—Aaron ordering for me, his dad's nonstop stories, Ken sneaking Hannah fruit snacks before her meal arrived. How was everyone chitchatting?

Back in the car on the way to the portrait studio, Aaron offered, "In a roundabout way, you are facing your fear."

"I don't want to face my fear; I want to know the future. I want to know that there really is nothing to be afraid of, that everything will turn out right this time." I shook my head and closed my eyes. "I can't do this, Aaron. I'm curious, but I don't think I can go through with the appointment."

"Yes, you can. You're not going to duck and hide; you're going to face this head-on. Now give yourself some credit. And we are doing this together, by the way."

I wheezed. The fullness of anxiety had worked its way into a thick mass in my lungs, and I struggled to breathe. "Am I having a heart attack?" Aaron drove on steadily, despite my hand pressed against my chest. "It hurts to breathe," I choked.

"Just think," he said, "you are going to see Eden."

"Oh, God!" I opened my mouth wide to suck in air.

"Maybe Eden will do this," Aaron stuck his thumb between

his lips and pretended to blow up his hand like a balloon. I swatted him playfully, feigning a grin. Aaron parked and paid the meter, eyeing the lot attendant who casually strolled between vehicles. We met our parents in the lobby and were joined by Aaron's middle brother and his wife.

Everyone talked as we rode the oversized elevator to the eleventh floor, but I heard nothing. Not even the *ding* before the doors swooshed open. The portrait studio's walls were covered in large photographs of grinning babies and pregnant women stroking their ballooning bellies. The door to the nearest exam room was closed, a session underway. The receptionist handed me a clipboard and pen, and I sat rigidly on one of the leather couches, filling out the form. I anticipated the questions: *What pregnancy is this?* Third. *Any complications with the previous pregnancy?* My second child died. I gave the clipboard back to the receptionist. "The basic package," I told her.

Bernie, one of the many ultrasound technicians at Baby Before Birth, was a jovial man with a stomach that drooped beyond his belt and a perfectly round bald spot on the crown of his head. He had been our technician for both Hannah's and Zachary's 3D portraits. Bernie poked his upper body out of an exam room and asked the receptionist something I could not hear. He looked in my direction briefly and smiled with coffee-stained teeth. Did he remember me?

An expectant couple emerged from Bernie's room and approached the counter to collect their DVD of images. Bernie was a step behind them and grabbed a chart from the counter and read my name. Springing to my feet, I rushed to the large man, with Aaron and his long legs just a stride behind me.

"One sec," I said to our family before addressing the technician. Bernie cocked his head to the side, confused. Aaron slipped his arm around my waist, and we spoke as one person, completing each other's sentences, finishing each other's thoughts. "You probably don't remember us," we began. "You did an ultrasound for us over a year ago. You found the issue with our son's heart and you phoned our doctor. Our son died."

Bernie straightened his head, tilting his chin up and inhaling deeply. "I remember." He narrowed his eyes, "What can I do for you?"

"Please, can you tell us if there is something wrong this time?"

"I can't. I will lose my license. I am not qualified to tell you— well, I'm not legally allowed to tell you." This time he dropped his chin, doubling it, and pursed his lips. "Sorry, folks."

"Last time we left and thought everything was okay; our whole appointment we didn't know there was anything wrong."

"I can't."

"What if you just hint? What if you just tell us if everything looks okay?"

"I'm sorry." Bernie was firm. "I cannot comment." He gestured to the darkened room behind him. "Shall we?"

Our family followed us into the dim space, and I reclined on the unrolled white-paper sheet and pulled my shirt up to the base of my bra. The translucent-blue gel Bernie squirted below my belly button was warm, and Aaron squeezed my hand and whispered something about enjoying myself, but all I could do was stretch my neck like a giraffe to watch the monitor.

Bernie narrated the unseen world inside me but not in the way Aaron and I had asked. "Here is your boy's hand on his cheek, see? See his fingers? His other hand is here, doing the rock-on gesture." Aaron was not far off in his earlier enactment. Bernie commented on Eden's chin and lips. "Strong and full. Definitely Dad's," he said.

We looked next at Eden's heart. The dense white tumor tissue I had come to recognize with Zachary was absent. Eden's chambers were unclouded and distinct, maintaining their rhythm, which we listened to through the computer speaker. Bernie clocked their tempo at the regular 150 beats per minute. I tipped my head in Aaron's direction and he returned my gaze through the dimness, his eyes reflecting the monitor's light. His smile was too wide, overcompensating in optimism for my sake. I turned away.

Bernie handed me large oval lollipops, grape and cherry, so I could wake Eden with a rush of sugar. It didn't work. Eden snoozed lazily, full after our lunch. His eyes were closed, and he held the umbilical cord like a stuffed toy. "He will be a good sleeper," predicted Bernie, whose nose and cheeks glowed from the monitor he studied like a crystal ball. I analyzed Bernie as much as I did Eden, but he had a fantastic poker face; he knew the script of acceptable topics and never deviated.

When the appointment was over, our family headed for the lobby while Aaron and I waited to collect our DVD of images from the receptionist. A moment later Mom returned to the counter where Aaron was paying. "Hannah has to go potty," she said, and she asked for the key to the bathroom down the hall. Just as Mom and Hannah left the studio, Bernie emerged from the exam room with a few printed photographs of Eden he passed to me quickly before picking up the next clipboard.

"Wait, please," I begged, despite the eager young couple sitting on the leather couch, ready for Bernie to read their names. I tried to meet the technician's eyes. "Are you going to call our doctor?"

Bernie backed away, his hands raised slightly. "I can't comment," he whispered, before turning to the couple in the waiting area and leading them into the darkened room. I looked at Aaron and he gave me a worth-a-try shrug. We stepped out of the studio and into the long white hallway to wait for Mom and Hannah.

It was the first time Aaron and I had been alone that day. "How do you feel?" he asked.

"It was nice." My voice cracked and I leaned into his athletic pullover, our hug a mess of fabric and briny tears. Just as we embraced, a door opened quickly, startling us, and I turned, expecting to see Hannah and Mom emerge from the washroom. Instead, the frosted glass door of Baby Before Birth swung halfway open. Bernie peeked through.

"I am not going to phone your doctor," he whispered. Aaron

and I stared blankly, speechless. "I'm retiring in a month anyway, so what does it matter. You happy? I am not going to phone your doctor." Bernie disappeared back into the studio.

Week 31: Silver Urn

The morning was grey. Ash-colored clouds overlapped themselves and stole away with the shadows beneath a blurring stream of rain. It was dark despite approaching noon. I was grey as well, my countenance mirroring the low-hanging sky like the pond behind my home: unruffled, its surface still like glass. Aaron was fortunate; he woke early for the gym, leaving before Hannah and I were up, avoiding my melancholy.

As my girl and I were en route to the grocery store that morning, on the small road between our residential neighborhood and an expansive farmer's field, the Jetta in front of us suddenly veered left. I soon did the same, dodging the spilling corpse of a large silvery hare. It looked like a reversible coat, unzipped and inverted with its insides on the outside, smeared across the pavement. The depth of redness, its vibrancy of hue, arrested my attention like a stop sign amid the grey of the day. The hare was fresh and raw, maybe still warm, and two large crows feasted like lionesses, faces bloodied, stabbing deeply with their beaks, tearing flesh from bone.

Death. I cringed and shivered. *Death.*

Animals were waking from their winter sleep and venturing out of the woods, like men and women in their cropped pants and sandals, testing the spring. People raised in Edmonton innately knew that the blossoming buds were deceptive and the city could just as quickly return to a blizzard within the hour. Just the day before I had seen a large deer sprawled on the grassy divide between

146

the northbound and southbound lanes on Terwillegar Drive. Its neck was broken and bent majestically backward, like a swan's. Natural and cyclical, death was a passing from one mystery to another, a changing of seasons.

I was thirty-one weeks pregnant. It was a milestone I had not reached with Zachary. The mystery of death was never far from my mind, overshadowed only by the mystery of life.

Once Zachary had died, and the doctor was still stitching my cut from the episiotomy, Aaron called the funeral director. "Five p.m.," he said. The funeral home had pressed us to set a specific time to pick up Zachary's body.

"How can we put a timeline on goodbye?" I asked, not expecting an answer.

Five o'clock came and went, as did five thirty, and then six and six thirty. Aaron and I said goodbye every minute for 135 minutes until the unapologetic funeral-home worker stumbled into our hospital room at seven fifteen. While I was thankful for every moment I had to rock my son, rage also burned savagely in my chest. I was not only furious at the man who claimed he couldn't find the hospital, but also at the whole scenario in which a stranger would take Zach for his first car ride—and that the destination was a mortuary instead of home.

When we arrived to collect Zachary's ashes one week later, I planned to rant. *How can you demand a time and then be two hours and fifteen minutes late? How do you think that made us feel? How are you people still in business if you treat your customers like this?*

A frail old woman with short bristly white hair and a crackling voice led us through the darkened hallways of the funeral home, past the chapel and the door to the casket display. She finally directed us into a cramped, musty office. The woman seemed as close to death as some of her clients.

Once we sat down she started the business transaction of collecting our son. She didn't apologize for the treatment we received and offered no condolences. It was all very quiet except for the *swoosh, swoosh, swoosh* of what was left of my baby boy. With one hand I rocked the minuscule amount of ashes in the heart-shaped silver urn. *Swoosh, swoosh, swoosh.* The weight of the object was clearly from the metal, not the ashes, which were likely no more than a tablespoon's worth we'd been told. Newborn bones were tiny, just a small collection of hope.

I did not yell. I barely regarded the woman who put a price of $90 on the container to hold my son. She rang in our order as if we had just purchased a scarf or a McDonald's Happy Meal. Indifferently. "Get me out of here," I whispered in Aaron's ear. Just like he did when I was overcome with emotion at Mourning Together, he made it happen.

Zachary was born on a Thursday, and we held his memorial the Wednesday following at Aaron's parent's church in its retro, brown-shag-carpeted sanctuary. Pastor Geoff, the one who had come to the hospital to dedicate Zachary, delivered a short message in front of more than eighty friends, family members, colleagues, and acquaintances who came to pay their respects and lend their support. Theresa's husband videotaped the service from the second-floor balcony, and a photographer volunteered to take pictures. Lisa played the piano. My mother-in-law and her church cronies made tiny sandwiches and squares for the tea-and-coffee time that followed.

Mom had found a free funeral program template online with a royal-blue sky and billowing, milk-colored clouds. I inserted the scan of Zachary's tiny footprints on the cover. His feet were virgins to the earth. They would never grow cold after splashing in a puddle or burn on the sand in the sweaty heat of summer. Zachary would never tickle me under the covers after sneaking into bed on Saturday morning, and I wouldn't get the chance to accidentally trim his toenails too short and atone for my mistake with a double scoop of ice cream after. Those feet replaced the stock image of a smiling, silver-haired woman with animated eyes peering out from behind thick wrinkles. The swap was unnerving.

One wrinkly face should have been exchanged for another, not for the folds of baby skin. *Where is the justice?* I still fumed 31 weeks into my third pregnancy, even as I bitterly, reluctantly acknowledged death's impartiality. *The deer. The hare. Why did they choose those moments to dash across the roadway?* They had lived each time preceding, but that day their entrails had been poured out like water, and who would remember them? One of our memorial readings, "Though I walk through the valley of the shadow of death," marked what should have been the thirty-first week in my pregnancy with Zachary.

At thirty-one gestational weeks in my pregnancy with Eden, I continued to find myself suspended between what should have been and what was, still trudging through the dense valley beneath foreboding, low-sweeping clouds.

Week 32: Meditation

My first attempt at meditation lasted fifteen seconds.
After eight months, my evening tea and steaming thermo-therapeutic compress had grown useless in calming my worry. I wanted a quick fix, but every book I read on meditation and mindfulness emphasized their *practice*. They were lifelong rituals, I discovered, developed by constant and diligent focus.

One day, when Hannah was visiting with Mom, I took my lunch out onto the dusty patio. Only a week before, Aaron had removed the winter tarps from our outdoor furniture. I slid the table back into place. My toes were cold in the wandering breeze that rippled the storm pond. I buttoned my sweater. A mother and her son, about Hannah's size, were out on a walk. Two large geese swam in the pond, their tail feathers wagging excitedly as they begged for bread.

In the sleepy lull of my surroundings, I decided it was the perfect time to try meditation. I closed my eyes and focused my breathing, imagining my lungs filling with the floral-smelling air and then emptying completely, exhaling my anxiety like a puff of smoke. One book had suggested choosing a word or an image to focus on, like staring at a poster on the wall when trying to balance on one foot at the gym. Some people say *Omm* or *Relax*. One single word came to my mind: *Eden*.

Eden became my *Omm*, my focus, my happy place, my mantra.

While my eyes were closed, the sun ducked behind the heavy-set clouds. Without its heat, the wind turned spiteful, pricking me through my sweater. I shivered and hurried indoors. Fifteen seconds had passed. *So much for meditating in nature*, I thought.

Once inside, I sat on one of our family's second-hand wing chairs reupholstered in black fabric stitched with a pattern of white leaves. I allowed my back to straighten and my feet to rest flat on the rug. I again began breathing slowly and eventually found a comfortable rhythm of in for five, out for five.

When exhaling, I hummed *Eden* for the whole release. I continued this way and felt my shoulders fall ever so slightly and my chest loosen. The literature I read about meditation instructed one to receive negative thoughts without judgment and to release them gracefully. I was not there yet; instead I snapped at these random intruders, harshly disciplining them and shooing them to bed without dinner.

I watched the darkness move like charred lava on the backs of my eyelids, the inconsistent light from the windows keeping me from total darkness. Relaxation seeped into my core, as each breath engaged my diaphragm, then moved into my arms and legs and then my fingertips and toes. I made every effort not to shuffle or adjust. My swollen feet throbbed objectionably, but I refused to move. Acknowledging their whines, I took another long suck of air then released the pain—and, to my disbelief, it went away.

As I became comfortable in stillness, Eden took note, or maybe he could sense the vibration of his name with each deliberate release of carbon. In response, my abdomen veered to the left and then to the right, followed by a cheeky streak of punts from my ribcage down the arch of my belly toward my public bone. I rubbed my taut skin above the little bumps I guessed were his heels.

Without noticing, entranced in the cadence of my breath and my mind nearly dislocated from my body, a subtle thought slipped stealthily beneath my consciousness. It was an image, a scene, and once formed—*snap!* My eyes flicked opened, and the meditation was broken.

The scene that came to me was familiar; I had seen it before.

Most of it. As though it were a film, I watched Hannah and me walk along a pine-and-birch-lined path not far from our home. The gravel trail curled through a small section of forest and passed beneath a canopy of woven leaves and needles. Suddenly, a large grey wolf stepped out from the shadows. The animal looked at us hungrily, saliva glossing its black gums behind retracted lips.

I first saw this scene in a dream shortly after Hannah was born. Back then I possessed strength and wildness all my own, the fierce love of motherhood the very plasma that flowed through my veins. In that scene, I was fearless and tore into the wolf with my teeth, ripping it to steaming shreds of skin and muscle and white cracking bone. I was the mother-protector, and nothing could touch my child.

Yet as I sat in the wing chair, I did not see myself respond as I had before. Instead I pictured myself grabbing for the bear spray I kept in the handlebar of Hannah's stroller. I pulled Hannah to my chest with one arm and with the other thrust the spray forward, firing a long burst of chemicals toward the wolf's oval eyes. But, wait—the nozzle head was facing the wrong direction. Instantly my eyes burned. My lungs and lips and skin were pricked with the red-hot iron of fire. I was helpless to protect Hannah and incapable of guarding myself or the child within me. My *Eden*.

Week 33: Failure to Repeat

The days leading up to Zachary's birth had been an incessant loop: the drive to the hospital, finding a spot in its parking garage, the freezing walk through the open-air pedway, the waiting rooms followed by the gradual revelation of an unforgiving genetic complex, and then the plodding slink through swollen roadways on our way home at rush hour. A year and a half later, as Aaron and I found ourselves heading to The Arthur Memorial Hospital for an echocardiogram of Eden's heart, one detail was dissimilar to all our previous visits. The difference was Hannah.

Hannah had not accompanied Aaron and me to hospital examinations during the month and a half preceding Zachary's delivery. She had, however, attended every prenatal appointment for both Zachary and Eden. She enjoyed tearing the thin paper that covered the exam table into a thousand pieces, which she then dropped to the floor like fluttering snow. She grew giddy at the sight of medical tools and the Doppler wand with its burping gel as it squeezed out of the bottle. She had been enraptured by the sound of both Zachary's and Eden's pulse. In those moments she lifted my spirits from worry, as only a carefree, soulful, and living child could.

Hannah sat in the backseat and was in a great mood, chattering about all kinds of random things. She squealed happily at the primary-colored balloons strung together above the car dealerships along Gateway Boulevard. She sang to herself as Aaron circled the hospital multiple times in search of a free curb, though he eventually resigned himself to our usual spot on the third floor of the parking garage.

Once in the hospital, the first thing I noticed was that the partially enclosed waiting area, with only a dozen or so chairs, was occupied by what looked like a junior resident meeting. The men wore coordinated suit pants, black socks, and white collared shirts tucked in at the waist. They took up space where they sat, ankles folded over knees and arms stretched across the backs of chairs. There was no room for Aaron, Hannah, and me. I stared at them, shaking my head. They were the second, but not the final, deviation from my conditioned experience of my previous pregnancy.

Aaron and I checked in with a sociable woman at the reception counter around the corner. The location of that station was inconspicuous, but we knew where to find it. "You can fill out the paperwork down in that direction." The woman gestured to three lonely chairs at the end of the hall, well away from the boys' club meeting and only a few steps from the wooden door of the small echo clinic. Somehow I was calm—strangely calm.

"How am I supposed to answer these?" Aaron slouched in his chair, scrunching his nose. "How many healthy pregnancies have you had? Were there complications in your last pregnancy? How many children do you have?" The questions mirrored those we had answered at Baby Before Birth just a few weeks before.

Hannah was standing on the tips of her toes, holding the umbrella-stroller's handles while merrily ramming the walls. *Bang, bang!* Then *click.* The echo clinic door opened. The technician was punctual and the hinges squawked at exactly 1:45 p.m. A black-haired woman poked her head out and welcomed us. We followed her to an exam room Aaron and I had visited many times before. Nothing had changed. The woman flicked off the lights.

I lay back on the slightly elevated exam table and lifted my shirt, pulling down the stretchy waistband of my maternity jeans. Hannah sat beside me in a tall swivel chair Aaron pulled over. She took my hand in hers, interlocking her petite fingers between mine. Aaron perched in a low '80s-style seat near my shoes, my notebook and pen ready in his hands.

"It's dark in here," Hannah observed in a whisper at my ear. She repeated this statement over and over as the technician lubricated her wand. "The lights are off," Hannah noted, her eyes scrutinizing every detail.

Staring up at the retro drop ceiling with squiggly lines looping across panels like script, I strained my eyes to read its handwriting. *What do you have for me today? More bad news?* Closing my eyes, I breathed in for one, two, three, four, five and then out to *Eeeedeeeen.*

The room created a calming lull with its darkened interior and ridiculous heat left unadjusted in the May thaw. The ultrasound camera clicked with low-decibel sounds like primitive music as the technician took pictures of my insides: my child, and his heart. Eden started to wiggle, and I squeezed Hannah's hand. My previous experiences in that room jumped in and out of my mind, but what lingered was the thought *My children are worth it all.*

The ultrasound monitor and its illuminated keyboard were my nightlight and, in between sleepy blinks, I stared up at the technician and tried to read her expressions. I was the only one who could not see the monitor. The technician smiled at Hannah and her serious face as she again informed everyone, "It's dark in here. The lights are off."

The technician's face suddenly morphed into a changed expression, her head tilted to the side, lips raised in a slight pout. It was the tiniest of shifts.

At last, I could bear it no longer. "Does everything look okay?"

"We need to wait for the doctor."

The technician finished and left the room. Hannah ate Cheerios from a green travel cup while we waited, and I spun the hospital bracelet with my name on it, the one wrangled around my wrist by the chatty woman at reception. I wished I could cut it off. Aaron's head bobbed, and he shifted to sit upright so he could fiddle on his phone.

"Playing a game?"

"No," he said, showing me the screen. "Just flipping back and forth; I'm nervous. This is stressful."

The technician had turned the lights back on at the conclusion of the exam, and when my eyes adjusted, I studied the room. A large illustrated poster held my gaze. It was pinned on the wall and depicted the cross section of a gestational sack cradling a full-term baby. The child's head was engaged in the mother's cervix, its legs curled in the fetal position. The expression on its face was serene and ready. Notes along the side of the poster described the stages of effacement. The corners of my mouth curled up at the peaceful face that grinned back at me.

The doctor entered the room, followed by the technician and two other people I assumed were residents. I knew the doctor immediately. "Your son's heart looks the same as any other baby's at this stage," he said.

"Really? That's wonderful," I said. Aaron continued, "That's such great news!" He and I turned toward each other, no longer sleepy in the heat. Aaron passed me the notebook and I scribbled down the doctor's words, exactly as he said them. I chose to believe each syllable of his declaration, letting them work their way through my body like a transfusion. The room suddenly seemed very large and the air cooler. I could breathe.

The doctor listed the conditions they could not detect, even at this stage, but his voice was a murmur in my head. All I could hear was that everything appeared normal. He passed us the report from the echo in a white envelope on hospital stationery. Below my medical identification number and particulars, there were a few decipherable words in the report, though they were packaged between complicated medical terms and abbreviated code.

NORMAL ATRIOVENTRICULAR ASSOCIATED, WITH A RATE OF 140 BPM . . . NORMAL SYSTEMIC VENOUS RETURN . . . NORMAL BIVENTRICULAR SYSTOLIC FUNCTION . . . NORMAL VENTRICULAR FLOW . . . NORMAL FETAL HEARTRATE AND RHYTHM . . . NORMAL . . .

Week 34: Mugo Pines

At the back of our yard, flanking the center gate in the green metal fence, stood our two Mugo Pines, or the Zachy trees, as Hannah called them. If we were out in the yard, I often noticed Hannah inspecting the stout evergreens, gently poking their sharp needles. She was about the same height as the trees. They were toddlers like her. We watered them together, and Hannah drenched herself, and my shins through my pants, but she didn't squawk about being cold or having squishy wet socks between her toes. She loved playing outdoors, and she loved the trees. "This one is the brother tree," Hannah reminded me, pointing with authority.

The week before, I had noticed brown needles on both the trees. It was a coming-of-age moment; it had never occurred to me that the evergreens would do anything but grow in the fullness of their name. I read up on the plants, technically called Columnar Dwarf Mugo Pines, baby versions of the full Mugo Pine that can grow to a span of fifteen to twenty-five feet both up and out. Our dwarf version would only reach three to six feet tall in ten years, almost like a person.

The majority of the needles were dark green, growing in loving pairs out of white, waxy buds. The left tree, however, had a small area turning a copper color, although these needles were mostly hidden. The right tree was worse off. A few branches near the bottom were fully transformed, starkly orange and unconcealed. I sat in our home office, appraising the trees through one of the large windows that framed our yard like a triptych. Searching online, I read about pruning techniques.

꙳

I had not realized the effect of my negativity until I visited my therapist, Dr. Haverson, who pointed it out so clearly. "What an exhausting way to live," she said. "You are overly critical."

"I can't help it. My mind jumps to the negative."

"Why?"

"Self-protection."

"It sounds more like self-sabotage."

I shrugged. Paused. "I don't want to get hurt again."

"Pain is a part of living."

"Everything with Zachary came as a surprise. If I think about the worst-case scenario now, then maybe when things go wrong next time—"

"*If.*"

"*If* they go wrong next time, then maybe I won't be so destroyed."

"Even if you knew from the beginning, even if you prepared yourself for the worst with Zachary, you would still have been devastated."

"I guess, I guess you're right. You *are* right." I thought for a moment then said, "But I don't want to tell myself everything is going to be okay with this pregnancy when I won't know until the end." My thoughts flashed to Laura, who was nearly full-term when Betty died without warning. Another story was fixed in my mind. A few years back I had heard about a girl I once knew whose baby died at birth because the umbilical cord had wrapped around her child's neck. There were no guarantees.

"Your negative thoughts are not truths," Dr. Haverson said, staring sternly into my eyes, almost chuckling. "You are not God. There are many gamuts to the rainbow."

"Yes, but what if—"

"Observe your language," she continued. "Recognize your

automatic thoughts. When you start thinking negatively, it snow-balls. Catch yourself thinking these things, then change your lan-guage. Affirm yourself."

"I don't know how to do that."

"Be good to yourself," she looked at me with compassion, slightly gesturing with her right hand. It was a good gesture, like the slow scattering of seeds into the wind or the tender stroke of a child's hair. "Speak the language of hope."

"I'm sorry. I wish I knew how to get there," I nearly whispered, realizing my native tongue was not hope.

"Be honest, be authentic, be true to yourself, communicate. You are worthwhile. Let that give you happiness, love, gentleness. Acknowledge that there is goodness in yourself. Tell me, what are your worries? Lay them all out."

"Where do I begin? Um, okay, well, I worry that when I don't feel Baby move, he will be stillborn. I worry that my baby won't be born healthy or that something will happen during delivery. I worry I am going to have a panic attack when I arrive in labor at the hospital. My family doctor is very laid-back, and I worry he doesn't take my concerns seriously. I worry I'll call this baby by Zachary's name . . . And I'm scared to death that all this worrying will negatively affect my child before he is even born."

"That's a lot to carry. Let's try turning a few of those around. You pick."

"Okay, so when I worry about a complication at birth with Baby Number Three and about him dying—how do I adjust that thought?"

"You tell me."

I doodled nervously in my notebook while I searched, against my natural instinct, to find the language of hope. "Maybe instead I could say something like, um, *I will trust my body and believe that the doctors will do everything in their power to deliver my baby safely. I've got access to excellent healthcare, and my son will be born healthy.*"

"Yes! Well done."

"Ugh—just saying that makes my stomach churn. Yuck. I don't fully believe it—"

"*Yet*. You don't believe it *yet*. It takes practice, Alexis Marie. Repetition. It may take an entire lifetime to shift your thinking."

My eyes went wide. Slowly I said, "That's a very long time . . ." as I contemplated the changes I needed to make and the outcome they would yield if I was successful. While I was afraid to further jinx my already-bad luck, there was also a small bloom of anticipation I wished to nurture.

In moments where I found myself alone, I crossed the threshold into the nursery and imagined holding my son. I traced the smooth lines of his face with my fingers, kissing each tiny knuckle, every joint. I then prayed over him all the good in this world I could conceive of. That hopeful person rocking herself in the glider, eager in expectation: she was the kind of mother, the kind of woman, I aspired to be—but I realized I would never grow into the full breadth of her without cutting away my urge for self-preservation. I was coming to appreciate that fear and disassociation were incompatible with vulnerability and love.

"This, right now, is a very special time in your life," said Dr. Haverson. "You need to do your art, you need to relax. You have, what is it? Five weeks to go?"

"Six."

"Six." She paused reflectively. "Your negative thoughts take up too much energy. Put that energy into the proper place right now." She looked down at my stomach, which I had hugged without realizing.

Dr. Haverson knew the vernacular of hope and it sounded lovely. Still, I worried my dreams for Eden would remain unfulfilled, as they had been with Zach. In one of my sessions, the doctor had shared that she chose to pursue her career over having children. In that vein, she never failed to empower my feminine identity; in motherhood, yes, but especially as an artist and professional. Dr. Haverson helped me see the value in my work. When we spoke of such things, it was easy to envision my short and long-term goals and all the steps I was eager to take in achieving them. In many ways, my unpredictable career in the arts provided greater certainty than my pregnancy.

The bereavement counselor at the hospital, who had children and had also lost children, spoke to me from experience when I bumped into her at one of my appointments for Eden. Through tears, I admitted my fears that many did not understand, not even Dr. Haverson. The counselor responded, "You will stop worrying when you have looked into the whites of your healthy baby's eyes." She was right. Until then, I could not fully surrender to sunny expectations for the future.

My research on Mugo Pines suggested the trees be inspected frequently and any damaged or infested branches be removed. When pruning, the branch should be trimmed slightly above the junction to the stump, cutting at a forty-five-degree angle. To avoid transference of the disease, the sheers must be cleaned thoroughly. Every source I read supported the same message: pruning was good; pruning encouraged healthy growth.

Week 35: Auntie Ruth

Aaron's maternal grandmother was ninety-two-years-old and smiled with her eyes whenever she saw us. She had a puffy head of frizzy white hair and gave Christmas cards without writing anything inside. Grandma Guthrie had never smoked a day in her life but was slowly dying of lung cancer and a failing heart. Her breaths had grown burdensome, and she was frequently winded. Recently she had been admitted to the small Mundare hospital; she was coughing up blood but had chosen not to undergo chemotherapy, operations, or any other types of intervention.

"I have lived a good, long life," she said once she had been discharged. She was back weeding her garden, sewing at her quilting table, and attending church towing an oxygen tank beside her. Not knowing how many days or months we had left with Grandma Guthrie, Aaron and I planned a trip to visit her.

The drive along Highway 16 paralleled greening prairies where plumes of dust and natural debris trailed air seeders and tractors as farmers tended their land. Rain was predicted in a few days, and a great deal needed to be accomplished to ensure the ground was ready for late-May seeding in a few weeks.

Hannah was oblivious to the scenery as she nibbled a chocolate-chip muffin, talking to herself and laughing hysterically at *Toopy and Binoo* reruns on the iPad. "We are almost there," Aaron said as he pointed to a tall red grain elevator. Hannah looked up momentarily. "That's the marker my parents used when I was a kid. Once you see it, Mundare is just a few minutes down the road."

We knocked loudly on the unlocked door of the russet wood-shingled bungalow just a few blocks off the main drag. No one answered, and we let ourselves in. "They can't hear us," Aaron said. Grandma Guthrie was almost deaf and had read lips the eight years I knew her. Aaron's family said it was because of her hearing that she always called me Alexa.

Grandma and Grandpa sat in their living room filled with mismatched couches and chairs and a collection of photographs sun-warmed in yellow sheens cuing their broad eras like carbon dating. Grandpa rose slowly to greet us, and Aaron and I bent over Grandma awkwardly to embrace her where she sat. Her right hand rested on the humming metal tank beside her.

Hannah clung to Aaron with her arms tight at his shoulders and legs bound around his chest, fastened at her ankles. Her boisterous personality was camouflaged as she blushed and buried her face in the curve of her daddy's neck. Whenever Aaron turned, Hannah flipped her head in the opposite direction so no one could see her face. Hannah's great-grandparents waved at her with hands lined in mountainous veins and wrinkles, like rivers that parted the Rockies, between their knuckles.

After an hour of visiting, we followed Grandma and Grandpa to their church. Aaron's mother had instructed us to drive them, but Grandma had backed their Chrysler Intrepid, which their kids called the *old-people car*, out of the driveway before we even finished buckling Hannah into her car seat. Aaron ran to their vehicle and tapped on the window, but Grandma smiled with equal parts innocence and mischievousness, fierce in her independence. She said, "No, no. We can drive ourselves, thank you," and sped off.

Aaron and I had not attended church in nearly a year, and I was strangely eager, albeit twitchy and fidgety in anticipation. It would be a spiritual litmus test, I decided. *Will my soul be stirred? Or will the experience result in the same blaring silence I knew after Zachary's death when I first began to question my faith?* I ached to believe and longed for something or someone to pray to in the final weeks leading up to Eden's birth.

We entered the church foyer through heavy glass doors and were welcomed by Aaron's family—his grandparents, Aunt Ruth and Uncle Lloyd; their son Ben's wife, Tiffany; and Ben and Tiffany's two daughters. The music began, led by young men in chunky black glasses with tornado hair and slim-cut jeans. After a few minutes they stepped aside for three baptisms that took place in a tank cleverly concealed behind a short wall and shrubbery at the back of the stage. Each person declared their love for Jesus before being fully immersed in the chest-deep water, receiving loud cheers upon resurfacing. As water dripped from the tips of their noses, they were declared new in Christ.

Baptisms once encouraged me. As a teen, testimonials bolstered my faith, but as I took in the humble country service I found myself coolly detached. The band started up again. To an impassioned melody, they sang about God's peace in the face of fear and his light in the darkness. The song championed the joyful life to be experienced in God, in the all-powerful Jesus, Lord and friend, who overcame the sting of death and was more than enough for his people. I had craved divine contentment for so long, but while the song was charming, I knew it was not true for me.

The youth pastor smiled through his round cheeks at the audience and delivered a sermon on the choosing of the twelve disciples. He posed the questions: "Do we believe Jesus is worth following? Do we believe he is the way, the truth, and the life? Can we give up our control and humbly follow?"

My heart said *No*.

The pastor continued, as if in tempo with the song, and asked if we who were gathered had the eyes to see that God was seeking us. "What is the condition of your heart?" he said, his brow furrowed in gravity for our eternal salvation.

The condition of my heart? I scoffed silently. *Well, it's enlarged for no apparent reason. How 'bout that?*

"If your heart's condition is off, it is more difficult to see God reaching out to you," the pastor continued. *All I want is the truth*; the words drummed in my chest. Taking a deep breath, I opened

myself to welcome the divine reach, the urge, the gut-level prick
of the Holy Spirit.

The service ended. I had felt nothing.

℘

We trailed Aaron's grandparents back to their house, which seemed
to be both in the center and on the outskirts of the dusty, wind-
whipped town. We'd brought shepherd's pies for lunch, which we
forgot to thaw adequately before baking. We were, luckily, joined
by Aaron's extended family, who had also attended the service.
They rescued our appetites with containers full of garden salad,
still speckled with earth, home-baked cookies, and jugs of juice.
Uncle Lloyd brought in a basket of glazed buns sprinkled with
oats. He was a farmer, like most men in the community, but he did
not believe in seeding on the Sabbath.

The adults filled their plates and ate off their laps in the living room while the kids—Hannah with Olivia and Rachel, Ben
and Tiffany's daughters, who were six and eight—and I sat at the
kitchen table. I ate across from Hannah, giving her space to enjoy
the company of her second cousins. She was perched between the
two older girls on a tall and badly nicked wooden stool. Hannah
grinned at the girls excitedly, her blonde pigtails bouncing as she
turned back and forth between them. She paid no regard to the
potatoes and corn that fell onto her lilac dress and bounced to the
floor.

Grandpa Guthrie had been encouraged to sit at the table with
the kids and me, but he had not said a word throughout lunch,
and I'd almost forgotten he was there. One by one the girls left the
table, and it was just Grandpa and me. All of a sudden he started
talking about World War II. He had served in the transportation
division from 1942 to 1946.

"They gave me special training to drive the ambulance. It was
a standard. No forgiveness for grinding the gears," he said, his long
eyebrows poking above his dusty metal-rimmed glasses.

Tiffany brought Grandpa a coffee, but he was focused.

"Sometimes a German would wave at us," Grandpa said. "They'd act like they needed help. Then another German would jump out of the ditch and shoot at us with a machine gun."

"That sounds scary."

Grandpa shrugged, not answering. His eyes gazed at another landscape beyond Alberta's prairies. He saw back to an era preceding the time in which we scratched his linoleum floor with the legs of our chairs and where his family filled every corner of the well-worn kitchen.

He told me how he met Grandma—Helen, as he referred to her—as we talked. "It was in Bible college before the war. She was a year ahead of me. We corresponded while I was deployed, but we had an understanding."

"That you would get married?"

He nodded. "I sent Helen a letter ahead of time, where and when I would arrive back in Canada. I rode a train into Calgary, and Helen was there, waiting for me on the platform."

"It must have been hard to be apart."

"I kept out of trouble. When I was off duty in England, I stayed with Christian friends, or friends of friends, and went to church."

When he returned from the war, he and Helen married and moved up north to Fort Nelson, British Columbia, where he pastored a small congregation. "It was a place I was warned not to go," he laughed, but he did not explain why.

Grandpa was gentle-mannered, unassuming, yet firm and sinewy from nearly a century of labor. He brushed his shaggy grey hair, tinged with wisps of dusty-amber, from his forehead like a shy youth. At times I strained to understand what he said, some words stringing together with stories hopscotching years ahead, others whole generations behind. My mother-in-law told me her father often shifted into states of dementia without warning or even a marked change across his face or in his steady voice. I studied Grandpa as he spoke, watching for cues, but all I could see was a man reminiscing about the woman he loved as she was on the cusp of death.

Aaron and I had chosen Royal, Grandpa's first name, to be Eden's middle name. *Eden Royal Chute.* I itched to tell Grandpa but kept quiet; Aaron wanted the name to remain a secret until Eden was born.

Grandpa continued to talk, most of his stories centering on his faith like the jeweled bearing at the apex of a compass's magnetic needle. Faith oriented every part of his being. I teared up. *What am I missing?* "I want to believe, but it feels like there is no one there," I said, and he struggled to relate. He offered more stories about people and places I did not know.

Aunt Ruth, who had been listening quietly, inconspicuously, from the other side of the kitchen counter, pulled up a chair beside me. "It's a journey," she said. "The trick is to not feel guilty. The search is not a sin."

"After Zachary died, I reached out to God, believing, but I felt so alone. People tell me I can't rely on my feelings, but I am an emotional person; I always have been. If God made me, shouldn't he know that I need to feel something?"

"I do think that's right," Aunt Ruth said thoughtfully. "Claim the Bible verses about God making you and knowing you while you were still in your mother's womb—and then wait. Maybe it's God's turn to respond."

"I agree. It's God's turn—and that's a liberating thought."

Aunt Ruth paused for a moment. "But God's time is different from our time. We were born into minutes, hours, years. God is not restricted to our clock. You have felt nothing for over a year, you say?" I nodded. "Maybe that is not long for God. The Bible says seek and you shall find—but it doesn't say when."

"The nothingness feels like it's gone on forever, but then it also feels like just yesterday that Zachary died, not a year and a half ago."

"It may be hard to see right now, but Jesus will find a way."

"Jesus?" I responded almost angrily. "I don't think I believe that Jesus is the only way to heaven." I cringed once the words had left my mouth, knowing I had likely offended every one of Aaron's conservative Christian relatives within earshot.

"I think we may be very surprised by who is in heaven." Aunt Ruth's open-mindedness caught me off guard, and I wasn't sure how to respond. "No one does faith the same way. That's too legalistic," she continued. "God reaches out to us in a million ways. Everyone is different. He reaches out to each one of us in the way that is best suited to us. Our churches tell us differently . . ." Aunt Ruth paused. "In the search for a deeper relationship with God, there is no wrong way.

"Freedom is key," she continued, and she told me about a young man she respected who had found peace with God outside the church. Aunt Ruth wondered aloud if structured religion was what Jesus had even intended. It was all I could do to sit quietly and listen, marveling at a woman so graceful and compassionate in her convictions. It was that very response I had hoped to find at Mourning Together more than five months before.

"It's all about loving God and loving people," Aunt Ruth concluded.

Later that night, back at home in Edmonton, I prayed for Hannah as I tucked her into bed and rubbed her back. I rested my hands on my stomach and prayed for Eden as well, who was just waking up for his evening wiggle-about. Even though I did not know the answers or what higher power, energy, or god I should direct my heart to, at that moment it didn't matter. Eventually God's time would catch up with mine, or the other way around. And if not, I realized I was okay with that, too.

Week 36: Worth It All

Margaret Pozzi, the provincial bereavement counselor of Alberta, the woman who had encouraged Aaron and me after Zachary died, asked if I would like to say a few words at the hospital's annual memorial service for families who had lost a baby. Since meeting Laura, a passion to support others like myself had been birthed inside of me, and I immediately agreed. For the event, I wrote an essay called "Love Is Worth It All."

"Don't change a word. It's perfect," Mom said after I finished reciting my final draft. "I feel I understand you better," she said. "Thank you."

Aaron, Hannah, and I arrived at the memorial fifteen minutes early and sat with Dad and his girlfriend, Jill, and Aaron's father, who slipped in a few minutes behind us. At that point, the chapel in the funeral home was only a quarter full, but as the service time approached every pew became occupied. Ushers began directing families to folding chairs in the room's addition on the east side of the building. Eventually the back of the chapel was crowded with people sitting on folding chairs or standing. Even the wide hallway toward the entrance was crowded.

At first the mood was somber. Before the program began, many women sniffled or openly wept, helped along by the harpist as she plucked dreamlike lullabies into the musty air of the chapel. Aaron fretted over shushing Hannah, who talked loudly in an animated dialogue, but soon there were many children chattering and laughing, slamming hymnals closed or pulling on the skirts of their mothers, pleading for snacks or toys. A dozen parents stood to rock wailing newborns.

There were people from every ethnicity in the room. Some were dressed in torn jeans and T-shirts, while others looked as if they had come straight from a business meeting. One man was covered with tattoos from his neck to his wrists. He held a tissue box on his lap.

The chaplain delivered a message of welcome, and a husband and wife followed with a poem. Another couple read from the Bible. Then Margaret Pozzi invited those gathered to participate in a candle-lighting ceremony. Families shuffled down the center aisle to the front of the chapel, lit a candle, and took a flower—pink, blue, or white. There was a microphone between the tables of candles and flowers. One by one, the mourners spoke.

"We remember our son, Timothy."

"For our daughter, Meghan."

"In memory of Bethany; we miss you."

Parents lifted their children to the microphone to say, "We remember our brother, Scott," and, "For my sister, Rose."

Aaron and I left Hannah cuddling her grandparents in the pew as we lined up in the aisle, our hands knitted together. Aaron lit a tea light and I took a blue flower. "We love you, Zachary." Aaron's deep voice trembled through the mic, and he tucked his bottom lip between his teeth.

When we had visited Margaret shortly after Zachary's death, she counseled us that the rawness of loss would fade over time. I didn't believe her. I felt that I would be like uncooked ground beef, bloody and grated, for the rest of my life. Yet, sitting back down in the pew beside Hannah and Aaron, as Eden wiggled and impaled my bladder with his heels, I could sense my healing had begun. The grief was not as fresh as it once had been—no longer the desolate brokenness I observed on the faces of many men and women that day.

It was my turn to speak. I approached the podium with Aaron, who held Hannah on his hip. "We are doing this together," I had told him earlier. Hannah sucked a lollipop happily, enjoying her elevated vantage point to watch the people gathered in the chapel. As I read, I did not weep, as I had when I practiced my speech for Mom, but the tears still came, like the spring rain that battered lightly against the stained glass windows that Saturday afternoon.

Love Is Worth It All

Did the world change overnight?
Food only hints at flavor. The sky is now a pale shade of iron. Friends seem distant, and career aspirations are awash with the tick-tock clockwork of mundane routine. Who is this person in the mirror? This battered soul with dreary eyes looking back at me? Who is this woman without her baby? This is not my life.
The world did not change.
I changed.
I changed the moment my son was diagnosed for death when I was twenty-five weeks pregnant with his life and twenty-six years expectant with his future. I changed at his birth, and I changed at our brief "Hello" followed by I-love-you kisses as he passed beyond my reach.
This is my new normal, *so they say.*
Yet, there is nothing normal *about life after the loss of so great a love as a mother for her child. Normal is waking up five times in the night to breastfeed. Normal is peanut-butter-and-jam sandwiches and preschool play. Normal is morning cuddles followed by breakfast arguments. Normal does not have to call itself normal, because it just is.*
I have chosen to replace normal *with life; instead of new normal this is my* new life. *I chose life because I have walked through the smoking embers of hell and somehow survived to tell the tale. Life because I have returned to the task of learning how to live each day,*

as a baby, born into a strange land where nothing is normal *but everything is new.*

In some way unexpected, death bore the gift of life and with it the appreciation of the world through young eyes, like a child. A warm sunrise, good health, riding a bike, wrinkles, a kiss, camping in the rain, reading by a fire, a puzzle, a laugh; what a privilege to re-learn these joys when grown. To learn, in the face of great sacrifice, that love, even in so small a form, is worth it all.

A child grows within me once more, but this is not then, this is not my normal; *this is my* new life. *My third pregnancy has become like the first, not in novel giddiness or eager anticipation but in awed wonder and nervous worry. Yet, I somehow feel equipped for whatever may come, the fire of loss having burnt to ash all doubt in my heart; yes, a child is worth the risk; love is greater than death.*

My son lives on in his new life *as well, in my heart, in the folds of God's hand, in the fortitude of the mountains, in the reflections of my husband's eyes. His name resides on my breath, and I will teach my daughter and however many children I am blessed to bear: you have a brother; there is more to life than what we can observe or experience; you are a part of a larger whole, a family, not unified by physical presence but by a love so mysterious that we all are bound by its thread across time and expanse and imagination.*

In this new life *I have found the meaning I've always searched for, the passion that I had never fully known, and the truest, purest, most holy and scared love. Love that is now and will always and forever be worth it all.*

Week 37: What Happens Here?

Nausea gurgled in my stomach whenever I thought about The Arthur Memorial Hospital, where Zachary had been born, where he had died. The unfamiliarity of St. Mary's Hospital, therefore, was a welcomed change. I had given birth to Hannah at St. Mary's almost three years earlier, but I was in so much pain from the contractions I had paid little attention to my surroundings, and I hadn't spent a month and a half in its hallways thinking about death. It was as if I were seeing the hospital for the first time when Aaron and I met there for an unconventional appointment.

"Where's her office?" Aaron asked.

"Let me see." I flipped through my notebook. "Unit 53."

Aaron scanned the directory and pushed the elevator button, stepping in after me. My palms were sweating and I wiped them firmly on the legs of my maternity jeans. Eden would be born at St. Mary's Hospital in approximately three weeks if my pregnancy continued to progress well.

A directory greeted Aaron and me as we exited the elevator. The four units on the fifth floor, all dedicated to the beginnings of life, were listed above an abstract image of a field of canola blossoms blowing in the wind. As we headed up the hallway, a tall scarecrow-thin man no older than twenty-five came around the corner. He was walking toward us and talking on his cell phone. "We named him Gabriel," the man was saying. "After the angel."

Once Aaron and I turned the corner, I recognized the unit where we had stayed after Hannah was born. It looked different. Like in a projected film, I watched my younger self carry the infant car seat with my day-old Hannah bundled beneath a blanket; it was bone-chillingly cold that November. The younger me headed toward the elevators on the same path the man on the phone had just traveled. In my memory, Aaron walked beside me, holding our bulging hospital bag. Our eyes were red-rimmed, our skin colorless, every muscle aching for sleep. I couldn't stop looking down at Baby Hannah, and Aaron too wore a smile that did not fade. We were incredibly happy then. *Will it be like that with Eden as well?* I nervously combed my long blonde hair with my fingers.

"Alexis Marie, this way." Aaron startled me from my memory.

A man in green scrubs behind the nursing station pointed us toward a door across the hall. We knocked, and the woman who greeted us introduced herself. "Hello, I'm Francisca."

Francisca was in her mid-fifties with handsome Dominican features and animated eyebrows. Her rich auburn hair folded in buoyant curls around her face and down to her shoulders. She was the main social worker on the fifth floor of St. Mary's Hospital. She welcomed us with a kind smile and shook our hands firmly as we entered her modest office. Francisca's manner was elegant and compassionate. Once we were all sitting, she asked, "So how far along are you, Miss Alexis Marie?"

"Thirty-seven weeks."

"Thirty-seven weeks! Oh, you look just great, my dear!"

"Really?" I made a face. "I've gained over forty pounds."

"Oh, nothing to worry about. You're healthy, I can tell." Francisca smiled and leaned forward in her chair. "Do you know what you are having?"

"A boy."

"Oh, fabulous! You must be just thrilled."

I began to cry. "I am, but . . . but . . . but I'm also terrified," I stuttered. Aaron put his hand on my arm. A wave of panic around the immediacy and uncertainty of birth—and my negative association with hospitals—crashed over my head. I imagined fleeing through Francisca's door like the Tasmanian Devil, leaving behind a hole in the shape of my short, round body.

"Tell me, Miss Alexis Marie," Francisca said calmly, passing me a tissue box. "What are you hoping for today?"

"I don't know exactly. Our son, our second child, passed away, and, well, I don't like being in hospitals anymore."

"Our doctor, Dr. Stilles, set this up. We thought it would be good if we got more comfortable with this place. Walk around. Know what to expect," explained Aaron.

"Yes, I see. You want to prepare yourselves. That makes perfect sense."

I nodded. "I don't want to arrive here and then . . . and then—" my chest heaved and wheezed like a hissing balloon as I strained to control myself. "I don't want to come here to deliver my baby and then react like this." I wiped away tears that had trekked all the way down my neck.

"It is far better to express yourself and get your feelings out," Francisca said, looking at me tenderly. "Too much time is spent trying to control our feelings."

I nodded and looked over at Aaron, who whispered, "I love you," with concern wrinkled across his forehead.

"Well, I think it is just excellent that you two are here. I will walk you through the floor, and when that boy of yours is ready for eviction, this place will feel just like home—well, almost." Francisca laughed so hard I could see the muscles along her jugular. Aaron and I couldn't help but join in.

"That would be great," Aaron said, squeezing my hand.

Francisca called the labor and delivery ward, or the case room, as she referred to it. "They're busy," she said after hanging up. "A nurse will call me back, but we may not be able to go in there. We will see everything else, though; I promise you."

Francisca led us through the postpartum unit where her office was located, showing us rooms like a tour guide. I wanted to memorize every square foot. The first stop was a semi-private room with two beds and a pale greenish curtain on a track that separated the space. Then we saw a private room with a large window to a view of a brick wall, which was the exterior of another part of the hospital. The beds were all made, and everything was clean and still. Whatever was happening in labor and delivery had not yet spilled over into Unit 53.

The hallways were lined with pictures of smiling newborns and Anne Geddes plaques of babies wearing pearl necklaces and popping out of giant eggs. Francisca showed us the nourishment center, as she called it, which was nothing more than a pass-through in the hallway with a small fridge, a few packets of soup crackers, and a loaf of bread.

"The hospital was renovated a couple years ago," she told us. "The theme is very calm now, don't you think? Relaxing?" The colors were indeed calming; pale goldenrod, muted spring green, and azure blue. The floor was also earth-themed, with tiles cut to mimic warm meadows of ripe canola touched by a blanket of velvety blue atmosphere above. Even the room numbers were embossed onto glass tiles lightly frosted with images of rural Alberta landscapes.

We passed recovery rooms with doors partially ajar from which the cries of fresh lungs escaped and reverberated down the hall. The sounds were all at once majestic and alarming, but I did not flee. Instead I took a deep breath and listened, eagerness overtaking fear as I thought of learning my child's own particular bawl. I told myself I was going to have a healthy baby and willed my heart to believe it. Still, I could not conjure in my mind the curves of a newborn face to look anything but swollen and taut. The dualities I had recognized so clearly in myself months before were again evident. There was the mom in me, who wished to skip down the halls, and her cynical and stubborn twin, who slunk along in the shadows.

Francisca checked her messages and informed us that the case room was still too busy; we could not visit there that day. She continued her tour with the other postnatal unit, a mirror to the one we had just seen, and took us into both family lounges, which were bright with colorful plush teddies, waist-tall plastic cars, and slides. Hannah's favorite channel, Tree House, was playing on the large TV, and I could already picture her ignoring Eden, pulling her grandmas and grandpas by the fingers to that room to plop down on the sofa.

"Would you like to see the nursery for preemies?" Francisca asked, pointing to a set of doors.

Aaron shook his head slowly and clenched his teeth. "Thank you, but I don't think that is a good idea for today."

"Well, that's about it," said Francisca cheerfully. "Anything else you want to see? No? Okay, then. I'll walk you two to the elevator. It really is so nice to meet you both. I'm sure everything will go just fine for you; I can feel it." All of a sudden, her voice faded in my ears and I no longer heard any sound. Aaron and Francisca were then whole strides away, but I stood frozen in the hall, staring. We had passed the labor and delivery entrance on the way to the elevator and, as someone approached, the heavy double doors had snapped open automatically. They hung agape for a solid minute as I peered in.

Nurses bustled about, charts in hand. A man pushed the wheelchair of a screaming, writhing woman. A doctor pulled off examination gloves while another discussed something across the counter at the nurses' station. The doors closed—but almost immediately swung wide as an attendant passed through. Again, they remained open.

Beyond the doors was a message written on the wall above the nurses' station. The lettering was large, black, and swirly. The message read,

Miracles happen here.

My eyes traced the curves of the words without pause. That message was all I had needed to see.

Week 38: Touch

Hannah and I talked about Baby Eden every day. She kissed my stomach, and I told her when Eden was kicking. She'd run over to rub my skin, sometimes pretending to pinch Eden through my protruding belly button. I'd yelp in pain, and she'd fall back on the couch, laughing and rolling until she cried.

Hannah played sporadically with the baby doll I gave her, taking off its clothes, carrying it around by the arm or the foot, and cuddling it tenderly while she sang "Rock-A-Bye Baby." A few weeks before, Hannah had settled on a name for her pink-clad newborn. *Tony.* I taught Hannah the actions to a song that we sang together: "Toe-knee-chest-nut-nose-eye-love-you, toe-knee-nose, toe-knee-nose." Tony sat on the floor between Hannah and me as we practiced pointing to our body parts.

While Hannah touched my stomach often, Aaron rarely did. When Eden was especially active right before bed, as Aaron and I were often lounging together talking about our days, I'd interrupt the conversation and tell Aaron where to place his hand. He would wait briefly and complain he couldn't find a comfortable position to lie with his wrist arced there in place. Five seconds later he'd shift away and resume the discussion about his work. *Is this a subconscious mechanism of self-protection?* The psychology books recommended by Dr. Stilles had broadened my vocabulary of self-analysis. *Or maybe is it a way for him to remain disconnected until the outcome is set, just in case?* My mind obsessed over Aaron's healing as much as my own.

Many things were coming to natural endings, or beginnings, and it seemed Eden's birth would be the culmination of them all. My art commissions were wrapping up nicely and, at the same time, my personal creative work was finding a sustainable rhythm. The biweekly prenatal appointments became weekly as my body ripened for action. At my last therapy session with Dr. Haverson she declared, "You really have come a long way, Alexis Marie, and it is very likely that when you give birth to your child any remaining conflicts in you will be eased." Aaron's work was winding down as well, the school year nearing completion, just as spring was gracefully easing into summer. As the sun grew friendly, I could sense my enlarged heart blossoming in anticipation.

"I'd like to make a plaster cast of my stomach," I told Aaron one night after Hannah was in bed.

"What are we gonna do with it?"

"I don't know," I shrugged, imagining a whole array of artsy-fartsy projects I could make. I knew to gradually introduce Aaron to my more abstract and conceptual ideas. "Not sure."

"All right, let's do it," Aaron replied energetically. I stared at him, confused.

"Yeah?"

"C'mon, Alexis Marie. Really? This isn't something we can put off for later." He feigned a snarky tone. "We are on a bit of a time clock here." He tapped the face of his watch.

I laughed and grinned at him, loving him tenderly in that moment for all the ways he tried so hard to make me happy. "All right, well, it'll only take you twenty minutes to put on the plaster clothes, then twenty minutes to dry. That's it!"

"You know how to do this?"

"I have notes, see. I watched a few YouTube videos on belly-casting. It doesn't look that hard."

Aaron closed the blinds, and I laid towels on the hardwood floor beside the island in the kitchen. I layered the towels so they were fourfolds thick and stepped on them, testing. I worried I would not be able to stand comfortably for forty minutes, as my feet were already looking waterlogged.

Pulling off my clothes, I began rubbing baby oil on my breasts, stomach, neck, and the tops of my legs. Aaron paused from cutting the plaster cloths into two-inch-by-four-inch strips, looking up. "The first thing I ever cast was my face back in high school," I said as I applied more oil. "I didn't put on enough lotion—the teacher gave us lotion instead of oil—and when I tried to take off the mask it pulled out chunks of my eyebrows and eye lashes. You could see two rows of black lashes stuck in the cast." Aaron didn't seem to be listening as he watched me lather oil into my pubic hair.

Aaron filled a bucket of warm water and placed it on the chalky corner of the island where the white strips of plaster wrap waited in a tall pile, shedding their white dust like baking flour. Following my instructions, Aaron dipped the first strip into the water and laid it tentatively on the arc of my stomach. "Great, now flatten it so there are no folds in the strip. Good job."

Aaron appraised his first piece with satisfaction and moved on to the next. I watched my stomach begin to disappear and savored each instance where Aaron's skin met mine. "Try blending them together. Well, that's sort of, um . . . can I show you?" I took Aaron's large hand in mine and applied delicate yet even pressure through his fingertips. The layers smoothed together, the porous holes filling with wet plaster, and the twelve or so pieces began to look like one.

Aaron moved his way up and down, sporadically laying new strips. I held a wooden spoon above my head with both hands, resting the handle on my temple to keep my arms out of the way. Aaron grew confident and placed new pieces quickly. White plaster water splashed on the floor and up the base of the island. As he started to sweat, Aaron pulled off his shirt and shorts and continued on in his underwear.

"What if you try applying the strips systematically?"

"Don't micromanage me," he snorted, emphasizing his point

with a quick and stern glance at me from the corners of his eyes.

I shifted uncomfortably on my feet. Half an hour had passed. Although Aaron was moving like an athlete, the area we had agreed to cast was large, from my neck to partway down my thighs. Already my feet throbbed.

"You are doing awesome," Aaron told me frequently. "This section is going really well."

"Talk to me. Distract me from my sausage toes."

"Hmm. Okay. Did you notice the date on the milk jug? No? Well, it says June 25, 2012."

"Eden's due date. Wow."

"I know, right?" Aaron was quiet for a few moments. "For some reason I thought we still had a month or more, but that's only two weeks from now." Aaron plastered up my torso to my chest. "This is probably the most unromantic way I have ever touched your breasts." We laughed. "These plaster strips remind me of teaching my students athletic taping in sports medicine. Plastering your boob is just like taping an ankle."

"Oh, thanks."

"It's a tough spot; the ankle, the breasts," Aaron continued. "You have to let the tape go where it wants to go." He did not look up as he said this. Aaron pursed his lips slightly, evaluating the placement of his last strip. He removed it and tried again, pulling one end slightly and adjusting the other. This time he rubbed the strip into the whole. "I'm doing my best on your breasts."

"That rhymes!"

Aaron cut more strips when the stack ran out. "Hang in there, babe." I cringed but did not move. He finished applying a second layer of plaster, and we agreed the first stage was complete. An hour and twenty minutes had passed. We turned on the TV, and Aaron flopped on the couch as I adjusted my grip on the spoon.

"Wouldn't it be funny if my water broke right now?"

"I'd tell you to hold still! That you are not allowed to move for another eighteen minutes!'"

We watched exactly twenty minutes of TV, not a second more.

"Ouch, oh fuck!"

"Sorry." Aaron winced as he helped me pull the cast from the skin on my neck. "Could have used more oil there, I guess." The rest of the hard white plaster pulled away easily. We laid a towel on the kitchen table and placed the cast on top, boobs and belly up. It was surreal to look at my own body like that, outside of myself. My stomach was huge and, because I was short, it seemed like my tummy ballooned right out from the base of my breasts.

It was almost midnight and we were both exhausted. I rushed upstairs to shower and scrub off the oil and plaster that was splattered down my legs, on my shoulders, and up my neck. I could see Aaron through the glass door, the shape of him coming into the bathroom and brushing his teeth.

"Did I get all the plaster off?" I asked, stepping out of the shower. Water trickled down my skin and steam escaped at my back. My nipples hardened in the cold. Aaron came over and checked me out, head to toe. He slid his hands from my chest to my stomach, pausing there without words, then up into my wet hair as we kissed.

Week 39: Ready, Set, Go!

Crossing my fingers Eden would come early, by week thirty-eight, all the laundry was done, the beds were made with clean sheets, and the house smelled like citrus thanks to the neighborhood carpet cleaner. Aaron's mother was on standby to watch Hannah, and Mom was showering before bed in case I called in the night. By week thirty-nine, though, dirty clothes were piling up again, the house was in disarray, and I'd grown antsy with too much free time. Hannah copied me and perfected twiddling her thumbs.

"Your cervix is posterior and closed, but I can feel the head," Dr. Stilles had told me at my last prenatal appointment, but I wished I was dilated, at least a few centimeters. My body felt ready.

One night, contractions began tightening the skin of my lower abdomen, shooting aches upward through my chest. The rhythm was annoyingly irregular. They began before bed and continued intermittently throughout the night. I let Aaron sleep, sneaking out of bed to sit on a chair by the window, where I could watch both the clock and the moon. Breathing deeply, I relaxed myself to feel the commencement and conclusion of each sharp pain, timing the calm between them. I tried to picture the whites of Eden's eyes as I nibbled my already painfully short nails, my brow creased with deep crevices as I focused. With each contraction, my worry multiplied, but so, too, did my excitement, which manifested in girlish giggles that required I bear down on my diaphragm to stifle.

Eventually I crept sleepily back into bed, hoping the contractions would grow in frequency and wake me, but the next thing I heard was a soft and dainty voice in my ear. Morning sunshine radiated through the curtains and pierced my eyes. "Mommy, I love you," Hannah whispered sweetly. I smiled at my girl and log-rolled out of bed to take her to the potty. After my own visit to the bathroom, where I experienced one of the best bowel movements of my life, the irregular contractions immediately halted. I felt great—and despondent.

In an email to Laura, whom I had kept in contact with since we had met to talk about Betty two and a half months before, I wrote, "This pregnancy is nerve-wracking, and I feel impatient to know that everything will be okay. I have mixed emotions—but for you, thinking about trying again, know that at thirty-nine weeks I am mostly excited. Mostly. It's a good thing that pregnancy stretches forty long, sometimes-unbearable weeks, because it forces you to work things out."

"In lots of ways I feel ready now," I said to Aaron, "but it could still be another two weeks . . ."

"Or tomorrow," he added before giving a day-by-day account of his year-end teaching schedule and his preferences for Eden's birth. "Keep your legs crossed tonight, because if Eden comes now I won't get my marking done. But a week from now I'll be all caught up and classes will be over. I could easily get out of exam supervision."

While walking outdoors with Mom and Hannah one day, I complained for fifteen minutes about my ballooning feet and by-then fiery-red and painful stretch marks. When Mom had tired of my whining, she pointed and said, "I'll give you ten bucks if you run to that garbage can up there."

"Ha ha, Mom, very funny. I really doubt that'll make me go into labor."

"Get movin'," she barked. "Ready, set, go!"

"You're serious?"

"Yep. You're going to jiggle that baby out of you. Now sprint!"

I began running, although *waddling* would be a more accurate description. I cupped my hands beneath my stomach to ease my aching muscles, as if I were carrying a bulging grocery bag. Hannah met my pace. "No stopping!" Mom yelled from behind us. We reached the garbage can at the top of the inclining path, and Hannah and I jumped around, raising our fists to the sky like Rocky Balboa.

That was the first in a string of little runs and long sweaty walks in June. I also added large cups of steeped raspberry tea as Lisa had recommended; Pizza Hut's flaming-hot wings, which Eden already craved; and blue dangly charm earrings from Mom to my baby-inducing strategy. Since labor for both Hannah and Zachary began late in the evening, it took a long time for me to fall asleep each night; I nearly leapt from under the sheets at every stomach gurgle.

"Your pregnancy has become real for me only in the last week or so," Aaron announced one day after we had checked on Hannah as she slept. We tucked ourselves into bed.

"Where have you been the last thirty-nine weeks?" I laughed, but Aaron was serious.

"I'm realizing," he cleared his throat. "I have a negative association with birth. Last time we went through this there were so many sad, depressing, negative feelings." He shifted uncomfortably, straining to express himself. "I need to break that association somehow. Do you know what I'm trying to say?"

"I do. Totally. I really, really do. If it makes you feel any better, I think I've been in denial about how far along I am as well—making my wood sculptures, applying for gallery shows . . . but Eden's coming, Aaron. Soon, I hope."

"We are almost there," Aaron said, shaking his head in disbelief. "I still remember when you went into labor with Hannah at our old house. The words that ran through my head were, *Wow, my life is going to change.*" His eyes were animated with memories. Aaron continued, "I said to myself, *I'm going to come home in a few days and nothing is going to be the same.*"

"And what about this time? Do you think everything is going to be okay?"

"I don't know." Aaron paused thoughtfully. "What I do know is that everything will change again."

Week 40: Living Fire

"Yeah, I'm tired, but we can't just hole up in the house and wait," I said. Aaron had suggested we skip that night's reception at a downtown gallery where two of my wood sculptures were on display. "I'd really like to go."

"All right. It will be nice to see your artwork." Aaron held up two ties to the breast of his dress shirt and raised his eyebrows at me. "Which one?"

I tugged on one of the last dresses that still fit my stomach and blow-dried my hair. Hannah mimicked me as she sat on the vanity counter beside the sink, watching my every gesture. I dabbed the small eyeshadow applicator in the pearly powder I had just used and gave it to her. After a moment, Hannah turned to inspect herself in the mirror, tilting her head slightly to the right, coyly smiling at herself.

Jake and Megan met Aaron, Hannah, and me for dinner at a gourmet burger restaurant on Jasper Avenue before the art opening. "Hey! Nice to see you guys—oh, wow, Alexis Marie—you look ready to pop!" Megan said, her smile full across her face.

We sat at a circular table at the back of the restaurant and chatted about work and summer plans while Hannah drew with crayons and hummed loudly. Suddenly, a familiar tightening diverted my attention. *Is it poop cramps again?* Without saying a word, I took a deep breath. The tightening was faint but distinct, and I held the lip of the table until it passed. Aaron and Jake were making golf plans, and Megan was helping Hannah draw a silly face on a napkin. No one noticed me, and that was fine until I knew for sure.

Before heading out that evening, Aaron had turned on the Tree House channel for Hannah, and he and I snuck upstairs to make love in a final effort to induce labor. Aaron's chest hair was like flint against my taut, aching skin, sending sparks of pain through my belly. We lubricated the fronts of our bodies and giggled like children on a Slip'N Slide. I told Aaron that if I did indeed go into labor that night he had a magic penis, but, alas, the contractions that followed were sporadic and proved uneventful, fading quickly to nothing before we resigned ourselves to the gallery instead of the hospital.

"Here you go." The server plunked tall water glasses with clinking ice in front of us just as the tightening eased. My mind raced as I strained to read the kids' menu and convince Hannah to stay in her highchair. Suddenly, I snapped back into a hyperaware state as another contraction began. Again, I intended to clutch the table subtly, but Aaron noticed my hand and the tension in my arched shoulders.

"Are you okay?" His eyes were wide. "A contraction?"

"I'm fine. Just a little one. Do you remember how bad it was with Hannah and Zach? This is nothing. Really."

Aaron began timing contractions while Jake and Megan, who were yet to have children of their own, watched silently. Hannah spilled her water and goofed off, slapping her hands in the puddle on the table, unaware of our conversation. A few contractions came and went. "Look, that was a weak one. I'm totally good for our plans tonight. 'Kay?"

"Uh oh . . ." Aaron breathed.

"What?"

"I think I messed up on the timing. I thought seven minutes had passed between the last two, but they're actually three minutes apart."

"Oh, shit! I thought so." Jake clenched his jaw, bemused.

"Oh my God!" our teenage waitress screamed through her

braces when Aaron told her why we needed our food to go. She looked at me with excitement and then disgust, as if I had delivered my baby on the order-up counter.

"That last one was three minutes, too," Aaron announced loudly, standing and shifting on his feet.

"Come on, Hannah," Megan coaxed my girl, struggling to slip Hannah's dancing feet back into her tiny pink shoes she'd kicked off under the table.

"Seriously, you guys, I'm fine." Aaron stared at me impatiently. "Look, I can talk through them, the pain is like, I don't know, a two maybe. We're totally good. Please, Aaron; don't make a scene."

"No, we're going," he said in a stern rumble.

"They are just going to send me home. Seriously, can you just trust me? This is not it. Okay? It's Braxton Hicks, false labor or something. Please sit down."

"This is kind of funny," Jake interrupted. "We were with you guys when Alexis Marie announced she was pregnant and now again as she's going into labor." He laughed heartily, but Megan elbowed him in the ribs. Aaron sat down slowly.

"I am not going into labor; I am going to the art gallery." I smiled and popped open my to-go box and ate a few fries. Hannah took a big bite of her kids' hamburger. The other three did not touch their food; instead they watched me like I was a bomb ready to explode a baby at any moment.

"Oh," the word escaped me like a punch to the gut. I clenched my jaw mid-bite.

"Like hell you're going to the art gallery," Jake barked.

We all howled, Hannah loudest of all as she again spilled her water and smeared it all over the table. "Don't make me laugh, you guys! It hurts my vagina!" I said, my jaw still locked tight on a fry.

"We are going—that's it, Alexis Marie. We are going!" Aaron said, and he phoned our mothers, calling them into action. Aaron's mom met us in the driveway at home so she could care for Hannah that night, while Mom joined us in the hospital parking lot. Aaron had attempted to drop me off at the door, but I refused, annoyed that the contractions had become irregular in the car and vocal about the absurdity of rushing to the hospital when I was clearly not in labor. We entered through the sliding doors and navigated the familiar halls that Francisca had led us through just a few weeks before.

"This is ridiculous," I said under my breath, but Mom was on Aaron's side, and neither of them would answer me.

"Hi, my wife is going into labor," Aaron said to the woman in scrubs at the nurses' station. She looked at me as I smiled at her calmly, bashful, and swayed girlishly in my evening dress.

"Are you sure?" The nurse raised an eyebrow but sent Aaron to do paperwork anyway and led Mom and me into a large room partitioned into eight examining stations. She directed us to a curtained cubicle on the right, a familiar spot, where I was first examined in my labor with Hannah three years before. It looked the same: dimmed lighting and starkly bleached bedding, a striped blanket at the foot of the hospital bed, and humming machines that muffled whispered talk among the other couples until one woman or another cried out mid-contraction.

"You are four centimeters dilated," the nurse announced, snapping off her green gloves. "We'll be keeping you." Every day for the full forty weeks of my pregnancy I had grappled with my feelings, anticipating that moment, but once it came, my first instinct was to cross my legs. I wrung the sheets in my hands and cracked every knuckle and my neck as well.

"My name is Stacy. Let me hook you up here." The nurse strapped the heart-rate monitor to my bulbous middle with a stretchy tensor. Instantly the speedy *bah bum, bah bum, bah bum* of Eden's heart stomped around us like a bull-chested marching band. Just as Stacy slipped away, Aaron arrived.

I must have been holding my breath, because short gasps suddenly burst through my teeth, and I grabbed Aaron's hand roughly. "How am I supposed to do this?" My words were shrill. I couldn't hear Aaron's answer as my body surrendered to sobs that rocked the monitor belted around me. With each whimpering shudder the monitor quaked, transforming the steady drumming into loud static and thunder in rapid, deafening bangs. Stacy hurriedly appeared in our cramped space and pulled the monitor an inch from my skin, to our ears' relief. The only noises that remained were my pathetic cries.

There was no look of disdain on Stacy's pale face or impatience in her brown eyes. Mom had earlier explained to the nurse, as she filled out my chart, that this would be my third delivery even though I had only one child at home. As Mom spoke, I couldn't help but see Zachary's face, as I had in the flare of light in the Greek Orthodox church forty weeks before during my last job in my Year of Distraction. I saw again the fullness of my first son's facial features and his tiny hands—delicate skin and small, frail bones. I felt the unnatural coolness of his body against mine. There, as I was being admitted, my skin goosebumped, and my chest deflated.

Stacy led our small party into LDR 2, Labor and Delivery Room 2, where a wooden crucifix hung on the wall across from my bed. The Jesus was made of a dull gold, his bleeding hands nailed to a splintering cross. Though repelled by the presence of the crucifix, I was also reminded to pray to my unknown God. It was the same aching plea of the last nine months: *Please, let my baby live.* Reluctantly, I accepted the watchful eye of the golden Jesus and his aged faith like voodoo, for Eden's sake. The evening light from the exterior window shone into the room, first a dusty-blue color that slowly faded to caramel with a hint of rose.

The anesthesiologist entered. He was about to prick my spine, which was bridged like an overpass above my baby, when an unfamiliar nurse raced into the room without knocking. "The woman in LDR 4 is ready," she declared breathlessly.

"I don't care," snapped the anesthesiologist. "I am not a cheap whore! You all can wait." The door clicked shut behind the nurse. "Ready?" he asked me sweetly.

"Yep," I chirped, and I followed his instructions obediently.

Distracting me from the needle, Mom, the natural storyteller, remembered aloud how she and my dad had packed bags of treats to snack on for her hospital stay at the time of my birth. "Why we brought candy is beyond me," she shrugged. She told me how my father, a sensitive man—and quite nervous, I presumed—gobbled one bag after another while Mom pushed. When I was born, they popped champagne in the hospital room and it spilled all over, but no one cleaned it up. Mom recalled her slippers sticking to the floor with every step to the bathroom.

With the freezing anesthesia quickly sloshing across my nerve endings, Stacy told me to rest and wait; the time for pushing had not yet arrived. Aaron fell asleep instantly and snored like a gurgling geyser. Mom reclined against a wall, her legs tucked up and ankles crossed on a short padded bench. She watched TED Talks on her iPad, listening through white ear buds until her resolve was spent and she leaned her head back in sleep.

The clock to the left of the golden Jesus, like a sun in his sky, ticked past midnight. I was restless. Sleep was beaten back by the footrace within me between longing and despair. Eden was kicking. I felt and heard through the Doppler each motion simultaneously. A song by Johnny Cash, written by John S. Hurt, ran through my head on repeat: *You Are My Sunshine*. Throughout the previous week the song had braided its way through my subconscious, and I found myself singing it at random times: on my long walks, while I bathed Hannah, and as I rubbed my stomach in the grocery store lineup.

I hummed the lyrics to myself in the dark room as Aaron and Mom slept and the IV dripped slowly like a rain-drenched gutter. Staring up at the ceiling, I imagined looking through it to the charcoal sky with its flecks of starlight. Above my feet, two giant spotlights were mounted from the white drop ceiling. Each light looked like an eye and was made up of a large glass dome with an inner sphere-like iris, reflective and ocean-blue. The eyes stared without blinking but were benevolent.

Stacy entered silently and added oxytocin to my IV. The machine purred and clicked. I imagined all kinds of magic as I dozed in and out of LDR 2. Eden's heartbeat was a tribal drumming. My soul danced outside myself around a fire that touched earth to cloud. Ritual movements quivered through my limbs in a celebration of life and its mysteries. Ancestral spirits danced with me: my paternal grandfather, Grandpa Robb, who I could remember only through pictures and by the smell of cigarettes; and Grandma Chute, who died six months after Zachary. Those present were the living and the dead, with me in spirit and finding shape in the fire's breath, in the orange sparks and flecks of white wafting ash. Zachary was with me, also. He was always with me, and I felt him so close in the sweetness of that sacred dance as I fell into sleep.

Stacy returned at 3:30 in the morning. Aaron and Mom did not stir when she examined me and said, "Not much change."

Alone again, I felt a droopy, downward pressure between my legs, like a raindrop growing on a windowsill. Then in all its fullness the drop fell to the earth; my water had broken. "You are nine centimeters!" Stacy said after I woke Aaron and he called her back into the room. She ran for the door to call Dr. Stilles, and her steps echoed down the hall.

Dr. Stilles arrived at four in the morning, sweeping aside the green curtain by the door and looking half asleep. "Well, thank you, Alexis Marie, for waiting until after the Lions and Eskimos game last night," he began. He instructed me to plant my feet in the stirrups and said, "Okay, team. It's time. Are we ready to go?" Aaron and Mom nodded. "Alexis Marie, when you feel the contraction, begin pushing down and hold your breath for ten seconds. Okay—push!"

I bore down, hardly believing how quickly my life was about to change.

The next contraction began and I pushed firmly, feeling the pressure and release of Eden's head passing through me. One contraction more and his body emerged into the light of the glowing robot eyes. The doctor laid my son on my chest. In that instant the intense pressure of pregnancy flowed out of me in an audible *slosh*. Instinctively I took the deepest breath I had inhaled in months; it seemed to fill every corner of my body.

"Is he alive? Is Eden okay?" I wheezed, the panic not yet abated.

"Look, see for yourself," said a disembodied voice, which I hadn't a care to place, for when I looked down at my child I saw that my final desperate prayer had been answered.

Eden is alive.

"I love you, oh my goodness, I love you, Eden, oh my goodness, I love you, I love you *so* much." I listened for his first cry, and it must have happened, but I forgot it the second it passed through my ears. Maybe I was not meant to remember, and I realized it didn't matter. Eden arched his back at the cold and sucked at the air, rooting for home. Ever so slightly, he parted his eyelids and revealed the gleaming whites of his eyes.

Week 41: Enlarged Heart

The summer solstice began in the northern hemisphere on June 20, 2012, at approximately 7:09 p.m. Eastern Daylight Time. On the twenty-first day of June I went into labor with Eden, and on the twenty-second he was born. Our new season had graced us. The grass was green, and the reeds at the pond's edge had shed their gold straw for tall, rich lemon sheaths with brown fuzzy caps. Full leafy trees were the amphitheaters for songbirds and crickets in the twilight. The sweet-smelling air buzzed with bees and dragonflies.

On sun-drenched and sweltering afternoons, Aaron and I sat entwined on a large quilt in the shade of our yard. Slowly, we were discovering each other all over again, as we had years before. I sipped Mother's Milk tea and hummed Eden his song as he dozed on my lap. He proved to be the perfect fulfillment of his name— *delight*. Hannah, my savior through dark seasons and my enduring joy, ran through the sprinkler and rolled in the damp grass. The warm breeze coiled around us, playfully, lovingly binding us together with its invisible thread.

Zachary was never far from my thoughts. Where cardiac ultrasounds and other tests made no sense of my enlarged heart, I came to believe it grew with my first son. It expanded to hold him, rock him, and cherish him in an eternal, untouchable place.

Acknowledgments

To Aaron Chute for always believing in me and my dreams. Thank you for your tireless encouragement and faith. I love walking this journey of life with you.

To my living children, Hannah, Eden and Luca – you are my greatest joys. You inspire my words and my paint brush, and I cherish you three more than you will ever know.

To Zachary, thank you. You taught me how to love in spite of fear. You helped me find my voice as an artist. I think of you always, and this book is your legacy to the world.

To my parents, Charlotte Robb, Robert Duke, Doug Robb and Nancy Reid – you have bestowed in me many beautiful dichotomies: how to be humorous *and* intense, street-smart *and* business savvy, and how to be passionate while also *com*passionate. Mom, you are my hero and my best friend. This book came to be while you babysat my kids. I couldn't have done it without you. Dad, thank you for taking me to the theater as a child and exposing me to great storytelling. Thank you Nancy for all the support over the years. And Bob, there is nothing *step* about your dadness. Because of you, I may take the LSATs one day – just for fun.

To my mentors at Lesley University, I am forever grateful. Rachel Manley, you are one of the strongest, funniest, wisest women I know. Pam Petro, you inspire me as a fellow hybrid writer-artist. And Jane Brox, your love was tough, but invaluable.

Thank you to my editors, Philip Sherwood and Joanne Haskins. Philip, you were the first to lay eyes on my book in its infancy and your counsel was spot-on. And Joanne, thank you for wrangling my exciting grammar. Also, a big thank you to Barrett Briske.

Thank you to my forward-thinking publisher, Brooke Warner, and to Crystal Patriarche, Julie Metz, and Lauren Wise. Thank you to my awesome publicity team of Janet Shapiro and Elizabeth Martins. Thank you also to Rachel Sentes, Warren Sheffer, Curtis Trent, Tom Lim, and Suzy Kassem – your poem moves me.

I want to acknowledge my writing communities: those in Edmonton, at Lesley University, the Lesley Posse, She Writes, and all my writer friends online.

To all the bereavement counselors, nurses, doctors, and support communities, again those in person and those online – thank you! You taught me that life after loss needn't be lonely. I specifically want to acknowledge Brenda Mann, Patti Walker, Cheryl Roberts and Lori-Ann Huot.

Thank you to all my friends and family for supporting Aaron and me and our children in life and on our journey of loss. If it wasn't for all the food you made for us leading up to and after Zachary's death, we would have starved. Your love and generosity sustained us.

To all the families who have included the real names of their precious babies in the "Seasons" chapter, thank you for allowing me to commemorate such important lives. These children live on in our hearts, forever, and will as well between the cover of this book.

Finally, to all my children, as I have told you from the very first day of your births:

"You are my sun, my moon, and all my stars."

–E.E. Cummings

Resources

Wanted Chosen Planned *http://wantedchosenplanned.com/*
Expecting Sunshine *http://www.expectingsunshine.com/*
Still Standing Magazine *http://stillstandingmag.com/*
Pregnancy After Loss Support *https://pregnancyafterlosssupport.com/*
Baby Center *http://www.babycenter.com/pregnancy-miscarriage*
The Compassionate Friends *https://www.compassionatefriends.org*
Pregnancy Loss and Infant Death Alliance *http://www.plida.org/*
Miscarriage, Stillbirth, and Infant Loss Blog Directory
  http://babylossdirectory.blogspot.ca/
Carlie Marie Project Heal *http://carlymarieprojectheal.com/*
Perinatal Bereavement Documentaries *http://www.bereavement-documentaries.ca/index.html*
Glow in the Woods *http://www.glowinthewoods.com/*
Grieve out Loud *http://www.grieveoutloud.org/*
Faces of Loss, Faces of Hope *http://facesofloss.com/*
Miss Foundation *http://www.missfoundation.org/*
Return to Zero Center for Healing
  http://www.returntozerohealingcenter.com/

About the Author

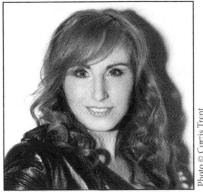

Photo © Curtis Trent

ALEXIS MARIE CHUTE is an award-winning artist, writer and filmmaker. She received her Bachelor of Fine Arts in Art and Design from the University of Alberta and her Masters of Fine Arts in Creative Writing from Lesley University in Cambridge, Massachusetts. Alexis Marie is a highly regarded public speaker and has traveled internationally presenting on art, writing, and the healing capacities of creativity. She is widely published in anthologies and magazines, and her artwork has been exhibited around the world. She lives in Edmonton, Alberta, Canada with her husband and their three living children.

For more information, please visit:
www.ExpectingSunshine.com
www.AlexisMarieChute.com
www.AlexisMarieWrites.com
www.AlexisMarieArt.com
www.WantedChosenPlanned.com

Follow Alexis Marie:
Twitter: @_Alexis_Marie
Instagram: @alexismariechute
Pinterest: pinterest.com/alexismarieart/
Facebook: facebook.com/AlexisMarieProductionsInc
YouTube: youtube.com/alexismariechute

SELECTED TITLES FROM SHE WRITES PRESS

She Writes Press is an independent publishing company founded to serve women writers everywhere. Visit us at www.shewritespress.com.

Three Minus One: Parents' Stories of Love & Loss edited by Sean Hanish and Brooke Warner. $17.95, 978-1-938314-80-3. A collection of stories and artwork by parents who have suffered child loss that offers insight into this unique and devastating experience.

Breathe: A Memoir of Motherhood, Grief, and Family Conflict by Kelly Kittel. $16.95, 978-1-938314-78-0. A mother's heartbreaking account of losing two sons in the span of nine months—and learning, despite all the obstacles in her way, to find joy in life again.

Make a Wish for Me: A Mother's Memoir by LeeAndra Chergey. $16.95, 978-1-63152-828-6. A life-changing diagnosis teaches a family that where's there is love there is hope—and that being "normal" is not nearly as important as providing your child with a life full of joy, love, and acceptance.

The Doctor and The Stork: A Memoir of Modern Medical Babymaking by K.K. Goldberg. $16.95, 978-1-63152-830-9. A mother's compelling story of her post-IVF, high-risk pregnancy with twins—the very definition of a modern medical babymaking experience.

Splitting the Difference: A Heart-Shaped Memoir by Tré Miller-Rodríguez. $19.95, 978-1-938314-20-9. When 34-year-old Tré Miller-Rodríguez's husband dies suddenly from a heart attack, her grief sends her on an unexpected journey that culminates in a reunion with the biological daughter she gave up at 18.

Changed By Chance: My Journey of Triumph Over Tragedy by Elizabeth Barker. $16.95, 978-1-63152-810-1. When her dreams of parenthood and becoming a career mom take a nightmarish twist, Elizabeth Barker has to learn how to summon her inner warrior—for her and her family's survival.

ENTRAPMENT

M. SPOONER

Margaret K. McElderry Books

New York London Toronto Sydney

MARGARET K. MCELDERRY BOOKS
An imprint of Simon & Schuster Children's Publishing Division
1230 Avenue of the Americas, New York, New York 10020
This book is a work of fiction. Any references to historical events,
real people, or real locales are used fictitiously. Other names, characters,
places, and incidents are products of the author's imagination, and any
resemblance to actual events or locales or persons, living or dead,
is entirely coincidental.

MARGARET K. MCELDERRY BOOKS is a trademark of Simon & Schuster, Inc.
For information about special discounts for bulk purchases, please contact
Simon & Schuster Special Sales at 1-866-506-1949
or business@simonandschuster.com.
The Simon & Schuster Speakers Bureau can bring authors to your live event.
For more information or to book an event, contact the
Simon & Schuster Speakers Bureau at 1-866-248-3049
or visit our website at www.simonspeakers.com.
Also available in a Margaret K. McElderry hardcover edition.
Book design by Mike Rosamilia
The text for this book is set in Gotham.
Manufactured in the United States of America
First Margaret K. McElderry paperback edition June 2010
10 9 8 7 6 5 4 3 2 1
The Library of Congress has cataloged the hardcover edition as follows:
Spooner, Michael.
Entr@pment : a high school comedy in chat / M. Spooner.
Summary: Two teenage girls assume false identities online in order to test the
fidelity of their boyfriends. Told in the form of chat room communications.
ISBN 978-1-4169-5889-5 (hardcover)
[1. Online identities—Fiction. 2. Impostors and imposture—Fiction. 3. Dating
(Social customs)—Fiction. 4. Online chat groups—Fiction. 5. Interpersonal
relations—Fiction. 6. Friendship—Fiction.] I. Title. II. Title: Entrapment
PZ7.S7638 En 2009
[Fic]—dc22
2008022944
ISBN 978-1-4424-0366-6 (pbk)
ISBN 978-1-4169-9493-0 (eBook)

✉ IM from the Author

meshikee: dedicated to the memory of Molly Spooner, who loved both opera and young people—*come scoglio* (like a rock).

meshikee: with many thanks to Syl and Isaac for the very idea, to Joyce and David for the lake effect, to Kylee and Jennifer for the feedback, and to Stephen and Lisa for believing in it.

meshikee: um, with apologies to Mozart and da Ponte.

YOUR UNCLE JERRY'S BLOG

Young Love
25 MAY

> *We will vow to one another*
> *there will never be another*
> *—Cartey and Joyner, lame old love song*

Peace and joy, camper. Spring has sprung, and young hearts have turned to thoughts of love—just as Your Uncle Jerry predicted. Young love. It's pathetic. Sad and sorry. Call it what you will, as long as it rhymes with "lame."

Now, don't jump to your keyboard, don't flame Your Uncle Jerry. Hear me out. Because I am just as fond of love's longing gaze as anyone. Uncle Jerry adores mouth-breathing and half-wit conversation. I *live* to hear young campers pour out the poetry of passion from their shallow, shallow souls.

Because Uncle Jerry knows what follows. And there is nothing—nothing—more entertaining than the flash of fury in a young girl's eye when she finds her boy in the arms of her own best friend.

Cruel, you say? Heartless? Not at all. I enjoy this only because I know it is the prelude to wisdom. Ah, yes, young lovers, I've had a love of my own. Worst eight hours of my life.

Pay attention—that's a joke. I say, that's a joke, son.

Oh. Sorry, camper girl, did you really think he could be true? Sorry, camper guy, did she say she'd save herself for you? Care to gamble on it? Turn your back and trust her if you dare. That's the only way to know.

Here's Your Uncle Jerry's wager (you know how Uncle Jerry loves a wager): I bet your lover will not love you still, young miss; your sweetheart will not sigh for you, young sir.

Young love will have another love next year.

Peace and joy.

CHAPTER 1
conspiracy

Ms.T has entered

Ms.T:	yo bliss, you there?
bliss4u:	hey T
Ms.T:	hey girl
bliss4u:	so what u guys do after the game?

gothling has entered

bliss4u:	hey annie
gothling:	**yo**
Ms.T:	we did nothing special. went to the mall
bliss4u:	again with the mall? <sigh sigh sigh>

Ms.T: ok, so he takes it slow. he likes the simple pleasures. i can totally live with it

gothling: who does? beau?

bliss4u: of course...

Ms.T: plus he's a little afraid of me. i like that in a boy toy. >:)

bliss4u: lol

Ms.T: you think it's the dreds?

bliss4u: or the grades =)

gothling: or yr death-2-the-oppressor politics

bliss4u: totally. i luuvvvv T, but i don't get half the stuff she says...

gothling: T is like alicia keys meets whoopi goldberg

Ms.T: oh great, i'm a sickly sweet soul singer and a saggy, middle-aged comic

gothling: but a leftist saggy, middle-aged sickly sweet comic soul star

bliss4u: what's leftist, anyway?

gothling: still, there's the beau boy. i thought brainy girls went for the star quarterback

Ms.T: we know what you think, dear

gothling: beau is what? like backup to the backup tight end? what's up with that?

bliss4u: lol. but he's a hottie in football pants. :->

gothling: but see: is he good enough for our Tamra? i'm just sayin...

Ms.T: he's a sweetie! and he's real. i don't need brilliant, and I sure don't need hollywood

gothling: u just like him because u can control him

Ms.T: ouch

bliss4u: not nice, annie

Ms.T: like with your record, you should choose
          a guy for me? i'm just sayin...

bliss4u: oh snap! i am so not getting between u 2nite

gothling: whatever

bliss4u: let's b nice, k? {{annie}} {{tamra}} k??

gothling: k, can we just not talk about boys right now?

bliss4u: sure. let's talk about me!

Ms.T: right. let's be nice to poor annie. she's all
          alone, and she's done her hair black again

**gothling: i'm not alone, prissy. i'm single. maybe u've heard
          of that**

bliss4u: well, um... certain people think ur bitter
          and cold. i don't know where i heard that

gothling: people get the strangest ideas

bliss4u: anyway, u were too good for... he who must
          not be named

Ms.T: well, and too intense, duh. what were you
          thinking, girl?

**gothling: wouldn't wanna be intense. the boys r SO easily
          threatened**

bliss4u: mitchie's not

gothling: we're not talking about boys, k?

bliss4u: sure, but who likes intense? who does
          that really work with, annie?

gothling: clearly, no one

Ms.T: anyway, annie hates all men this year. you said a
          year, right annie? :)

gothling: **back off, u**
listen, i am not a man-hater. i am simply willing 2
learn from experience. unlike some people

Ms.T: and you've learned what? um... tattoos, black
nails, and a tongue stud attract men of intellect
and refinement?

gothling: **no, dred-girl. i have learned that none of that**
matters. u can't trust em, anyway. the wretches

bliss4u: ok, sugar. but we can't all stay as angry as u

gothling: **ok baby. but i'm just wiser, not angry. see me**
smile : -

bliss4u: now see? that's really nice. she doesn't hate
anyone

Ms.T: she only finds them wretched

gothling: **oh, gimme a break. i LIKE lots of guys. i just think**
they're dumb as a box of rocks

bliss4u: puhleeeze. mitch is really really smart

gothling: **not about what matters. oh sigh, what do i know?**
i'm the one who fell for what's his name. voldemort

Ms.T: seems like i was just making that point

gothling: **shut up, u. but that's it. never again. u just can't**
trust em

Ms.T: any of them?

gothling: **any of em. any of em**

bliss4u: but he was only 1, annie

gothling: **sure, but they all... forget it. u guys are just**
pushing my buttons today

bliss4u: {annie} what?

gothling: **i dunno. they're just morons. geeks and jocks**
and gangstas and all of them. i hate how easy
they have it

Ms.T:	how easy?
gothling:	**easy peasy. they don't even know—that's why they can't be trusted. the world revolves around them, and they can't even see it**
Ms.T:	that's what i'm talking about. institutional sexism
gothling:	**if they could even SEE it, i could cut them some slack**
bliss4u:	mitch isn't that way. he treats me really nice
gothling:	**ok, listen, sugar, 1) ur da perky blonde bomb of the universe**
bliss4u:	awww
Ms.T:	but how can you stand those airheads on cheer squad? brrr.
bliss4u:	come on. they're fun!
gothling:	**2) mitch is like chief geek of the chess club (though i admit he cleans up good)**
bliss4u:	ok, he didn't WANT to be president. that was Mrs Fafner
gothling:	**therefore 3) he would be insane not to worship u**
bliss4u:	well, true... =)
gothling:	**but 4) if yr worst enemy breathed in his ear, he'd follow her right 2 the backseat**
Ms.T:	maybe...
bliss4u:	u mean kami day? she wouldn't dare!!
Ms.T:	ROTFL. i just sprayed coke on my keyboard
gothling:	**um, bliss? u may be missing my point, dear**
bliss4u:	besides, 5) mitch doesn't even like her, so there!
Ms.T:	lol <cough cough cough>

bliss4u: what? WHAT??

Ms.T: no, i'm with u. mitch and kami? never happen

bliss4u: that's what i'm sayin

gothling: T, ur not helping

Ms.T: or mitch and frankie? no worries there, either, am i right?

bliss4u: totally. my 2nd worst enemy

Ms.T: lol

bliss4u: WHAT already???

gothling: okay, chickies, listen up. u people need 2 learn a lesson here

Ms.T: yes, mum, we listening

gothling: i'll make u a little wager, my pretties, 2 see who's right about the dumber sex <rubbing hands evilly>

Ms.T: annie loves a wager

bliss4u: what wager?

gothling: let's just test yr 2 handsome units. see how much u can really trust them

Ms.T: ah... velly interesting. please to go on

gothling: but u have 2 put yrselves totally in my cynical scheming hands. understand? u must do exactly as i say, or u lose the bet

bliss4u: wait wait. what do u mean "how much we can trust them"?

gothling: trust means trust

Ms.T: i think annie's going to steal your boyfriend, honey

gothling: eww

bliss4u: that can't be legal... =)

Ms.T: both of ours. she'll woo them away from us

gothling: **sick bags on standby**

Ms.T: no seriously, u think i can't trust beau tanner, star backup to the backup tight end?

gothling: **that would be the general idea. u in or u out?**

bliss4u: but i still need 2 hear the bet

gothling: **well, it's obvious, isn't it? u guys disappear, and 2 mysterious young hotties slide in 2 take yr places**

Ms.T: TRY to take our places

gothlIng: **whatever**

bliss4u: wait. who r they?

gothling: **who?**

bliss4u: them

gothling: **them who?**

bliss4u: them! who r THEY??

gothling: **what? they're u, duh!!**

bliss4u: what??

gothling: **YOU**

Ms.T: annie, let me do this.

bliss. darlin. here's the deal

you and i PRETEND to go away. mitch and beau are heartbroken, right?

bliss4u: right...

Ms.T: we make them promise to be good till we come back, ok?

bliss4u: sure. k. then what?

Ms.T: then we PRETEND to be someone else,
               and try to break them down

gothling: **there u go**

bliss4u: but how do we...? i mean, if they see us...

Ms.T: true. um, Annie? online? we make up identities
               and hit on them from there?

gothling: **exactly**

Ms.T: e-dentities

gothling: **whole new personalities. like costumes and masks
               and foreign accents. see, bliss?**

bliss4u: oooo, i c now. this could be fun...

Ms.T: yeah, i know just how to get to beau baby

gothling: **oh, ahem. not so fast, sweetie**

bliss4u: now what?

gothling: **er, well, just that it won't be ms. tamra gray and
               beau baby.**

               it will be... <ta daa> BLISS and beau baby!

bliss4u: excuse me?

gothling: **as a different person, of course**

bliss4u: what r u talking about?

Ms.T: niiiiice. so bliss goes after beau, which leaves
               me available for... oh NO.

gothling: **now ur gettin it**

bliss4u: help!! I'M not gettin it

Ms.T: what's not to get?

gothling: **u trade boys u trade boys u trade boys**

bliss4u: now i'm gettin it...

Ms.T: this'll never work, annie

bliss4u: i don't get it

gothling: **of course it'll work**

bliss4u: we trade boys?

Ms.T: they'll never go for this

gothling: **\<slamming forehead on desk once, twice, three times\>**

             ok listen up, campers. everybody take a deep breath

             here's the deal

             so, bliss's grandmother is sick and bliss needs 2 go help her. tamra, official best friend, gets 2 go along 2 keep her company

             u with me so far?

bliss4u: but my grandmother is fine

Ms.T: pretending...

gothling: **what u really do is hole up at home 4 a couple of days. we'll be in chat mode constantly**

bliss4u: yay! we could do a sleepover!

gothling: **or not.... anywho, while ur "away," 2 very interesting chicks chat up yr boys online**

Ms.T: kewl

gothling: **lemme see. chessmaster mitch gets his king row invaded by... oh let's say Tatiana. yeah, Tatiana del Capo, some kind of genius gurl from italy— or no: albania**

bliss4u: where's that?

gothling: **and this tatiana chick is played by our very own tamra gray**

Ms.T:	gee thanks. Ta-tyahn-a from Al-bahn-ya. like a lady wrestler
bliss4u:	lol. i like it
gothling:	**mitch is smart, T. but u got world stuff in yr 47 AP classes, right? of course u did. everything is politics 2 u**
Ms.T:	i could look it up...
gothling:	**good. so then beau boy hears from a certain... Bridget... or Bonnie... or... lil help with the last name, tam**
Ms.T:	grindstaff, a banker's daughter from london
gothling:	**oooo, yes. and portrayed, of course, by the lovely and talented bliss taylor**
bliss4u:	i still don't get this. why me and beau?
Ms.T:	we trade boys... it's crueler that way. more like annie
gothling:	**it just keeps u... honest. ho ho**
Ms.T:	nice one, annie
bliss4u:	but me and the hottest boy in the state? i don't think so. u do it yrself, annie
gothling:	**don't make me come over there**
Ms.T:	come on, bliss, you can handle this
bliss4u:	but he's so... what would i SAY 2 him???
gothling:	**i'll tell u what 2 say**
Ms.T:	oh, you just go: beau, i am utterly muddled by what you americans call football, and you seem like just the chap who could help a poor english girl understand
gothling:	**perfect**

bliss4u: hmmm. well, but we have 2 actually see them
             sooner or later

Ms.T: true. annie?

**gothling: not really. bridget and tatiana just have 2 set them
             up online**

bliss4u: but...

**gothling: we wing it, k? the point is, they agree to hook up,
             and then guess who appears?**

Ms.T: bliss and tam, of course

bliss4u: i don't know. this whole thing is kinda sketchy

**gothling: what sketchy? it's a sting. llke cops and a
             speed trap**

Ms.T: spies and a politician

bliss4u: but it's setting them up. how twisted is that?

**gothling: law-abiding citizens have nothing 2 fear.
             don't u trust him?**

bliss4u: oh puhleeeze. i trust mitchie completely

Ms.T: i have a question. what are the stakes here?
             what do we lose if you win, annie?

gothling: oh, u lose plenty

bliss4u: come on. what does that mean?

gothling: yr innocence, for starters

Ms.T: annie thinks we're naive. <sigh> no faith, no
             faith

gothling: well duh

bliss4u: but why, annie?

gothling: o, just listen at u. "i trust mitchie completely."

bliss4u: well, i do. so there

gothling: i rest my case. so there

Ms.T: ok ok, so if we lose the bet, we lose our innocence and our faith in men. that's the best you can do?

gothling: what? u want a money bet? make it 10 bucks. make it 20. i'll be rich

bliss4u: yikes. 20??

gothling: u don't want 2 bet money?

Ms.T: no money. and we need a timeline. this isn't going on forever

gothling: fine. how bout this: we scam them for 3 weeks. WHEN u lose, no matter how mad u are, u have to take them back, where u have to deal with their hurt little egos, knowing u'll never EVER trust them again

bliss4u: yowtch

Ms.T: so dark, annie. tsk tsk... and what do we win when we prove you wrong?

gothling: u say

bliss4u: she has 2 kiss em both—like in middle school :-D

gothling: whatever

Ms.T: eww. no, she has to do something serious. like apologize

bliss4u: 2 us?

Ms.T: to them. she has to confess the whole thing and admit she was wrong about guys. the hardest thing in the world. especially for annie.

gothling: have i mentioned my new black nail polish? not a chip anywhere

Ms.T: girlfriend, these guys aren't like him

bliss4u: ...who must not be named...

gothling: **come on, campers. they're all like that. the ones who don't cheat r the ones who never got a chance. so do we have a deal or not?**

Ms.T: deal

gothling: **bliss? u in?**

bliss4u: annie, that is so not true about guys. mitch would never ever ever, and i'm sure he's had chances

Ms.T: really? i haven't noticed the cheer squad hitting on mitch...

bliss4u: very funny, my former friend

gothling: **seriously. when were all these chances 2 cheat?**

bliss4u: i don't know, k? i just know he would never do it

gothling: **then ur in, right? nothing 2 lose**

bliss4u: i'm thinking. there's something about this that is a little bit sick and wrong

gothling: **and yr point is?**

Ms.T: lol

gothling: **seriously, gurl. if u trust him, then where's the risk? it's just a game**

bliss4u: i know, but still

gothling: **plus, u get 2 know beau a LOT better : ->**

bliss4u: lol

Ms.T: hey, easy with that

gothling: **think of it as a chance for mitchie 2 PROVE that ur right about him**

bliss4u: hmm... well...

Ms.T:	come on, blissie. it'll be fun. like wearing costumes to the dance
gothling:	**a masked ball**
bliss4u:	yeah... i do like a costume
Ms.T:	a formal dress, a foreign accent, a shiny little mask on a stick
gothling:	**or cowgirl boots and a lone ranger mask**
Ms.T:	it'll be fun...
bliss4u:	yeah, it could be
gothling:	**so ur in?**
bliss4u:	ok ok, i'm in

CHAPTER 2

premonitions

THE DAWG HOUSE

MAY 27 08:15 PM

chessman has entered

chessman: bo. u there?

BoBoy: dude. sup?

chessman: nothing really. paper for history

BoBoy: no way. that's due tomorrow???

chessman: relax. it's not due till wednesday.
i'm just getting a head start. the
last paper of the year. ahhhh

BoBoy: mitch, u kill me, man. this is sunday night

chessman: i know. but see, if i'm done early,
then i have time to bail u out at the
last minute

BoBoy: lol. that's why i keep u on the payroll

chessman: so what did you guys do after
the game?

BoBoy: me and T? no mucho. a little smoocho.
winkwink, know what i mean?

chessman: go to the mall again?

BoBoy: lame, huh? <sigh>

chessman: not really

BoBoy: it is. i know it is

chessman: whatever dude

BoBoy: what can i say? i'm scared 2 put the big move on her

chessman: it'll happen when it's right. don't
let the team shine you about that

BoBoy: nah... they think it's impassive 2 be going out
with her at all

chessman: impassive?

BoBoy: u know, like: whoa, dawg, impassive touchdown!

chessman: oh. impressive

BoBoy: impressive! my bad. i knew that

chessman: close enough. well i'm just
checking in

BoBoy: hey. sometimes tamra's too much for me.
know what i mean?

chessman: too much?

BoBoy: nah. i mean, it's just like, what's she doing with me?
of all people?

chessman: i figure she likes you. why fight it?

BoBoy: i hear ya. but really, dawg, that girl has a brain on
her. she can think circles around me

chessman: ok, but you gotta ask yourself,
would she waste her time on a moron?

BoBoy: i guess not

chessman: seriously. besides, you're a gentleman, which women always dig

BoBoy: true. well, what about johnson? he's no southern gentleman

chessman: dude, get real

BoBoy: no u get real. he hooks up with tons of chicks

chessman: tons of skanks, you mean

BoBoy: true... still

chessman: you think johnson would ever, in his wildest dreams, have a chance with T?

BoBoy: ha. not so much

chessman: exactly. so you, my man, have GOT something

BoBoy: well... i gotta say yr logic is perfect, once again

chessman: that's why i'm the geek around here

BoBoy: my dad says for guys like us, there r 2 rules with women—treat em like a lady, and make em laugh

chessman: guys like us?

BoBoy: me and him. u know, not the sharpest bricks in the load

chessman: good advice. sharp isn't necessarily what women look for

BoBoy: lol. if it was, my man, T would be with u

chessman: yikes. no way. too much pressure for me

BoBoy: pressure?

chessman: way too much. i would totally freeze if i had to hook up with her

BoBoy: get out

chessman: no, she's impressive, but i like
her right where she is—with you.
at the mall

BoBoy: lol. u can just keep yr distance then. i'm not
complaining. but that is so weird, dude

chessman: why?

BoBoy: nah. i just mean she's nothing 2 fear, man. she's totally
not a competitive person

chessman: glad to hear it. i always liked her.
but take it from me, she kills in
AP classes

BoBoy: k sure, AND she totally imbues her politics

chessman: she what?

BoBoy: no, she totally does. but then she's got this happy little
way of hooking my arm around her. it cracks me up

chessman: i've seen her do that

BoBoy: like some kinda dance move, and boom,
she's tucked in tight

chessman: that's what i'm talking about.
she likes you

BoBoy: but hey. doesn't bliss do that kind of stuff?

chessman: bliss is great. really fine

BoBoy: she's awesome, dude

chessman: but she like, waits for me to move,
i guess. i dunno

BoBoy: yeah

chessman: i mean she's real cozy, but when we
go out, it's like, whatever you
wanna do, mitch

BoBoy: right. traditional girl

chessman: which is cool

BoBoy: it is

chessman: as long as what i want to do keeps her happy. :-)

BoBoy: lol. u worry about that?

chessman: definitely

BoBoy: so ur like—well, what do U wanna do?

chessman: yep

BoBoy: but that's cool. give and take

chessman: right

BoBoy: yeah.... i was saying 2 johnson... nah

chessman: what?

BoBoy: aw nothing. u know how he is

chessman: what did he say?

BoBoy: nah, he was just messing

chessman: come on...

BoBoy: nah, he was like, what does a hottie like bliss see in old mitch?

chessman: <snore> he says that stuff to me, too

BoBoy: i go, dude, the woman's in love. show some respect

chessman: i don't mind. johnson's cool

BoBoy: yeah

chessman: a little random, but he's cool

BoBoy: smart guy. jokes with all the teachers, but then he blows off classes. loves the women, but treats them like ho's... i dunno. hard 2 respect that stuff

chessman: witty, creative, sexist, underachiever. what's not to like?

BoBoy: lol. true. but he also calls u our nerdy friend

chessman: sure. but with capitals: Our Nerdy Friend. like it's a title or something

BoBoy: i don't like him talking that way. where's his loyalty?

chessman: see, this is why Coach doesn't start you. you don't want anyone to get hurt

BoBoy: lol. u got me

chessman: it's fine about johnson. let it go

BoBoy: no it ISN'T fine. dude, he'll be lucky 2 graduate. ur like on yr way 2 harvard and stuff

chessman: whatever

BoBoy: seriously. that is so far out of reach for anyone i know

chessman: no, it's cool. i AM your nerdy friend. so what?

BoBoy: get out. but hey if it's cool with u, i'll let it alone. i just think he should... i don't know

chessman: show some respect

BoBoy: something like that

chessman: nah. i'm just glad to hang with you guys

BoBoy: hah. u have serious issues, dawg

chessman: you have no idea how boring it gets in geek land

BoBoy: LOL. i know i'll never see harvard

chessman: stick with Ms. T

BoBoy: oh, i get it. good one

chessman: that girl is way smart. and she does it without getting called a nerd. gotta admire that

BoBoy: bliss is no dummy either

chessman: true true true. but... well...
bliss doesn't really live in her head

BoBoy: like she should act smarter?

chessman: nah, i just mean she really likes
her thing with the cheer squad and
all. she's smart about social stuff,
you know?

BoBoy: u saying that's bogus?

chessman: no, i totally like it. bliss is
popular. good for her. i'm just
not part of that crowd

BoBoy: oic

chessman: i'm her boyfriend and like this
third wheel at the same time

BoBoy: no, i get it

chessman: no you don't. you're one of the
popular gang. how could you get it?
;-)

BoBoy: jocks and chicks. it's a beautiful thing

chessman: lol. so it's like you say tam can
think circles around you. bliss can
TALK circles around me

BoBoy: she does have lotsa friends...

chessman: tell me. she's always calling
somebody, or texting somebody,
or just WITH somebody

BoBoy: dude, ur jealous!

chessman: nah. i'm just... ok, you got me,
i'm jealous

BoBoy: i knew it. u tell bliss?

chessman: nah, i don't complain

BoBoy: tell her, man

chessman: no way. i'm lucky just to be going out with her. i mean, look at me

BoBoy: true

chessman: lol. and btw? your history paper is toast

BoBoy: no really, i get ya. i'm totally insecure about the same thing

chessman: what? like someone's going to move in on you?

BoBoy: u know it

chessman: get out. Ms. T's too smart for that

BoBoy: no, i mean it. i get these prepositions

chessman: ??

BoBoy: when something's gonna happen...

chessman: oh, premonitions. sure. i get those

BoBoy: i'm like running scared half the time

chessman: really? so what's your premonition lately?

BoBoy: i don't know. she could change her mind, i guess

chessman: i hear you. there's always the chance

BoBoy: i guess

Big.J has entered

Big.J: yo. anybody home?

BoBoy: what up, J?

chessman: hey Johnson. how's it goin?

Big.J: omg, it's da both of dem. frick and frack doing their after school thang chessman: i told you he was witty, didn't i?

Big.J: it's mickey and goofy. popeye and
bluto. death and destruction.
delight... AND instruction

BoBoy: he works on this stuff. gotta respect the discipline

Big.J: dudes, it is hard 2 believe,
and i don't like 2 brag, but once
again, i am the gingerbread on
the smorgasbord of love

BoBoy: u what?

Big.J: smother me with lemon sauce and
serve me sizzlin. yowza!

chessman: how do you do it, johnson? always
the women

Big.J: ah, my poetic spirit. they cannot
say me nay

BoBoy: get outta town

Big.J: one look into these soulful eyes,
and their sugary pink hearts just
melt 2 goo

chessman: it's a gift, bro. no 2 ways about it

BoBoy: LOL

Big.J: it's a gift... and a curse

BoBoy: what curse? u always have a lady at yr side

chessman: so do you, but with johnson it's
a different lady every time

Big.J: yr friend has a brain on him, i c

BoBoy: so wattup today, J?

Big.J: what indeed? care 2 guess?
anyone? anyone?

chessman: hmmm. love is on his mind, and...
let's see, it's been...

BoBoy: u met tiffany's mother and she's stolen u
from tiff?

Big.J: i'm thinking not

chessman: oh no. it's tiffany. she's lost
that new car smell

Big.J: now, that's why u the king of the
nerds. u figure things out....

BoBoy: what r u saying, johnson? i've heard none of this

chessman: ...plus there's a new car on the
street

Big.J: check and mate. the chess dude
wins again

BoBoy: wait a minute. what happened to tiffany?

Big.J: moving 2 woodstock as soon as
school's out. her dad is changing
companies. and i'm not driving up
there every other day. that's 1
thing...

BoBoy: dude, that's a drag

Big.J: u'd think. but somehow... i dunno.
it wasn't going 2 work out with
tiff anyway

chessman: something about the poetic soul
getting restless?

Big.J: there u go. i need variety.
i need stimulation. challenge.
i have needs

BoBoy: um, does tiff know?

Big.J: know what?

chessman: about variety

BoBoy: about yr needs, big J

Big.J: she'll get the picture

chessman: what are you going to tell her?

Big.J: i'll think of something. she texted me a minute ago. crying about having 2 pack her stuffed animals 2nite

BoBoy: bro, that's cold

Big.J: get a grip, dawg. i'm too young to marry. and hey, i always let em down gently. i'll write her a poem

chessman: it's a shame, though. tiff was the best you've hooked up with so far

Big.J: if u don't mind a muffin top and constant gum snapping

BoBoy: get out

Big.J: and cherry lipstick. but i rather like cherry lipstick

chessman: come on J. she's who she is...

Big.J: she's a skank. u know that. a sweet skank, but still

BoBoy: aw man. where's yr heart? u keep it in a box somewhere?

chessman: well, um, nobody thought you'd be with her long

Big.J: yo, check it out, my brothers. i'll write her a poem right b4 yr eyes: lets see, my image will be... k, a bird. yes, a bird migrating. title? anyone? no, i have it:

"farewell in spring"
for tiffany, on moving to
woodstock

my little bird, i know
that you must fly
—as birds in spring
are wont to do—and i
must set you free
to go where you must go
and be what you must be.

my little bird, i know
the universe
is calling you, and i
must be as strong
as i can be, and must not cry.
for though i long to fly
with you, my little bird,
and you to stay with me,
we know that I must let you
go.

my little bird, we
know the universe
is calling you
—as it, in spring
is wont to do—and i
must set you free.

that's it, dudes. what do u
think?

chessman: you've written this before

Big.J: no i haven't. i swear!

BoBoy: u just made this up?

Big.J: dude, this stuff just comes
           2 me. i tell u, it's a gift

chessman: and a curse...

Big.J: lol. now ur a dead man. u don't
mock an artist

BoBoy: dude, i don't know if it's good or bad, but u knock out
a poem in 30 seconds and ur going to toss it at her
like ttfn? shouldn't it cost u?

chessman: i think tiff would say it should, yes

Big.J: bro, that's just how it happens.
i can't help it when the lightning
strikes

BoBoy: u are truly cold, J

chessman: at least tell her to watch that
screen door

BoBoy: really, johnson, she'll cry about this for a month

Big.J: boyz boyz, chill. hey, she's the
1 leaving

chessman: and hey, easy come, easy go

Big.J: lay off, nerdman. she'll rebound
in a week. i know this girl

chessman: no, it's cool. for the girls are
calling you, and you must do what
you must do

BoBoy: LOL, mitch. u guys crack me up

Big.J: look, very few guys can stay with
1 chick forever. it isn't normal,
man. play the field. hey, it's
what they do

BoBoy: not me, dude. i'm totally staying with the 1 i got

chessman: it's what THEY do, johnson?

Big.J: zackly. every chick i know has
had like 3 dudes this year. tiff

will find someone in woodstock,
and probably tomorrow

chessman: so, but let me just follow the
logic here. you think all women
are ho's, basically, is that
about it?

Big.J: u make it sound like a bad thing

chessman: ok, so they're all ho's. and that
makes you want to be one too? dude,
i hope that works out for you

Big.J: wellllll. looky here, looky here.
brittney's sending me a lil ol
text message on my lil ol cell
phone

BoBoy: oh, man. now brittney??

Big.J: i know. she's a ho. i'm weak.
i'm weak

chessman: and you must fly...

Big.J: btw, i will totally get u for
this. never mock a man's poetry.
an artist channels the universe.
if there's anything more important
than cherry lipstick, art would
be that thing

BoBoy: focus johnson! brittney on line 2, remember?

Big.J: k. i gotta bounce, dawgs.
check u 18r

the setup

BoBoy has entered

BoBoy: yo mitch

chessman: hey

BoBoy: dude, what's this about bliss leaving?

chessman: ??

BoBoy: yeah. annie told me. she didn't say anything 2 u?

chessman: totally in the dark

BoBoy: dang. i saw annie, and she said something about B's mom or grandmom is vegetating

chessman: she what??

BoBoy: really sick in the hospital. like had a stroke or something

chessman: got it. but not her mom?
she's too young

BoBoy: mom or grandmom. she didn't know which.
just that B's gotta leave 4 a while. bummer

chessman: totally

BoBoy: so u haven't talked 2 B?

chessman: not since lunch. she had cheer
squad meeting, last day of school
stuff. then something with Tamra.
you know. she was going to IM me
later tonight

BoBoy: u better ask about this

chessman: absolutely. did annie say
how long?

BoBoy: she said it could be awhile. like months or longer

chessman: months? like all summer?

BoBoy: dude, i don't know. annie was just rattling
stuff off. she's like o it could be forever or it
could be just a weekend. all depends on the
hospital or something

chessman: where's the hospital?

BoBoy: tallahassee. i'm really sorry about this, bro

chessman: i'll check it out

BoBoy: dude, how can u be so chill? i'm freaked,
and it's not even my girlfriend

chessman: no, i'm plenty freaked. but i just
don't have enough information

BoBoy: i'm ballistic, man. i'm epileptic

chessman: lol. oh, wait. bliss checking in

✉ IM from bliss4u

JUNE 01 04:19 PM

bliss4u: mitch, honey, can we talk?

chessman: sure. hey, beau says there's something going on with your mom?

bliss4u: no, my grammy

chessman: what's happened?

bliss4u: i'm not sure. mom says she fell

chessman: did she have a stroke?

bliss4u: yeah. she totally freaked

chessman: no, your grandmother. did she have a stroke?

bliss4u: oh, right. i'm so dumb. no, she just fell. or, i mean, she could have... we don't know 4 sure yet. that could be it

chessman: that's a drag

bliss4u: i know

chessman: so what's going to happen?

THE DAWG HOUSE

BoBoy: **dude, what's she saying?**

chessman: it's her grandmother. she's fallen.
            maybe had a stroke

BoBoy: **i knew it. i knew it**

✉ IM from bliss4u

bliss4u: we have 2 go down there

chessman: you and your mom?

bliss4u: yeah

chessman: where is she? i mean where's
the hospital?

bliss4u: oh, jacksonville. or no, it's lauderdale. silly.
can't remember anything

chessman: wow, ft lauderdale's a long way

bliss4u: i know

chessman: why do you have to go?

bliss4u: um? cuz she's my grammy?

chessman: sorry. that was a selfish question.
i just mean, if your mom is going, and all...

bliss4u: no, that's ok. i just have 2

chessman: i'll just miss you. totally

bliss4u: ur a sweetie. but don't worry,
i'll come back

chessman: i'm not worried

bliss4u: mom needs my help with stuff

chessman: yeah...

bliss4u: like moving her back home, and helping her
walk, and taking care of her, and yeah

THE DAWG HOUSE

BoBoy: oh man, i knew this was gonna happen. i knew something was gonna happen. it's my permutations. they been coming all the time lately. something's gonna happen. i knew it. this could be what they were telling me

mitch boy, what's she saying now?

chessman: she has to go down there to help her mom

BoBoy: **dude**

chessman: yeah

BoBoy: **how long?**

chessman: good point. i'll ask

✉ IM from bliss4u

chessman: does your mom say how long?

bliss4u: how long what?

chessman: how long you'll be there

bliss4u: oh. no she doesn't know 4 sure. it could be awhile, i think she said

chessman: what about cheer camp this summer? and then school? i mean, it's going to be our senior year

bliss4u: oh it won't be THAT long! school isn't till the end of August

chessman: eleven weeks

bliss4u: oh, silly, we'll be done with this in a week or 2. u'll see

chessman: really? beau made it sound like you're never coming back

bliss4u: beau? how would beau tanner know a thing about this?

chessman: from annie

bliss4u: yikes

chessman: and she was saying, like, indefinitely. maybe 3 weeks. maybe forever

bliss4u: well, k, maybe 3 weeks. but i don't think so. i don't think i could stand 2 do this that long

chessman: well, but it's your grandmother

bliss4u: sure. i know. um, but i just meant i couldn't do this 2 u. i told annie i didn't want 2 do it at all

THE DAWG HOUSE

BoBoy: i mean, u know how long it takes old people 2 get better. annie was like, it could be forever. that would be the worst, man. coming into your senior year and yr girlfriend like disappears

and who knows what she'd be doing all that time. those old boys in tallahassee know how 2 court a woman too. college town and everything

prepositions premonitions permutations. now i forget which 1 is right. dang. it's the stress

chessman: she thinks less than a month

BoBoy: dude. k. well, not as bad as it could be

chessman: not tallahassee. ft lauderdale

BoBoy: oh wait. here's T

chessman: see ya...

✉ IM from Ms.T

JUNE 01 4:30 PM

Ms.T: hey handsome, you there?

BoBoy: check it out, speak of the devil

Ms.T: whatcha doing?

BoBoy: thinking of u. what else?

Ms.T: lol. listen. we have to talk

BoBoy: totally. there's some weird stuff going on

✉ IM from bliss4u

chessman: so when do you have to leave?

bliss4u: i'm not sure what the plan is 4 that. i mean, it's up 2 my mom. she's the 1 driving and everything

chessman: you're driving to ft lauderdale? that'll take a while

bliss4u: or maybe we're flying. i can't remember. i am such a ditz today

chessman: well, you have a lot on your mind

✉ IM from Ms.T

Ms.T: there's something i have to tell you

BoBoy: sounds serious, T. fire away

Ms.T: don't mean to be that way. but it is kinda serious

BoBoy: i'm listening

Ms.T: well, bliss's grandmother has fallen down. it sounds like she might have had a stroke. they've put her in the hospital

BoBoy: hey, i've heard about this from annie. saw her after school

Ms.T: annie? she wasn't supposed to... well never mind

BoBoy: wasn't supposed 2 say anything?

Ms.T: sort of. anyway, it doesn't matter

✉ IM from bliss4u

chessman: but you think it could be soon? like this week you're leaving?

bliss4u: yes. oh. today. i'm just starting 2 pack

chessman: wow. that's quick

bliss4u: well, in a way. but who knows how long she'll last?

chessman: true. didn't think of that

✉ IM from Ms.T

BoBoy: when does she leave?

Ms.T: who?

BoBoy: bliss. 2 go help her granny

Ms.T: oh. right away. tonight

BoBoy: yeah. makes sense. gotta be there 4 those we love

Ms.T: yeah. has she told mitch?

BoBoy: um, yeah. he's chatting her right now. poor guy. this'll be rough on him

✉ IM from bliss4u

chessman: ok. but let's think positive. let's believe she'll be better soon, and THAT will help make it happen

bliss4u: o ur such a good guy

chessman: and you'll be back in no time

bliss4u: i really hate 2 do this 2 u

chessman: B, you're not doing it to me. you're helping your grandmother. that's important work.
i know lots of people who wouldn't even go.
she'll think you're an angel

bliss4u: ur right. it's important. still. i'm gonna miss u

chessman: and i think you're an angel too

bliss4u: i don't deserve u, mitchell saunders

chessman: but you'll call me or something?

bliss4u: i will. oh. um, grammy doesn't have internet

chessman: really?

bliss4u: but i'll call when i can

chessman: ok. wow. we've only been apart that one time

bliss4u: i know. 2 whole weeks away from u. and that jerk at disney world hitting on me. i hated it

✉ IM from Ms.T

Ms.T: bo, um, there's something else

BoBoy: what's that, miz T?

Ms.T: i need to tell you... how shall i put this?

BoBoy: oh no.... i know what ur gonna say

Ms.T: you do?

BoBoy: well, k... i'm guessing it's like... well, this isn't easy but maybe it's like...

so, now that school's over, u like want 2 see other people, don't u?

Ms.T: what? OMG no!

BoBoy: really?

Ms.T: REALLY. TRULY

BoBoy: whew. u were so serious

Ms.T: get that outta your head, bubba. you are totally stuck with me

BoBoy: T, that's such a relief. i was really sweatin there

Ms.T: what even made you think that?

BoBoy: dunno. just a hunch, i guess. i get these prepositions sometimes

Ms.T: well, that one totally steered you wrong

BoBoy: great. man, i was scared

Ms.T: really, beau. there's no man alive who could tempt me away. and don't you forget it

BoBoy: awww. i feel just like that about u, miz T

Ms.T: shucks

BoBoy: um... oh, dang it! it's not preposition, is it? :)

Ms.T: nope. <grin>

BoBoy: i knew it

✉ IM from bliss4u

chessman: i hated that guy too, and i wasn't even there. :-D

bliss4u: u had nothing 2 worry about

chessman: lucky for him... because i'd have come down there and... and given him a computer virus!

bliss4u: my hero <sigh>

chessman: hey, um, bliss? seriously?

bliss4u: yeah?

chessman: there aren't any guys down in ft lauderdale, are there?

bliss4u: ft lauderdale?

chessman: yeah. there aren't... oh never mind.
i was just thinking of something johnson said

bliss4u: johnson? mr. sleaze?

chessman: i know. he's a little sketchy... but

bliss4u: but what?

chessman: well, sometimes he thinks you're
nuts to be hooked up with a nerdster like me

bliss4u: listen, mitchie, i'm just an airhead cheerleader,
but i know what i've got in u

chessman: you're not an airhead

bliss4u: and i would never mess that up.
not in a million zillion years. u got that?

📧 IM from Ms.T

Ms.T: but listen, big sweetie

BoBoy: yes ma'am?

Ms.T: i have to go with bliss

BoBoy: say again?

Ms.T: when she goes to tallahassee

BoBoy: no way

Ms.T: way. i gotta go with her

BoBoy: i knew it. i knew something was coming

Ms.T: i know. you always do

✉ IM from bliss4u

chessman: so you're packing?

bliss4u: guess i better

chessman: this is so sudden. i'm going to miss you big time

bliss4u: don't worry, i'll be back b4 u know it. just...

chessman: what?

bliss4u: well, i know u

chessman: true

bliss4u: so i know this isn't a problem, but...

chessman: but what?

bliss4u: oh, just promise 2 be good while i'm gone, k?

chessman: lol. like the chess club girls are lining up. both of them

bliss4u: stop it. girls like u, mitchie. i hear them talking. ur smart and funny and wonderful. ur a real... oh what's my mom's word... a catch. ur a real catch. u just don't know it. and that's probably my fault. i should tell u more often

chessman: sweet. i can't wait to be mobbed at the mall. ;-)

bliss4u: i'm being serious, k? just shut up and promise

chessman: i promise. i swear. no messing around

bliss4u: good. better not

chessman: i would die first

bliss4u: well, let's not get carried away =)

chessman: you mean you'd miss me if I died?

bliss4u: hah. only at first. oh, my mom is yelling something

chessman: i'll swing by tonight to say bye, ok?

bliss4u: k. gotta run. luv u! miss me?

chessman: you too. i will. bye

✉ IM from Ms.T

BoBoy: k. i can deal with this. deep breaths, beau boy. take it easy big guy

Ms.T: you're too funny, you know? you always make me laugh

BoBoy: yessir. make em laugh, that's what my daddy says. but really, why do u have 2 go with her?

Ms.T: well, because i'm the best friend. that's what girls do

BoBoy: i was afraid of that. btw, it's lauderdale

Ms.T: what?

BoBoy: ft lauderdale. that's what she told mitch

Ms.T: no, it's supposed to be... well, never mind

BoBoy: what?

Ms.T: no, i could have remembered it wrong

BoBoy: no way. maybe she told u wrong

Ms.T: maybe

BoBoy: so r u packing right now?

Ms.T: yeah. listen, beau

BoBoy: tell me

Ms.T: you'll be good while i'm gone, won't you?

BoBoy: be good?

Ms.T: yes, duh. while i'm gone? get it??

BoBoy: oh that! oh man. trust me, miz T,
i'm yrs alone

Ms.T: {{bo}} you i trust. girls, i don't trust for
a minute. you're such a big handsome unit

BoBoy: u crack me up, girl

Ms.T: but don't evade the question. you promise me

BoBoy: i promise promise promise

Ms.T: once is fine. i trust you, but... well, thanks

BoBoy: no problem, lady. and hey, u gonna call me
or anything?

Ms.T: <sigh> i'll try, but her grandmother has like no internet, and we'll be at the hospital a lot, where you can't use a cell phone. and i don't know when we'll be free, you know?

BoBoy: drag

Ms.T: hey

BoBoy: what?

Ms.T: you're not worried about ME, are you?

BoBoy: nah. yeah. a little

Ms.T: beau honey, i promise you there's nothing like that to worry about. i'm trusting you, and you gotta trust me back. you put your premonitions to rest

BoBoy: can do, ma'am. that's what i needed 2 hear

Ms.T: :) you are really the find of the century, darlin. come say goodbye tonight, but i gotta run pack now. xoxo

BoBoy: k, T. i'll think of u all the time. xoxou2

THE DAWG HOUSE

BoBoy: dude, u still there?

chessman: still here

BoBoy: guess what T just told me. she's going with bliss

chessman: really? why?

BoBoy: girl stuff. best friend stuff

chessman: got it

BoBoy: u ok, dude?

chessman: i guess

BoBoy: i know. i'm totally bummed. ur thinking about what johnson said, aren't u?

chessman: not really. well, yeah. pretty much totally

i mean, i trust bliss. but i know what guys are like around her. makes me feel... i dunno. helpless

BoBoy: hey, hang in there. tam will be with her

chessman: yeah

BoBoy: and hey, not many guys to see in the hospital

chessman: true. i just can't believe how long it's going to be

BoBoy: a long road to hoe, but at least we're in the same boat on this

a little help

 TXT to Johnson

June 02 02:30 pm

From: Gothling

IM me

 TXT to gothling

June 02 02:31 pm

From: Johnson

1 sec bz rt nw

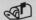 **TXT to Johnson**

June 02 02:32 pm

From: Gothling

tk yr tm...

GURLGANG ROOM

JUNE 02 02:33 PM

Ms.T has entered

Ms.T: hey kids. sorry i'm late

bliss4u: where were u?

Ms.T: so i had to laugh. i'm innocently stocking up at the video store, cuz i don't want to be out while we're "gone."

              i come out the aisle with an armload of dvds, and i nearly dump em all down mitch's back

gothling: **omg**

Ms.T: did a quick u-turn and ducked behind the dollar rentals. (how embarrassing)

bliss4u: what was he doing?

Ms.T: honey, he looked so bummed. he was flipping through the black-n-whites, just staring at the covers

bliss4u: that's my guy. he came over last nite 2 say goodbye, and i'm like, oh it's going 2 be so long, and he's all, i'm going 2 miss u so bad. it was sweet

Ms.T:	i know. beau was a little panicky. like hyperventilating
gothling:	**lol. he'll cope**
Ms.T:	be nice, annie. you didn't talk to these boys
gothling:	**i don't need their talk. i know their tiny black hearts. back shortly**
Ms.T:	so bliss, did your mom see him?
bliss4u:	she made me tell her the plan, or she wasn't going 2 disappear when he came by
Ms.T:	yeah, well. bound to happen
bliss4u:	mom was like why ARE u doing this 2 poor mitch? don't u think he has feelings? stuff like that. she totally likes mitch
Ms.T:	what did you say?
bliss4u:	i blamed annie, of course >:)
Ms.T:	lol
bliss4u:	no really, i said oh it's just a test bla bla bla. so finally she said whatever, but if i lose mitch, she will definitely kill me
Ms.T:	i know. i got the same thing
bliss4u:	really?
Ms.T:	mom just said "i won't lie for you." but my dad was totally pissed. "you're just playing him cause he's a white boy, aren't you?" no, daddy, no. "i thought i raised you better. yadda yadda." he thinks beau treats me really well.... which is true. <sigh>
bliss4u:	<sigh>

TXT to Johnson

June 02 02:36 pm
From: Gothling
still WAITING

📧 IM from Big.J

JUNE 02 02:37 PM

Big.J: yo annie, wattup?

gothling: johnson, how dare u keep a lady waiting?

Big.J: annie, ma petite, so sorry. but i have another <ahem> lady on my screen at present

gothling: why am I not surprised? which skank is it this time?

Big.J: um, well... in fact, it's brittney. i think u know her. heh heh?

gothling: eww. brittney now???

Big.J: u don't care 4 brittney?

gothling: johnson, what is yr problem? ur not really a moron, so is it like a hormone imbalance, or what?

Big.J: can i get back 2 u on that?

gothling: whatever

Big.J: thx

gothling: hey, johnson. i have something going here, and i thought you might kick in. a lil help, u might say

Big.J: why would i EVER want 2 help u? inquiring hormones want 2 know

gothling: because it's evil

Big.J: ah yessss... our 1 weakness. please 2 tell us more

gothling: mitch and beau are going 2 be very lonely very soon

Big.J: so i hear

gothling: tam and bliss think the boys will be good while they're away

Big.J: it's possible

gothling: depending on who they meet in the meantime

Big.J: of course. so?

gothling: well... i have a couple of prospects 4 them

Big.J: already? no way!

gothling: yes way. so i need u 2 play a little puppet master with me

Big.J: puppet master! u sweet talker. hmm... and i do owe them a small payback

gothling: good

Big.J: but wait. who are these so-called prospects?

gothling: bliss and tam

Big.J: ummm...

gothling: surely u knew the whole gone-2-grandma's bit was a fiction?

Big.J: be still my heart

gothling: u really didn't know?

Big.J: nobody here suspected nuffin! ur a genius, gurl

gothling: true, true. still, if u missed it, things worked better than even i had hoped

Big.J: a compliment??? oh, u really MUST want something

gothling: shut up, J

Big.J: so... then the next step would be 2 bring the "prospects" onstage?

gothling: right

Big.J: but they can't appear in person, obviously. so that means... ah, invent characters 4 them online, yes?

gothling: correct. we're settling on names and personalities now

Big.J: excellent. this is really inventive, annie dearest. so we just need 2 get them chatting 2 the lonely boys club

gothling: i knew u'd find this amusing

Big.J: amusing? gurl if this works, it will be historic. and u know i don't exaggerate

gothling: never in a zillion yrs

Big.J: i may have 2 write an epic 4 u when this is over

gothling: if it's like what u wrote tiffany, we can just let it go

Big.J: shh, i'm scheming.... it happens that i owe the school some tech work this summer. this could work... yes, i may be able 2 help u

gothling: awesome. oh, um, btw... did i mention that my gurls r switching?

Big.J: not sure i see.... they switch?

gothling: think, my man. tamra takes the chessman as her pawn, and little bliss shakes the tree called big beau

Big.J: they switch!... omg. it's shakespeare. it's mozart! i'm all in a dither.... just get a load of yr bad self

gothling: flatterer

Big.J: oh cruella de ville, marry me this instant, i beg u, and end my misery

gothling: we'll see, we'll see. today i'm busy

Big.J: oops. 1 sec. brittney on line 1 again. heh heh...

gothling: ok, but make it snappy this time, jasper. we got schemes 2 scheme

GURLGANG ROOM

Ms.T: i dunno, bliss, i may be feeling guilty... ish

bliss4u: about this whole thing? totally

Ms.T: but then, i dunno, it's also kinda fun

bliss4u: bliss and tamra's excellent adventure

Ms.T: it will be interesting for sure

bliss4u: well, it will be fun 2 prove annie wrong =)

Ms.T: sure. but i mean it's like a two-way mirror. i
             kinda want to see what beau will do when he
             thinks i'm not watching

bliss4u: oh he won't do anything

Ms.T: you're so sure?

bliss4u: i just know he won't. besides, eww

Ms.T: what?

bliss4u: T, ur my best-est friend. how am i going
             2 make a move on yr boyfriend?

Ms.T: true. the yuck factor

bliss4u: plus, we only win if he's a good boy, so
             why would i?

Ms.T: to find out

bliss4u: get real

Ms.T: well, i guess i'd like to know for sure

bliss4u: i won't do it, T

gothling: oh yes, u will

bliss4u: hi there, annie =)

**gothling: yes u will make a move on beau boy,
             and u know why?**

bliss4u: come on, annie. ur so serious all the time

**gothling: because tam is going 2 find mitch totally,
             totally, fascinating**

Ms.T: now THAT was cruel, miss annie

gothling: call me cruella, but prove me wrong

✉ IM from Big.J

Big.J: k. i'm back

gothling: finally

Big.J: man, brittney is a whiner. her mom this, her sister that. why don't i come over? why don't i take her 2 the mall?

gothling: johnson, ur wasting yrself with her. u know that, right?

Big.J: i know, i know. she's temporary

gothling: it's pathetic, dude

Big.J: oh look, there she goes again. whatever

gothling: whatever. k, listen up. here's the plan

Masks and Mask-osity

03 JUNE

The mask is *the face.*
—Susan Sontag, lame old philosophy quote

Peace and joy. Lately, some campers have written Your Uncle Jerry to ask about avatars. Avatars. Are they more than pictures? When should you change them? Do they cause a twitch or rash? May you have more than one? Should you talk with your parents about them? So many questions.

In Your Uncle Jerry's dictionary, young camper, "avatar" comes right after "mask," which comes right after "face." Now, a mask is something You put on, to put on a new You. But a mask is not JUST for Halloween. Think of how many masks you wear in RL. You have a mask for home, a mask for school, a face you wear to Grandma's house, a face for that party at your friend's house. Those are avatars of you, dontcha see. Different incarnations, different sides of you. And sometimes you make one up online so you can be someone totally new.

On social sites such as the wasteland known as MySpace, camper girls and boys should *never* show their home faces; they should *always* don a different mask. "Yes, my parents work at the embassy. I spend most of my time in Paris."

But then the question is, who am I when I wear a mask? Am I still myself, or am I a new identity? Is a mask dishonest? This brings us to ---->

Your Uncle Jerry's Rules of Mask-osity

Rule 1. Your face is a mask.

Rule 2. A mask is your face.

Rule 3. There is no rule 3.

Rule 4. There is no point in trying to figure this out.

Can you wrap your head around this, camper? If you ever allowed the Real You to appear, we both know how that would look: a huge blob in a diaper, flopped in front of the tube, pounding gummy bears and pizza with four hands. In short, you'd be your little brother. To cover their shame at creating such a monster, your parents make you adopt an avatar called Good Manners. Are good manners dishonest? Yes. But won't you be glad when your brother learns them?

Peace and joy.

CHAPTER 5

lonely hearts club

THE DAWG HOUSE

JUNE 04 06:55 PM

BoBoy has entered

BoBoy: dawg, u there?

chessman: yo

BoBoy: spirits up, my man?

chessman: sure. not a prob. you?

BoBoy: u bet. shootin hoops all afternoon

chessman: helps to stay busy

BoBoy: shootin hoops till my hands are raw

chessman: lol

BoBoy: i mean, it's still the first weekend, but i totally cannot let it rest chessman: yeah

BoBoy: i keep turning it over in my mind. maybe a week. maybe 2. maybe 6. maybe maybe maybe

chessman: yeah

BoBoy: how long's it been? like 3 days or something?

chessman: 46 hours

BoBoy: dude, i need a hobby

chessman: tomorrow coming soon. you got that thing set up?

BoBoy: with the lawn care guys. yep. how bout u?

chessman: starting wednesday

BoBoy: what was it again?

chessman: phone surveys

BoBoy: kewl. so u'll call at dinnertime and piss off my dad, right?

chessman: right

BoBoy: sweet. always a bright spot in the evening

Big.J has entered

Big.J: ding dong

chessman: johnson. word up

Big.J: word

BoBoy: dr. J! what brings u out of the contumelious dark this evening?

Big.J: listen, dudes and dudettes.
(what he say? never mind.)
a small proposition

chessman: contumelious?

BoBoy: my new word. i even looked it up

Big.J: i do hate 2 come 2 u in time
            of need. however...

chessman: kewl. what's it mean?

BoBoy: now THAT i don't know. i just know it's in the
            dictionary

Big.J: hellooooo? click-click-click.
            i called information, but i got
            the drug abuse hotline...

chessman: sorry dude. bo's wordsmithing tonight
            :-D

BoBoy: so, Big.J. u need something? like from us?
            hard 2 believe

Big.J: touching, isn't it? like best
            friends

BoBoy: exactly like that

Big.J: actually, no. i don't need
            anything like a favor. more like
            an exchange. both sides have
            something of value. a trade

chessman: i'll just go get my boots on

Big.J: u know what? is it better if i
            come back later? u girls seem 2
            be out of the mood right now

chessman: no, please. give us the pitch.
            this is great

Big.J: bubba?

BoBoy: present

Big.J: i was saying. ahem. we all have
            something of value. u have,
            well, a certain ability with
            the keyboard. plus u have
            evenings free

BoBoy: that's cold. evenings free. like we're not totally aware of that

chessman: true though...

Big.J: put it this way. the women r gone, the dawgs r restless, and u need something 2 keep u from prowling

chessman: fair enough. and you have?

Big.J: i have a small technology project related 2 my, um, "summer scholar" program

BoBoy: dude. u got summer school? i thought u were such a talent. poetry and all

Big.J: i am a fair student, but there was the small matter of afternoon absences during the month of may

chessman: oh yes: the Tiffany Era

Big.J: zackly

BoBoy: say no more

chessman: so this project is for a tech class?

Big.J: 4 the eminent dr. bartolo

BoBoy: the contumelious bartolo. why do they put the 90-yr-old dude in charge of tech?

chessman: everyone else has a life...

Big.J: he wants me 2 test a new program

BoBoy: hey, no fair. i wanna do that

Big.J: well, now's yr chance 2 do that. unfortunately, my project has 2 be school friendly and useful 2 other students

chessman: a website

Big.J: actually, a chat room

BoBoy: yeah. way easier

chessman: so, but useful to students? how lame
             is that?

Big.J: true. still, if it's gotta be lame,
             i wanna push it off a cliff

chessman: hyper-lame. nutrasweet

Big.J: u do catch on. i don't care what
             they say about u

BoBoy: what's our part of this?

Big.J: well, here's the thing. it will
             be a chat room 4 exchange students
             coming in the fall

chessman: exchange student, you mean. there's
             only one. but hey, you can't get
             lamer than a one-man chat room

Big.J: there are 2, actually. but dr.
             bartolo doesn't know that. i told
             him 4. he thinks i'm after like a
             citizenship award

BoBoy: are these dudes or chicks?

Big.J: why do u care? oic.

             no, they're 2 guys from albania or
             somewhere. don't worry about little
             bliss, little tamra. they will
             approve

chessman: so what's for us to do? as if i
             didn't know...

Big.J: oh hang on. here's brittney IM-ing
             me. tee hee. back soon

✉ IM from gothling

JUNE 04 07:17 PM

gothling: johnson

Big.J: yelloooow?

gothling: are u talking 2 them?

Big.J: trying 2, yes, and i need 2 get back. i told them u were brittney

gothling: wait. what are they saying? bliss and T are here

Big.J: they're nibbling

gothling: reel em in, dude

Big.J: listen, it's not that easy with guys

gothling: jeeze i hate a whiner

Big.J: i am not whining. i'm telling u that dudes are not as easy 2 persuade as chicks. u had the easy part. i'll get back 2 u in a minute. now let me do my work

gothling: oh, yeah, dudes r genius. they see right through things

Big.J: mitch actually is a smart 1. u can't rush him

gothling: he's a pansy. if u can't handle this job, i'll do it myself

Big.J: just u back off, girlfriend. we'll do this my way or i spill the beans—all of them

gothling: well, just DO it. they're only a couple of guys

Big.J: real men take finesse, darling…. as u would KNOW if u had ever DATED one!!

gothling: oh, johnson. ouch. i love it when ur rough. now will u GO??

Big.J: viper

gothling: toad

THE DAWG HOUSE

Big.J: k, i'm back. but u know what, nerd
            boy? forget it. if ur too busy
            these summer evenings, i'll get
            someone else

BoBoy: but 2 do what? just out of curiosity

chessman: to chat, i'm guessing. so johnson is
            free for brittney

Big.J: brittney does have needs

BoBoy: and yr other babes

Big.J: perhaps a summer love. who knows?
            a poet is much in request

chessman: have you started your poem for
            brittney?

Big.J: har har... k look. so there's this
            new thing on the school server.
            i'll do the setup and give u and
            the foreign dudes a sign-on. then
            we chat at set times every evening.
            u with me?

chessman: hypothetically, yes...

BoBoy: contumeliously

```
Big.J:      in the off times, u can also
            email inside the same program,
            or chat, whatever. got it?

chessman:   sure

BoBoy:      k

Big.J:      point is, it makes a transcript
            that i can dump 2 bartolo as my
            project. he doesn't care what's
            in it, as long as it looks like
            we're giving the exchange students
            a good impression of the school,
            the flag, and atlanta (pearl of
            the sovereign south)

            plus, i have 2 show him how 2
            run the software

BoBoy:      i still can't believe u have summer school

Big.J:      i'll ignore that

            anyway, i just thought that if i
            build the chat room, locate the
            players, and wake up bartolo once in
            a while, i would be doing my share

chessman:   and in return for being good buddies
            about this, we get what?

Big.J:      helloooo?? u fill yr lonely
            summer EVENINGS! u light up the
            dreary architecture of yr SOULS!
            u r 16 and WITHOUT WOMEN this
            summer, r u NOT??!!!

BoBoy:      but what's the catch?

Big.J:      u exhaust me

chessman:   well, in fairness, there's usually
            a catch with you, johnson

Big.J:      one sec. brittney again...
```

GURLGANG ROOM

Big.J has entered

gothling: **yo johnson.**
    still can't get them 2 take the bait, can u?

Big.J: almost there

Ms.T: well, i guess we win

bliss4u: great. that was quick

gothling: **lol. i have plenty of tricks left**

Big.J: ladies, PLEASE. a little faith

gothling: **did they go 4 it?**

Big.J: they will

gothling: **ok. i'll take over from here**

Big.J: WILL u chill out? they'll do it.
    trust me

Ms.T: yeah. no rush, annie. let him take his time

gothling: **what have u tried? threats? bribes?**

Big.J: i'm using reverse psychology.
    surely u've heard of finesse,
    darling

gothling: **only from u, johnson. and every time u write it,**
    my screen goes a sickly green...

Big.J: witch

gothling: **troll**

Big.J: ogress. medusa... harpy

THE DAWG HOUSE

Big.J: dudes, i can see this isn't going 2
           work. well, i tried

chessman: i'm pretty sure there's a catch, but
           i don't see it yet

Big.J: u make it so difficult. why? what
           have i done?

BoBoy: nah, we just shining u, dude

Big.J: there's no trust anymore. no trust
           and no respect

chessman: true true. but we might do it anyway

BoBoy: yeah, i think i'm in

chessman: any prepositions on this, beau?

BoBoy: no, it's good. i'm in

Big.J: no, no... please don't be
           impulsive. give it some thought

chessman: ok, johnson

Big.J: you're online 24/7, but this will
           mean opening 1 more window...

chessman: ok big J

Big.J: it will mean putting down yr book,
           typing a word or 2...

BoBoy: lol. u don't read, do u mitch?

chessman: only when i'm chatting johnson

BoBoy: rotfl

chessman: wouldn't want to waste my time
           completely

Big.J: that's fine. i'm used 2 disrespect
          from the nerd patrol. my poetry
          isn't up 2 his standards

BoBoy: so when will u set up the room, J?

Big.J: it's ready. i just have 2 email the
          exchange dudes

BoBoy: k, send us the sign-ons

Big.J: ur sure?

BoBoy: sure

chessman: yeah, why not?

BoBoy: just make this fun, k? i am feeling contumelious lately

Big.J: my man, u have no idea how much fun
          this will be

chessman: see, i hate it when he says stuff
          like that

Big.J: g2g dudes. ttfn

GURLGANG ROOM

bliss4u: i can't believe u have johnson in on this

gothling: why? johnson's our inside connection

bliss4u: because he's a sleazeball, maybe?

gothling: don't be such a prude

Ms.T: yeah, johnson's in. we need him

Big.J: yo check it out, annie dearest

gothling: johnson, did they bite?

Big.J: they are eager 2 meet with
             a pair of lovelies from a
             foreign land

bliss4u: no way

Big.J: we should have u ladies outta
             exile by wednesday

Ms.T: i can't believe it

gothling: told u...

Ms.T: told us what?

Big.J: that i could get them on board,
             i'm sure. <ahem ahem>

gothling: that men r all the same

Ms.T: agreeing to join a chat room isn't exactly
             messing around behind our backs

Big.J: all in good time, sugar

**gothling: whatever. we're set. good work, J.
             i knew u could do it**

Big.J: brrr. i get such shivers when
             u patronize

gothling: though it took u long enough

CHAPTER 6

foreign affairs

GURLGANG ROOM

JUNE 06 10:59 PM

Big.J has entered

Big.J: k, kids, ready 2 go?

gothling: just waiting 4 u, johnson. ur 14 mins late

Ms.T: where oh where could he have been?

Big.J: i have a life too, peanut

gothling: no time 4 brittney stories. let's go

Big.J: fine. the boyz r just signing
            on now. u go first tatiana, then
            bridget, then me

gothling: don't forget i'm here if u need me, kids. bliss?

bliss4u: present

gothling: i'm here if u need me

EXCHANGE STUDENT ROOM **UNION HIGH SCHOOL**

JUNE 06 11:00 PM

chessman has entered

BoBoy has entered

BoBoy: sup mitchie

chessman: just got here

BoBoy: albania, where's that?

chessman: by italy

BoBoy: u look it up?

chessman: nerd patrol

BoBoy: so these r italian dudes?

chessman: no. it's like halfway to greece. across the water. totally different but nearby

BoBoy: got it. like miami 2 cuba

chessman: sorta. whatever

Tatiana has entered

Tatiana: hallo?

BoBoy: union high chat room

Tatiana: excuse? me?

chessman: he said this is the union high school chat room. for exchange students

Tatiana: of atlanta, usa?

BoBoy: u got it

chessman: that's correct. this chat room is for exchange students at union high school

Tatiana: yes, that's who i am

BoBoy: **ur an exchange student?**

Tatiana: yes, for high school union. atlanta, usa

chessman: oic

Tatiana: sorry, what means "oic"?

BoBoy: **means he understands now**

chessman: it means "oh, i see." american slang

Tatiana: oic

BoBoy: **right**

Bridget has entered

Bridget: hello, good morning

BoBoy: **union high chat room**

chessman: this is a chat room for exchange students at union high school in atlanta

Bridget: brilliant... everything worked. hello, everyone. i'm bridget

BoBoy: **so, ur like an exchange student, too?**

Bridget: very much like 1

Big.J has entered

Big. J: yo, group, it's me. everyone here yet?

BoBoy: **sup J**

Tatiana: hallo, johnson

chessman: been looking for you...

Bridget:	hello, good morning
Big.J:	good good good. so everyone's already getting 2 know each other. have we done introductions?
chessman:	not as such. but i have a question for you
Big.J:	hold that thought, mitchie. let's do intros. i'll go first
	my name is johnson. i'm the 1 who brought u all together. i've set up the chat room, and i'll be logging the chat for my summer educational project.
	who's next?
Tatiana:	yes, i will be next. my name is tatiana del capo. i am living since many years in tirana, albania. it is beautiful mountainous country on adriatic coast
BoBoy:	adriatic? mitch said it was by italy
chessman:	the adriatic sea is between italy and albania
Tatiana:	ah, you know of my beautiful country?
chessman:	a little. i looked it up
	i'm mitch, by the way. mitchell saunders. i go to school at union high in atlanta, and i used to be a friend of johnson's
BoBoy:	beau tanner. i need to speak 2 johnson too
Bridget:	so. well. my turn, then. hello, good morning, i will be coming 2 atlanta as an exchange student from london. my name is bonnie grindstaff

BoBoy: bridget, u mean

Bridget: beg pardon?

≣⃗ IM from chessman

JUNE 06 11:06 PM

chessman: johnson, what gives?

Big.J: hello, good morning

chessman: these aren't guys, johnson. you said they'd be guys but they're chicks

Big.J: wait a minute. ur saying i knew? that i deliberately put u in a chat room with foreign women?

chessman: sure looks like it, J

Big.J: dude, chill. i just found out this morning when i emailed them

chessman: gimme a break

Big.J: go ask the office. the names they gave me were Bret and... something else. sounded like dudes 2 me. i only found out their real names an hour ago.

chessman: i don't think i can do this

Big.J: ur complaining?

chessman: i just wouldn't feel right. i promised bliss

Big.J: u promised her not to mess around. u didn't promise 2 sleep through the summer. besides, these chicks r overseas, dude. where's the danger?

chessman: we'll see...

BoBoy: u said bonnie just now, but yr name is really
            bridget, right?

Bridget: is it?

            i mean, did i? oic. yes i surely did. i'm such a dunce.
            my little nephew calls me aunt bonnie. just learning
            2 talk, u know

chessman: that's funny. i have a little
            niece who calls me uncle mick

Bridget: u do not

chessman: seriously. it happens with names.
            speaking of which, there was this
            thing about your name at union
            high school

Bridget: my name?

chessman: yes, funny thing. they have you
            with a boy's name on your record

GURLGANG ROOM

Big.J: bliss, quick, tell him u go by
            bret

bliss4u: what?

gothling: **what happened?**

Big.J: mitch is suspicious

gothling: bliss, no, just say the letters have been coming 2 u as Bret

Big.J: yes, better. and say "how dreary"

bliss4u: what r u guys talking about???

Big.J: quick!

EXCHANGE STUDENT ROOM **UNION HIGH SCHOOL**

Bridget: oh, that. how dreary. all the papers from atlanta have been addressed 2 bret grindstaff. like they lost 3 letters in my name

BoBoy: no way. bret? like bret the guy's name?

Bridget: i guess

Big.J: well, THAT certainly solves a mystery

BoBoy: i like that word. dreary. how dreary

Tatiana: i am feel very interested to be hearing this. since the first letter from atlanta, they are calling me as tim. does anyone know what means tim?

GURLGANG ROOM

Big.J: beautiful catch, tamra. very nice... love the accent, too

Ms.T: the accent sounds russian to me. gotta work on it

gothling: russian, albanian, transylvanian, it's all good

EXCHANGE STUDENT ROOM **UNION HIGH SCHOOL**

chessman: in english tim is a short name
for timothy. strange, though. it's
not even close to tatiana

Tatiana: oic. well, starts with T. includes I.
when does school office get everything
correct?

chessman: true...

Tatiana: you should see italian bureaucracy.
i am saying oic correctly, mitchell?

chessman: absolutely. and please call me
mitch

BoBoy: **but ur from albany, right? not italy**

Tatiana: albania. my mother, she is of italy.
so from a child i can speak the italian
and also the albanian

chessman: and the english

Tatiana: also the english. is true. but only those
three. i no have greek or serbian. not
a good language student, sorry

Big.J: this is fascinating, i must
say. so few americans know any
language besides english. heh heh.
and the english don't even think
we can speak that 1. right,
bridget?

Bridget: i have a question about names

Big.J: right, bridget??

GURLGANG ROOM

bliss4u: annie, i don't like this

gothling: **what??**

bliss4u: johnson is too bossy

Big.J: oh, puhleeeze.

Ms.T: come on, bliss! play along. you're doing great

Big.J: i'm only trying 2 get us off the
         name thing. ur gonna blow the
         whole game

EXCHANGE STUDENT ROOM **UNION HIGH SCHOOL**

Bridget: i was just sitting at my desk here in london, u know, and
           i wondered why they call u Johnson. don't u have a proper 1st
           name?

Big.J: oh dear. proper first name.
         so english. oh my

BoBoy: **lol. well, see, the thing with johnson is that his
           mother couldn't think of a name 4 him**

chessman: he was too ugly

BoBoy: **they didn't have a baby name that ugly**

Big.J: ignore them, ladies. american humor
         is so shallow

chessman: he was so ugly that when he was
           born...

BoBoy: **the doctor slapped his dad**

Bridget: rotfl. nice 1, beau

BoBoy: thank yew. thank yew very mush <hand to heart>

Tatiana: a good team, if i am understanding this joke

Big.J: ah, we're all so giddy tonight. what fun we're having in america

📧 IM from gothling

gothling: johnson, how goes it?

Big.J: i hate these people. hate em

gothling: r they teasin u, baby?

Big.J: morons! if they knew what i know...

gothling: let it go, wuss

Big.J: wuss?! now ur turning on me too?

gothling: u can take it, johnson. grow up

Big.J: arrrrgh... i hate it when ur right

gothling: get used 2 it

Big.J: if u weren't so evil, i'd hate u too

gothling: they'll get theirs

EXCHANGE STUDENT ROOM **UNION HIGH SCHOOL**

Bridget: slapped his dad. i just love american humour

chessman: seriously? i've always liked british

Tatiana: is very dry, the english humore

chessman: exactly. more satire, more absurd

Bridget: maybe. i like the 3 stooges, myself

BoBoy: **the stooges rule! and tom & jerry**

Tatiana: mitchell saunders, please to tell me
what your town atlanta is in august.
am i to wear the warm clothing?

Bridget: i love tom & jerry!

chessman: very hot in august. you do not
want warm clothing

BoBoy: **on guard, monsieur pussycat!**

Tatiana: so somethings cooler. understood

chessman: in fact, most of us go naked in
august

Bridget: u do not!

BoBoy: **lol. well, mitch does, but u wouldn't wanna see it ;-)**

Tatiana: who knows? perhaps i would join him. <a
joking>

Bridget: and what do u wear in the summer, beau?

BoBoy: **aw man. by august i'm in pads and practice jersey**

chessman: beau is a football player. this year
he may even make second string

Tatiana: i am sure he is very fine player

BoBoy: **mitchie's teasing me, but he's right. i'm not hard
core enuf 2 be any good**

Bridget: beau, sometime maybe u would explain the game
u americans call football. i get all muzzled

BoBoy: **muzzled?**

Bridget: puddled

chessman: lol

Tatiana: muddled, i am sure she means!

Bridget: right, sorry. it muddles me, rather. know what i mean,
                guv?

BoBoy: hey no prob. yeah, i can teach u that stuff easy

chessman: wait... "it muddles me, rather."
                i've read that somewhere

BoBoy: i mean, i can tell u the basics

chessman: are you sure you're from england?

Tatiana: mitchell, what in your spare time do
                you do on summer?

Bridget: of course i am. but me mum is irish a little. a wee bit
                of the irish there

Big.J: well, group. i said that this
                would be a short session since
                i know that tim and bret—i mean
                tatiana and bridget—have 2 be
                going. the day starts early on
                the other side of the ocean...

Tatiana: is very true. i have almost 7 of the
                clock now. in the morning

Bridget: o my yes. look at the time

BoBoy: well, hey. u'll check in again tonight, right?

chessman: tomorrow

BoBoy: doh. tomorrow morning

Bridget: oh, i was thinking the same thing. i'm such a ditz

BoBoy: a ditz? they say ditz in england? kewl

Tatiana: the american television is in everywhere, my friend

Big.J: listen, we'll meet at the same time every day. but u can chat each other lots in between. this server runs 24/7, and school wants us 2 be best friends by the end of summer. heh heh

chessman: see bro, there he goes again...

Big.J has left the room

BoBoy: **what?**

Bridget: well. good nite. or good morning...

Tatiana: ciao to everyones. very nice to have meeting you, mitchell

chessman: tell ya later

BoBoy: **prepositions?**

Bridget: cheers cheers

Bridget has left the room

BoBoy: **cheers, bridge**

Tatiana: goodbyes, mitchell?

chessman: right. cya later

Tatiana: cya?

chessman: sorry. see you later.

Tatiana: oic! goodbye for now

Tatiana has left the room

CHAPTER 7
facing the alter ego

GURLGANG ROOM
JUNE 06 11:55 PM

gothling: so, ladies?

bliss4u: brrrr...

Ms.T: mitch is onto us

gothling: **don't be paranoid. johnson sent me the transcript and u done gr8!**

bliss4u: i was so nervous!!

Ms.T: i think he knows something

gothling: **johnson will take care of it**

bliss4u: but i thought i made a pretty good english girl...

gothling: **u killed, girlfriend**

Ms.T: i about wet my pants when mitch said there's this thing about your name

gothling: who cares? it was johnson he didn't trust. u 2 were in the clear

bliss4u: i hate johnson

gothling: we need johnson

bliss4u: i don't like johnson telling me what 2 do

gothling: i'll talk 2 him

Ms.T: mitch knows he was lying

gothling: come on. u should be flattered

Ms.T: why flattered?

gothling: duh. johnson told them u were dudes because THEY didn't want to chat up foreign WOMEN

bliss4u: <sigh> true love

Ms.T: still, mitch is dangerous

gothling: get a grip, T. the point is, u guys did great

bliss4u: how dreary. beau thought that was cute. i have to remember that. i'll make a list

Ms.T: can johnson really handle mitch? can i even handle mitch?

gothling: it's fine. jeeze, u worry so much

bliss4u: cheers. i thought of that 1 myself. and spelling humor like humour

Ms.T: you did great bridget. i mean bliss

bliss4u: lol. u think so?

Ms.T: yes i do. just don't get too attached to my man ;-)

bliss4u:	beau? please, i'm just playing him...
gothling:	**break his heart, girl**
Ms.T:	hey!
bliss4u:	i'm a player =)
gothling:	**tam, u were awesome with yr tatiana accent**
Ms.T:	these accent? oh, is nothing
bliss4u:	u were like, i dunno, a different person totally
Ms.T:	i kinda FELT like a different person
bliss4u:	it's funny, isn't it? i did too
Ms.T:	like i didn't know those guys at all
bliss4u:	i could say stuff as bridget that i would never say in RL
Ms.T:	yeah, like you would never stare down johnson in real life
bliss4u:	don't u have a proper name? i don't know what made me say it
Ms.T:	except he's so crude with his name
gothling:	**u took a big risk doing that, bliss**
bliss4u:	i know i did
gothling:	**if u slipped and let on that u know johnson...**
bliss4u:	i dunno. if it had been me taking the risk, it would have blown up in my face. but it was like not me
Ms.T:	like bridget was doing it
bliss4u:	there was just this other voice in my head
Ms.T:	me too. i like opened a room somewhere, and there was tatiana talking away in a foreign accent

gothling:	\<snore>
Ms.T:	what?
gothling:	**u campers need 2 get a grip. haven't u done this before?**
bliss4u:	done what?
gothling:	**u know. worn a mask online. had a different e-dentity**
Ms.T:	have you?
gothling:	**all the time**
bliss4u:	oh right. like when?
gothling:	**like ur talking to uncle jerry clarkson of bloomington minnesota**
Ms.T:	you have a guy avatar? you made up a whole life for him and everything?
bliss4u:	why would u do that? ⊙www...
gothling:	**oh u have 2. especially on myspace if ur a female. so many losers hitting on u**
bliss4u:	i know. that's why i quit going
Ms.T:	so who's jerry clarkson?
gothling:	**u can call me Uncle Jerry—camp counselor, online preacher, amateur psychic, and broom-straw philosopher**
bliss4u:	how do u think this stuff up?
Ms.T:	psychic? cool
gothling:	**totally. he reads tarot cards**
Ms.T:	what?? you like tell people they'll inherit a fortune or meet a dark man with a family message?
bliss4u:	u really love 2 mess with heads, don't u?

gothling:	**no, it's kewl. jerry wouldn't hurt anybody**
Ms.T:	jerry wouldn't. annie would ;-)
gothling:	**heh heh heh**
bliss4u:	but really. tarot cards and boy scouts? that doesn't go
Ms.T:	so annie, read my cards, ok?
bliss4u:	eww. no!
gothling:	**u don't need it, girl. tatiana needs it. she's the 1 courting disaster**
Ms.T:	nah. she's only courting mitch
bliss4u:	if she catches him, it will be a disaster 4 u. i'm serious
Ms.T:	hey, you're after my beau boy. i gotta defend myself
bliss4u:	i am not after beau
gothling:	**no, dear, but bridget is...**
bliss4u:	get real
gothling:	**"there was this other voice in my head"**
bliss4u:	that doesn't mean...
gothling:	**"it wasn't me taking the risk... it was bridget"**
bliss4u:	that doesn't mean i would do anything
Ms.T:	play nice, annie
gothling:	**i'm just saying u never know what yr alter ego will do**
Ms.T:	ok, we get it
bliss4u:	do u think that's so true?
gothling:	**totally. u never know. just like 2nite**

bliss4u: i think we were still in control

Ms.T: well, but we were improvising like mad

bliss4u: i just know i didn't say anything i'd regret
                later

gothling: **not yet, but u will**

Ms.T: don't listen, bliss. annie's in a dark phase
                this year

bliss4u: she totally is

gothling: **i just want our bliss 2 be clear on what
                she's doing and what could happen**

bliss4u: like what?? i can bail anytime if i don't
                like how things r going. u can play yr little
                game all by yrself

gothling: **don't u believe it. ur in this 2 deep 2 bail
                on me**

bliss4u: i'll bail if i want 2. i swear i will

Ms.T: kids, kids. let's not argue

gothling: **really, bliss? did yr grandma get well all
                of a sudden?**

bliss4u: maybe

gothling: **because that's going 2 look fishy 2 mitch**

bliss4u: so?

gothling: **so he'll want a real explanation, and i happen
                to have 1**

bliss4u: u wouldn't

gothling: **yes, sweetie, i would. and johnson would
                back me up**

bliss4u: mitch wouldn't believe johnson

gothling: **the question is, can mitch believe u after this?**

Ms.T:	come on ladies...
gothling:	**i don't even have 2 make up a story. u lied about yr grandma. u cried false goodbye tears. and u came back as bridget 2 hit on his best friend. how can he trust u now?**
Ms.T:	ok annie, you've made your point
bliss4u:	ur truly an awful person, annie
gothling:	**ur too, but i still luv u...**
	so here's the thing: nobody bails until we see who wins the bet
Ms.T:	come on. bliss won't bail. she was just talking. it's late and we're tired
bliss4u:	rude, hateful, and mean-spirited

bliss4u is off-line

gothling:	**oh, fine. <sigh> she has no staying power in a fight**
Ms.T:	you cannot be rough with her, annie
gothling:	**she's a wuss**
Ms.T:	you play it too dark
gothling:	**she'll be fine**
Ms.T:	listen, if you break with bliss, then everything comes apart
gothling:	**whatever. it's her own throat she's cutting**
Ms.T:	you think she's weak, but she'll surprise you. and—just so you know—i won't take your side
gothling:	**okokok, i'll fix it tomorrow. jeeze**
Ms.T:	just remember you like this game more than anyone else does

like a rock

THE DAWG HOUSE
JUNE 07 05:30 PM

BoBoy has entered

BoBoy: so dude. chat room 2nite?

chessman: i guess

BoBoy: u not sure?

chessman: no, it's cool

BoBoy: kewl

chessman: yeah. hey, you like them?

BoBoy: bridget and...

chessman: tatiana

BoBoy: right. she's harder 2 understand.

chessman: well, non-english

BoBoy: yeah. albany

chessman: albania

BoBoy: really? oh, right

chessman: bridget was a little... i dunno

BoBoy: what?

chessman: i dunno. kind of not so bright,
           i guess

BoBoy: she was nice tho

chessman: definitely. i'm just saying

BoBoy: yeah

chessman: yeah

BoBoy: u like tatiana better?

chessman: a little. why?

BoBoy: no reason... but, well, would u like take her
           out or anything?

chessman: get real. we just IM'd a little.
           besides -> bliss

BoBoy: i know. i'm just sayin

chessman: sure

BoBoy: yeah

Big.J has entered

Big.J: dawgs and dawgies!

BoBoy: wazzup, J?

chessman: zup

Big.J: just passing on a message.

           i saw annie at the mall, and
           she talked 2 bliss last nite

chessman: cool

Big.J: yes. btw... something about phones.

chessman: um... mine is temporarily out of service

BoBoy: dude. u run up the phone bill again?

chessman: bliss likes to text. what can i say?

Big.J: whatever. bliss doesn't have her
           phone. she called from granny's
           landline

BoBoy: no way

Big.J: that's what annie sez

chessman: what about Ms. T?

Big.J: same same

BoBoy: left her phone? oh like i believe that

chessman: hmm

Big.J: well, that's the story... anywho,
           a message: more bad news 4 youse

chessman: what's that?

Big.J: another 2 weeks in tallyhussy

BoBoy: another... man, i need a hobby

chessman: okay. tell her i'll write. oh wait.
           i don't have the address. i'll call
           from somewhere. does annie have the
           phone number?

Big.J: never fear. i'll give annie a
           message of love and mournfulness.
           ur pining. ur wasting away. i'll
           take care of it

chessman: gosh, johnson, what a pal

BoBoy: lol

Big.J: on the upside, the chat room
            is doing very well

BoBoy: it's flowering

Big.J: u know, mitch, between us, i don't
            get half of what our bro says

chessman: it's flourishing

BoBoy: see? no worries. mitch can translate

Big.J: so i was saying. chat room again
            2nite, dudes?

BoBoy: we're there

Big.J: what do u think of the
            euro-hotties, eh?

chessman: what do you mean?

Big.J: nice ladies?

BoBoy: yeah, nice

chessman: whatever

Big.J: u should really lighten up,
            mitch boy

chessman: how is brittney, johnson? started
            your farewell poem yet?

Big.J: brittney is... well, 2 be honest,
            brittney is needier than i expected

chessman: ahhh

BoBoy: Big.J, say it ain't so

Big.J: alas and alack, tis true,
            i greatly fear

BoBoy: alack?? what's that mean?

chessman: same as alas. our Big.J is a
            literate man

BoBoy: well, i knew that

Big.J: gentlemen, u flatter me

BoBoy: i mean, goes 2 the opera and everything
                     <smirk>

chessman: and look at his poetry...

Big.J: okok, ahem, i was saying

chessman: and all that summer school

Big.J: the search 4 knowledge, my brother,
                     does not end with the school year.
                     nay, the quest goes on unto the
                     edge of doom, or at least till
                     june 19

BoBoy: lol. dawg, i can't keep up

chessman: so J. any news on the summer love
                     front?

Big.J: 4 lil ol me? perhaps...

BoBoy: perhaps. see, mitch, u gotta love a dude who
                     can say perhaps

chessman: perhaps one of the euro-girls?

Big.J: dude, no. those women r spoken 4

chessman: how do you know?

Big.J: ur kidding, right? right?

BoBoy: mitch, what's he talking about?

Big.J: get out. u didn't feel it?
                     don't tell me u didn't feel it.

chessman: what i felt was you trying to
                     pull something

Big.J: me? dude, ur totally up in
                     the night

chessman: i don't think so. i've got this
            preposition

Big.J: ?? now it's mitch with the word
            disease. i'm worried

BoBoy: he means permutation. no, wait...

Big.J: seriously, dawgs. u need 2
            cut loose. u've been away from
            yr women too long

BoBoy: dude, that's the truth

chessman: another 2 weeks now

Big.J: well, i don't know everything,
            but i can tell u what works 4 me

BoBoy: what's that, J?

Big.J: love the 1 ur with

chessman: predictable, really

Big.J: hey those foreign ladies r coming
            in the fall, and all u need 2 do is
            cultivate them a little now

BoBoy: cultivated. now there's a word

chessman: like opera, like farming

Big.J: don't start on opera

BoBoy: lol

Big.J: serious, they'd be soooo grateful 2
            have a friend they can trust
            in a strange land

chessman: johnson, you don't seem to get this:
            i am not available

BoBoy: me neither. i'm a rock 4 ms.T

Big.J: gimme a break. ur dying here

BoBoy: **mitch is a rock 2**

Big.J: yes, ur both COME SCOGLIO

BoBoy: **we're what?**

Big.J: co-may sco-lio, dude. like a rock.
              ur straight outta "cosi fan tutte"

BoBoy: **kewl**

chessman: what's your stake in this, johnson?

Big.J: <sigh> dude, it's nothing 2 me.
              have it yr way

BoBoy: **or wait. mitch is a rock—i'm a brick**

Big.J: i'm just saying u 2 r wrapped
              a little tight these days

chessman: ok. and i'm just saying bliss and
           i have an understanding

Big.J: no, that's cool. so she understands
              u and u understand her

chessman: something like that

BoBoy: **it's a cultivated understanding**

Big.J: why is there always 30 seconds of
              silence after he writes anything?

chessman: lol

BoBoy: **what i say?**

chessman: i'm still working that out, bro.
           but i think it was profound

Big.J: here's a thought. suppose u heard
              something that made u doubt yr
              faraway ladies?

BoBoy: **u got something on bliss and tamra, dude?**

chessman: no, he doesn't have anything

Big.J: just suppose i did

chessman: whatever

BoBoy: doesn't matter. i wouldn't listen

chessman: ok, so, hypothetically. what kind
            of thing would it be?

Big.J: what would make u doubt her?

BoBoy: like the worst that could happen?

chessman: seems obvious what that would be

Big.J: going out with another dude,
            right?

BoBoy: i'm gonna lateral this 1 2 mitch

chessman: going out with Big.J

BoBoy: rotfl <high 5s all around>

Big.J: well. i can c u boys r hard core

BoBoy: i'm a rock. what can i say?

Big.J: i'll just tell tatiana and bridget
            2 forget it

chessman: forget what?

Big.J: forget any ideas they might have
            had about cultivating dudes in
            atlanta. unless... well, sure. i
            can always dig up some other guys

BoBoy: get real

chessman: johnson, don't try and play us, ok?

**BoBoy: besides, those women have their own dudes back
            in albany. euro-dudes**

Big.J: sure they do

chessman: albania

Big.J: but look. they're going 2 be
            away from home, in a strange
            country. the euro-dudes will be far
            far away 4 a long long time

chessman: what's your point?

Big.J: they're in the same place u r
            right now. the point is simple
            friendship. online companionship.
            perhaps a trifle more

BoBoy: perhaps a summer online love

Big.J: perhaps. and seriously, why not?

chessman: don't even, beau. T would cut
            you into dog meat

Big.J: perhaps she would

BoBoy: no, she would definitely

Big.J: perhaps it would be worth it

peach

Tatiana has entered

Tatiana: hallo mitchell? no one else is here?

chessman: hi, tatiana. just me, so far

Tatiana: mitchell, is good to see you

chessman: lol

Tatiana: i mean read you. well, what does one
            say for this in english?

chessman: no, it's cool. just funny, because
            no one can actually see online

Tatiana: yes, i understand. however, i would like
            to see you :)

chessman: um. yeah. hey, you know that joke about the dog?

Tatiana: a joke?

chessman: yes. 2 dogs at the keyboard. one says to the other: on the internet, nobody knows you're a dog

Tatiana: lol. is very true joke!

chessman: yeah, i like it

Tatiana: you have a good humore sense, i think

chessman: thanks

Tatiana: but excuse. how do i know you are who you say? lol?

chessman: nice one. how do i know your name is tatiana?

Tatiana: yes! ha, because i might be a dog!

chessman: :-) no, i don't think you could be a dog

Tatiana: well, you must to wait and see when i come to atlanta usa, no?

chessman: um, well, in albania, what would you say for "good to see you" online?

Tatiana: ah, in albania, one doesn't have the internet so much

chessman: oh right. not a wealthy country, i hear

Tatiana: is true. i am being very lucky because of this exchange with the america school

chessman: well...

Tatiana: mitchell, you have read something of
              my country, yes?

chessman: sure. i mean, well, just a little.
              i looked you up online

Tatiana: you are very sweet to do this

chessman: not really

Tatiana: sweet is correct, is it no?

chessman: um, yes, that would be correct. nice
              is another way to say it

Tatiana: no i am think sweet is what i mean

chessman: ok...

Tatiana: you make me feel important to read of my
              country, mitchell. usa is such important
              nation. for you to look up me online is great
              compliment

chessman: well i'm sure albania is important
              in many ways

Tatiana: we have very rich history but also much
              sorrow. a crossroads of empires. is correct,
              crossroads? where roads do cross?

chessman: yes correct. what are the people
              like in albania?

Tatiana: ah, we are a passionate people. passion
              is in the water, i think. lol

chessman: i see

Tatiana: especially the women are so very full
              of passion. the men are brilliant and
              handsome but they go to other country
              for working

chessman: i read about that

Tatiana: about our passionate women, lol?

chessman: um, about the men looking for work in western europe

Tatiana: you are also brilliant and handsome, mitchell, i think?

chessman: lol. actually beau is the brilliant and handsome one

Tatiana: except he cannot remember the name of my country. albany, he calls it

chessman: well, that's a point. but i remind him

Tatiana: thank you, my friend. a very sweet thing for to do

chessman: nah

Tatiana: you remember albania because you think of me, yes?

chessman: well, not really

Tatiana: you not think of me??

chessman: no. i mean yes. of course i think of you. but...

Tatiana: there. i knew it. i have instincts of this thinking

chessman: what do you mean?

Tatiana: instincts? is not correct?

chessman: i'm not sure. like a preposition? i mean premonition? like a dream? an intuition?

Tatiana: an intuition, let me say. i will tell it you like this.

late in the night, i am look to the stars
over my beautiful sad country of albania,
and i am thinking yes, somewhere,
somewhere in atlanta usa is brilliant
and handsome young man who is think
of me this very minute

chessman: that's... um, well, that's very
             nice of you to tell me

Tatiana: a sweet man on whom these same stars
             will shine tonight

chessman: um...

Tatiana: and this man is you, i am so sure

chessman: you are?

Tatiana: in my heart, i know this

chessman: you do?

Tatiana: an intuition. so for you to say of course
             you think of me—oh, mitchell, i have
             not the words in english to say it, how
             beautiful this to me is

chessman: well... um

Tatiana: this is fine for me to tell you?

chessman: i think so. but...

Tatiana: not too much of the passion?

chessman: um, tatiana, i should explain
             something

Tatiana: of course. please to explain me. i listen
             to all that you say with my open heart

Bridget has entered

Bridget: hello, good morning

Tatiana: bridget! hallo my english friend

Big.J has entered

Big.J: johnson's here, ladies and germs.
             what up what up?

Tatiana: johnson, you are the late one, i think. 15
             minute

Bridget: hello, mr. johnson

Big.J: is it that late already?

chessman: johnson, listen. beau's here in a
             minute, and i really gotta bounce

Tatiana: you really bounce?

Bridget: lol. i think he means he needs 2 leave early

chessman: um, right. sorry. leave early.
             gotta go

Big.J: whoa whoa, hold on there, young
             feller

Tatiana: wait mitchell. you were to explain
             me something, i did think?

Big.J: yes, leave us not in contumelious
             haste

Bridget: contumelious?

BoBoy has entered

BoBoy: word up, dawgs, sorry i'm late

chessman: dude. there you are. hey, sorry gotta
             go

BoBoy: i beg yr stuff?

Big.J: mitchie's trying 2 bail on us

chessman: yeah, remember? i have that thing

Tatiana: a thing?

BoBoy: what thing, dude?

chessman: see you later all

Tatiana: but i thought you were to explain

chessman has left the room

Tatiana: ah, there he goes

BoBoy: weird. he doesn't have a thing. it's the middle
            of the nite

Big.J: he's escaping. what did u say
            2 him Tatiana?

Bridget: oh, that IS 2 bad. how very tiresome.

Big.J: what was he going 2 explain?

Tatiana: he didn't say

BoBoy: how dreary

Tatiana: he only say he must explain to me something,
            and i say i am listening
            to hear what it is

Bridget: really? i didn't catch any of that

Tatiana: it was only before you entered the
            chatting room

Bridget: oic

Tatiana: i will have to, um, ask it out of him in another
            day

Big.J: zackly. slap him around 18r.
            there's plenty of time

Tatiana: slap him? that would be difficult

Big.J: a figure of speech

Tatiana: how strange a thing of you to say

BoBoy: lol. mitch might just like a little spanking now and then

Bridget: beg pardon? whatever do u mean?

Big.J: well, a man does like a woman 2
show some fire

Bridget: really

Tatiana: in my country, i was telling mitchell,
women are full of the passion. is unusual for
america?

Bridget: yes, is it unusual?

Big.J: um no, not unusual. not at all

Bridget: 4 example, i'm sure mitch has a very passionate girlfriend

Tatiana: he has girlfriend? he say nothing of her
to me

Big.J: u'd have 2 ask him how passionate
she is. let's just say that some
american women r a little reserved

Bridget: is that a fact?

BoBoy: not my girl, dude

Tatiana: no? your girl is passionate one?

Big.J: tamra's a fine person. very fine

BoBoy: passion like a racehorse. like a steamroller

Tatiana: excuse? your girl is a horse? and she
rollers over you?

Big.J: dude, <cough cough> if she heard u
say that, she'd dope-slap u into
next week

Tatiana: she slaps, too? you don't say

Big.J: no no no. just kidding around.
         ms. T is a peach of a girl

BoBoy: lol. she's a peach all right. yum

Tatiana: i am so confused. she is this horse first,
         then a road equipment, now a food. if you
         not like this girl, why you would keep her?

Bridget: tatiana, did mitch say his girl isn't passionate?

Tatiana: no no, my friend, he said nothing of
         complaint about his girl to me. unlike
         Mr. BoBoy here

Bridget: u must know her, beau?

BoBoy: bliss is a peach too

Tatiana: a peach

BoBoy: mitchie don't complain, i guarantee

Big.J: yes, a real peach, that girl.
         what a sweetie

Tatiana: sorry, sorry. excuse me very much.
         but peach is fruit, correct?

Bridget: yes, that's right

Tatiana: so. the girl is something to chew up?
         and then—how do you say?—to spit
         away the center

Big.J: oh please. it's just a figure
         of speech

BoBoy: yeah

Tatiana: meaning?

Big.J: ok. meaning, um, creative,
         generous, kind, yet... full
         of character

Tatiana: hmm

BoBoy: **and delicious ;-)**

Tatiana: excuse me?

Big.J: he means delicious to the spirit!
to the heart

BoBoy: **what?**

Tatiana: is how you see a woman this way, beau?
a fruit to be sliced and swallowed and spit
away? how extraordinary

Big.J: really, tatiana. it's not
offensive. it's a southern
thing. hard 2 explain

BoBoy: **yeah, southern**

Big.J: yeah

Tatiana: and other times a horse beast for racing and
breeding, and other times a truck machine
for flattening the road?

BoBoy: **u make it almost like degratory**

Tatiana: ah. now you begin to see.

Big.J: please please, tatiana, all this
about peach? peachy? peach-i-tude?

Tatiana: i cannot say it's something i would like to be
called

BoBoy: **dude, my grandmother says it all the time, and
she doesn't have a degratory bone in her body**

Big.J: not a bone

BoBoy: **yeah**

Tatiana: hmm, and sometimes to you i am even dude,
which is, i think, a casual BOY acquaintance?

Big.J: bro, u just painted us into a corner

BoBoy: **what i say? what i say?**

Tatiana: excuse me so much, but, talking of
            grandmothers, mine is on the next room calling
            to me. i must say goodbye for today

Tatiana has left the room

Bridget: oh, she's gone away mad. how dreadful

Big.J: that was weird

BoBoy: **we ticked her off, didn't we?**

Bridget: u think????

BoBoy: **now i feel bad**

Big.J: aw man. she can't really be
            offended by "peach" can she?
            how lame is that?

Bridget: i thought u liked yr women passionate

Big.J: i like em reasonable too. jeeze

Bridget: she's lame because u offended her?

Big.J: no, because she's a femi-nazi

BoBoy: **it didn't offend u, did it?**

Bridget: maybe i'm not passionate enuf

BoBoy: **i can't believe that**

Bridget: she's smarter than me. that counts

Big.J: whatever. uh, listen, bro. britt
            just popped up. can u hold down
            the fort 4 a while?

Bridget: another passionate woman, mr. johnson?

BoBoy: **lol. u just got dissed in england, J**

Big.J has left the room

Bridget: can i just say yr friend johnson is a difficult person
            2 like?

BoBoy: **really?**

Bridget: really

BoBoy: **aw, he's all right. a little sketchy, but he's cool.
            that's what mitch says**

Bridget: i get this feeling when i talk 2 him

BoBoy: **what feeling?**

Bridget: like my teeth r grinding and something is twisting in
            my stomach

BoBoy: **hey that's serious**

Bridget: i know i shouldn't feel that way

BoBoy: **no, that's ok. johnson can be hard 2 take**

Bridget: like he's not lying, but he twists words. like a politician

BoBoy: **he's a poet**

Bridget: whatever

BoBoy: **hey no problem. how u feel is how u feel**

Bridget: i don't know...

BoBoy: **u won't offend me, that's 4 sure**

Bridget: well, i'm glad of that

BoBoy: **totally**

Bridget: thanks

BoBoy: **take some deep breaths now. that always
            helps me**

Bridget: helps u? u get this way sometimes too?

BoBoy:	sure. well, i mean, usually i'm a tank, a rock. but sometimes...
Bridget:	sometimes u get steamrolled?
BoBoy:	i shouldn't have said that, huh?
Bridget:	no it's ok. she'll get over it
BoBoy:	it's just, well, it seems like my girl is way ahead of me half the time
Bridget:	yeah
BoBoy:	like, i dunno. well, i'm not what u'd totally call smart and handsome
Bridget:	oh please. i happen 2 know u r
BoBoy:	dude! don't make fun of me
Bridget:	i'm not
BoBoy:	here i am getting all girly...
Bridget:	i'm not!
BoBoy:	whatever
Bridget:	no i mean it, k? i just know ur plenty smart and really handsome
BoBoy:	lol
Bridget:	seriously. i can tell these things
BoBoy:	well anyway...
Bridget:	yeah?
BoBoy:	i just mean... k, i'm not complaining about ms. T, but sometimes i just feel like she's too smart 4 me
Bridget:	i know. i totally feel that way
BoBoy:	she really is—and gorgeous too. and, well i get these feelings like... i dunno. like she might find someone else

Bridget: absolutely. me too

BoBoy: **but really i'm like in awe of her**

Bridget: right. i have the same fear about my... chap

BoBoy: **seriously?**

Bridget: sure. he's totally beyond me sometimes, and i just get desperate when i think someone else might snatch him away. u know

BoBoy: **yes, i do know**

Bridget: so what do i do?

BoBoy: **no worries. there's nothing 2 do. just keep being yrself**

Bridget: that's it?

BoBoy: **sure! keep growing, keep loving him. he's with u 4 a reason**

Bridget: i guess

BoBoy: **i learned that from my man mitch**

Bridget: mitch said that?

BoBoy: **when i worry about T, he says, dude, she chose u, and she wouldn't hook up with a bonehead**

Bridget: that's a nice thing 2 say

BoBoy: **yeah**

Bridget: u really like this girl, don't u?

BoBoy: **she's a real... oh, oops, i'm not going 2 say that again**

Bridget: lol

BoBoy: **ha**

Bridget: ur a funny guy. i never knew that... about americans, i mean

BoBoy: **oh sure. keep em laughing, that's what i always say**

Bridget: it's so easy 2 talk 2 u

BoBoy: **well...**

Bridget: how i feel is... what did u say?

BoBoy: **it's how u feel. can't blame yrself 4 that**

Bridget: ur nice. ur a nice boy, beau... beau boy.

BoBoy: **:)**

Bridget: well...

BoBoy: **what u thinkin?**

Bridget: dunno... i shouldn't say

BoBoy: **come on. i won't tell**

Bridget: it's just... listen, um...

BoBoy: **i'm listenin**

Bridget: ok, what if i felt... oh i don't know

BoBoy: **what?**

Bridget: oh, i'm too comfortable with u. it's like i could
             tell u anything. anything at all

BoBoy: **u CAN tell me anything, bridget. of course
             u can**

Bridget: i really shouldn't

BoBoy: **no, what? seriously**

Bridget: well, like what if i felt something 4 u?

BoBoy: **wow. really?**

Bridget: i mean, nothing that would get u in trouble. but...

BoBoy: **but what?**

Bridget: well. put it this way. if a certain american chap was
             ever free to look around...

BoBoy: yes?

Bridget: then he wouldn't have 2 look far

BoBoy: sweet. just over in england?

Bridget: maybe england's not that far :) but seriously, is that ok?

BoBoy: bridge, honey, that is just the nicest thing 2 say

Bridget: so ur ok with it?

BoBoy: well, it's like u say, IF a person was available

Bridget: yeah

BoBoy: which i'm not, technically

Bridget: technically?

BoBoy: well, T is gone all summer it looks like

Bridget: oic

BoBoy: but can i tell u something?

Bridget: what?

BoBoy: if i really was a single dude, i'd be looking at england in a heartbeat

Bridget: awww, u know what, beau boy?

BoBoy: what?

Bridget: ur a peach

CHAPTER 10
grounded

THE DAWG HOUSE
JUNE 08 07:30 PM

Big.J has entered

BoBoy: j-man, sup?

Big.J: mitch boy, u bailed on me.
            that ain't right

chessman: i had to. sorry

Big.J: HAD 2? what's HAD 2?

chessman: it is what it is. get over it

Big.J: dude, i gotta tell u this is
            totally TOTALLY against the code

chessman: what? there's no code

BoBoy: yeah, mitch. the code of the south

Big.J: never give up. never surrender

chessman: get outta town

Big.J: may the farce be with u

chessman: i didn't give up. i made a decision

Big.J: decision 2 give up, u mean

BoBoy: so, mitch. ur out?

chessman: looks like it, bro

BoBoy: dude, i thought u were the stable 1

chessman: yeah, well

Big.J: u can't bail, mitch

chessman: watch me

BoBoy: but why? what happened?

Big.J: we had a deal

BoBoy: no really, what happened? i show up, and ur
            gone right now

chessman: i don't know. i was just getting
            a feeling

Big.J: wait a minute...

BoBoy: u got the BRAINS, dude. I'M sposed to get the
            feelings. this isn't fair

Big.J: wait a minute. he and tatiana
            were there b4 us

BoBoy: as in alone?

Big.J: what i'm sayin

chessman: not my idea

Big.J: bro, she hit on u, didn't she?

BoBoy: tanny from alBANNy? hit on ol mitch?

Big.J: that's what i'm thinkin

chessman: albania

BoBoy: u dawg u!

chessman: hey, i did nothing!

BoBoy: u stinkin dawg. way 2 go!

Big.J: that's it, isn't it, mitchie?

chessman: maybe

BoBoy: what a hound

Big.J: k listen, dude, that's no reason
2 bail

BoBoy: what did she say?

chessman: she was just, i dunno. she said
some stuff

Big.J: gimme a break

BoBoy: like what? what did she say, bro?

chessman: nah, man, i'm not going there

Big.J: whatta wuss

BoBoy: come on, mitch boy, u gotta give us something

Big.J: seriously, how bad could it be?

chessman: i'm honestly not sure. but bad
enough

Big.J: but i mean she's in freakin italy
or somewhere

chessman: ALBANIA. would someone tell me why
it's SO hard to remember ALBANIA?

BoBoy: ...oh he likes her

Big.J: oh man

BoBoy: **k, now u really gotta tell us what she said**

chessman: talk to the hand

Big.J: no, that's cool, bro. we can
            fill in this part ourselves

BoBoy: **yeah, we know what she said. let's see... johnson?**

Big.J: no, i got it. she talked about...
            oh, dude. passion, right?

chessman: maybe

Big.J: k, stop me if u've heard this 1.
            ahem: ALBANIAN women r passionate.
            they're VERY passionate. they
            basically have passion in the water

BoBoy: **nice**

Big.J: and she's in fact been having
            some thoughts lately about mitchell
            back in (how does she say it?) back
            in atlanta usa

BoBoy: **no way. is he right, bro?**

chessman: he isn't wrong

BoBoy: **oh u dawg**

Big.J: first she gets misty <sigh>,
            then she comes on like a little
            strong 4 u. she says, hmm,
            something about... stars

chessman: bite me

BoBoy: **amazing, J. how do u do it? <fist bump>**

Big.J: it's the poetry. nothing 2 it

BoBoy: **mitch boy, did u even tell her about bliss??**

chessman: i tried... honest i did

BoBoy: **dude, ur toast**

chessman: she wouldn't listen

Big.J: course not. she's a poet. no...
no, that girl is poetry itself

chessman: it was like holding off a team
of girl cousins

BoBoy: **lol**

chessman: i'm like, dude, i need to tell
you something, but she's all
mitchell, mitchell you're so sweet
to think of me. you DO think of me,
don't you mitchell?

BoBoy: **oh man**

chessman: and i go, um, i wasn't really
thinking of you that way, ok? and
she's like what?? you never think
of me?? i break-a you fingers. and
i go, no no, i DO think of you,
just not like THAT, only she doesn't
hear the "not like that" part

BoBoy: **oh man**

chessman: then she's all, oh mitchell, i
knew it, and then, THEN, she
goes totally over the top. oh at
night I am look at the stars over
my beautiful passionate freakin
homeland, and I am think of you
thinking of me thinking of you, and
i pray for the stars to be shining
on you in usa... and i'm like, oh
please, this canNOT be happening

BoBoy: **oh man oh man oh man**

Big.J: did i nail it, bo boy?

BoBoy: u da man, J

Big.J: oh, wait, so that was what
she meant about he was going
2 explain something

chessman: i guess. did she say that?

BoBoy: oh yeah. she kept on that 4 a while

Big.J: until bubba pissed her off

BoBoy: hey

chessman: you did? what did you say?

BoBoy: not me! it was johnson

Big.J: u wish, dude. i wasn't the 1
objectifying all the women in
the room

chessman: aw man

BoBoy: objectionizing? i don't know nuffin bout this,
mitch, i swear

chessman: come on, what happened?

Big.J: funny how i remember it so
differently...

BoBoy: mitch, she's wild. u know what i'm talkin about.
when she gets her teeth into u, she's totally a steam—

oops

Big.J: a steamroller. see, mitch?

chessman: man, you can't say stuff like that

Big.J: zackly. a steamroller with
teeth? mixed metaphors r totally
out of line

chessman: no dude, you can't call a woman
things that are... well, THINGS

Big.J: oh that. right

BoBoy: i know i know i know. i know NOW. tatiana
            totally went cold on us

chessman: man

Big.J: she had the nerve 2 cross-examine
            me. ME of all people

chessman: about what?

Big.J: totally uncalled 4

BoBoy: left the room in a snit

chessman: about what?

BoBoy: just don't call her a peach, that's all i can say

chessman: well, duh

BoBoy: come on. my granny says that all the time.
            now he was a nice man—a real peach. do u
            hear dudes complaining? i don't think so

chessman: but it's different with guys

Big.J: the english chick didn't seem
            2 mind

BoBoy: yeah. i was talkin 2 her later

chessman: man, i hope you didn't say chick
            to her

BoBoy: well, u know what i mean

chessman: how long did you talk to her?

BoBoy: i dunno. awhile after johnson left

chessman: you tell her about tamra?

BoBoy: um?

Big.J: ooo la la, i knew it

BoBoy: no i did. i think i did

Big.J: of course he didn't

chessman: aw, beau... what were you thinking?

Big.J: oh u people need 2 get over
            yrselves

chessman: easy for you to say, poetry man

BoBoy: **skanks aplenty, skanks galore**

Big.J: i mean, why WOULD he tell her
            about T?

BoBoy: **um, wait. i think i know this one**

chessman: because ms. T isn't brittney.
            show some respect

BoBoy: **thanks, man**

Big.J: brittney? easy there, cowboy

chessman: or what, skank boy?

Big.J: chill, mitchie. brittney is
            very fragile right now

chessman: we know. she's needy, you keep
            saying

BoBoy: **wait. she's fragile?**

Big.J: fragile i said, and fragile it is

BoBoy: **dude, what have u done?**

Big.J: let's just say i won't have u
            dissin my ex-girlfriends

chessman: oh man

BoBoy: **i knew it. i knew it**

Big.J: chill out, boyz. she'll be fine

BoBoy: **what is that—like 9 days?? bro, yr license 2
            love is hereby revocated**

```
chessman:  totally. you're grounded, J

Big.J:     get out

chessman:  no, you are
```

BoBoy: **it's outta control**

```
chessman:  you get no more cooperation from
           us until you straighten out

Big.J:     slow down, dudes. as much as we
           appreciate yr concern 4 the J man,
           we must say ur crossing a
           line here

chessman:  dude, say nothing. you've lost
           all credibility
```

BoBoy: **and now ur startin 2 reflect on yr bros**

```
Big.J:     well mercy me. we're worried
           about our reputation, r we?

chessman:  we're worried about YOU, man
```

BoBoy: **dude, ur a train wreck on wheels**

```
chessman:  you can't use people up and toss
           them aside like... i don't know
```

BoBoy: **like peach pits**

```
Big.J:     lol

chessman:  seriously, J. you don't want to
           do people that way

Big.J:     aw man, he's gone 2 church on
           me now

chessman:  you don't want to be carrying
           all those broken hearts

Big.J:     i always lay them down gently,
           thank u ;-)
```

BoBoy: nah. u carry them. i can c it, dude

chessman: you don't have to agree with us, J

Big.J: thank u

chessman: but here's the thing. we're out of the chat room unless you grow up

Big.J: is that so?

BoBoy: u got it

chessman: he needs to... what, beau? totally stay away from women?

BoBoy: except in the chat room

chessman: where we can supervise you

BoBoy: that's it

Big.J: sure... that could happen

chessman: and with them, you have to pay attention, you have to show some class, and... let's see...

Big.J: u done yet, mother mitchell?

BoBoy: u have 2 make em like u

chessman: those are the terms, johnson. make em like you

Big.J: ur such little girls

BoBoy: J, ur messin up their life and yr life too

Big.J: it's MY life. if i want 2 mess it up i will

BoBoy: no, that won't work, bro. sorry

chessman: we know you don't like criticism, so take it as a challenge

BoBoy: sure! it's just retraining the mind. u have a
           strong mind

Big.J: and u people have me confused
           with someone who cares

chessman: come ON, johnson. for your own
           good. you know it's a problem

BoBoy: even annie said it's a problem

Big.J: no she didn't

BoBoy: she totally did

chessman: well, annie's hard core, beau.
           can anyone please her?

BoBoy: he's afraid he can't do it. especially with annie...

chessman: he's too used to skanks

Big.J: k. u can just chill with that,
           mitch

BoBoy: it's a poet's challenge, J. c what u can do

Big.J: that is so lame

chessman: seriously, bro. bottom line is
           we're outta here unless you
           buy in

Big.J: whatever

chessman: ok sure. you'll hardly miss us

BoBoy: just makes yr summer school a little tougher.
           that's all

Big.J: @#$%!*

BoBoy: really J. friends don't let friends self-destruct

Big.J: ur SO over the line with this

BoBoy: oh nooooo! we crossed the line...

chessman: so move the line, J. i know you can
           see SOME way this will work for you

BoBoy: or not. either way is cool with us

Big.J: don't bluff me

chessman: nobody's bluffing, bro. WE don't
           have summer school

Big.J: okokok

BoBoy: aight then

Big.J: just hold up a minute

chessman: ok, here's where he tries his
           own bluff...

Big.J: look. it's true that i still
           need u bozos 2 finish the chat room

BoBoy: there u go, J boy

Big.J: that's the only reason i would
           do this yr way

BoBoy: c... he needs us

chessman: i can live with that

Big.J: plus, well... honestly... i've
           <ahem> got my eye on a very
           interesting number lately who may
           require a different approach

BoBoy: aw johnson...

chessman: no, that's ok. different approach
           is good. but not till after the chat
           room is over, got it?

Big.J: whatever. fine

BoBoy: fine

chessman: fine

Big.J: but here's MY condition

chessman: he's incorrigible

BoBoy: **he's what? that's not good, is it?**

Big.J: the condition is that NOBODY
            bails until this is over. got
            it girls? no mitchie running away.
            no bubba getting cold feet. for
            2 more weeks, i belong 2 summer
            school, and u punks belong 2 me.

chessman: <sigh> fair enough, bo?

BoBoy: **i'm there**

Big.J: after that, skanks of the
            world unite. Big.J is back in
            circulation!

CHAPTER 11
politics

GURLGANG ROOM

JUNE 08 08:30 PM

gothling: now THAT was good work last night, ladies.
i read johnson's transcript. very very nice.

bliss4u: did u think so?

gothling: i thought u were especially good with beau this
time

bliss4u: really?

gothling: awesome. nice back and forth. u stayed a step
ahead, then u left him with a sweet little wink

Ms.T: really? what was that? i left early

bliss4u: oh, i said he was a peach

Ms.T: you didn't!

bliss4u: well, bridget did. and besides it was true

gothling: **it was excellent. true or not, it worked**

Ms.T: worked? i spent like 50 lines telling them not to say that stuff

gothling: **exactly why bliss should say it**

bliss4u: i just thought it would make him feel better

gothling: **right. u soothed the male ego**

Ms.T: stab me in the back, why don't you?

bliss4u: why?? what's wrong with calling him a peach?

Ms.T: what's wrong is i don't want him saying stuff like that. duh...

gothling: **tam, ur outta line. bridget isn't yr lil yes-gurl. besides, he didn't know he was talking 2 u when he had that convo**

Ms.T: that doesn't matter

gothling: **it matters because he doesn't take his housetraining from tatiana—only from tamra**

bliss4u: housetraining? that's cold, annie

gothling: **oh, he does whatever T says. and hey, i was giving u props, girl. don't u come after me now**

bliss4u: i'm just saying

Ms.T: he needs to see that women agree on this

gothling: **well, tam, women DON'T agree on it. so he learns 2 read the signs**

Big.J has entered

Big.J: allo allo?

gothling: **johnson, what up? nice of u 2 break in**

Big.J: word. hey i just wanted 2 say how well lady bridget, lady tatiana did last night. well done well done

Ms.T: johnson, frankly, i'm not feeling approachable right now. so before you compliment me, do me a favor?

Big.J: at yr service, miss

Ms.T: change your username

bliss4u: lol, tam. gotta agree with u on this one

Big.J: beg pardon?

gothling: oh 4... johnson, u really caught her in a mood this time. sorry

Ms.T: i am not in a mood, annie. i've always hated his username. it's offensive

Big.J: yeah, but i really don't get it. my username? ah. oh, NOW i c. heh heh. never thought of that. hmm. well, k. give me a moment

Big.J has left the room

gothling: tam, this is uncalled for, don't u think?

Ms.T: oh, like he should get to be crude to us, just because he's your friend?

gothling: no. but he shouldn't have 2 toe any line u just happen 2 draw

bliss4u: i'm with tam. it's an offense 2 all womankind

gothling: u chicks r totally putting me off. i thought we were going 2 have a nice evening of bonding and affirming. gurl stuff

Mr.Jeeves has entered

Mr.Jeeves: better?

gothling: oh, johnson, i don't know...

bliss4u: lol. much better

Ms.T: puts a whole different leer on your face

gothling: i just don't like it, J

Mr.Jeeves: really? what's wrong with it?

gothling: well, in a nutshell, ur not their butler

Mr.Jeeves: ah. true... is that important?

Ms.T: but he could stand to play the role for a while :)

gothling: i don't think so

bliss4u: now who's being picky?

gothling: ur nobody's servant, johnson. be a man

Ms.T: leave it, johnson. we like it

gothling: absolutely not

Mr.Jeeves: not a problem, annie dear. be right back

Mr.Jeeves has left the room

bliss4u: u guys r kinda pushing him around

Ms.T: yeah. the irony of this is lost on no one, annie

bliss4u: what irony?

Ms.T: "ur nobody's servant. now go change yr name"

gothling: at least i don't force my politics on people

Ms.T: you just did! everything is politics, annie. you know that

bliss4u: not 2 me. somewhere u stop and it's just people

Ms.T: people are never just people

bliss4u: ur SO twitchy 2nite, girl

gothling: **she's mad because she can't control beau when he's outta sight.**

Ms.T: i'm FINE. lay off

gothling: **grow up. this all started when u found out that bliss and beau r getting along**

bliss4u: hey, i didn't do anything. i just said he was a peach

gothling: **which he is...**

Ms.T: oh, shut up, you two. i wanna know why johnson is being so... whatever he's being

gothling: **he's being friendly. maybe u've heard of that?**

bliss4u: lol annie

Ms.T: he's being TOO friendly

bliss4u: well, u did say u wouldn't talk 2 him if he didn't change his name

Ms.T: his name was crude. i just didn't expect him to give up without a fight

gothling: **listen, T. this has 2 stop. u can't just dictate 2 everyone**

Ms.T: i didn't think i was dictating. i thought we all wanted to get along

bliss4u: we do!

Ms.T: then we have to respect each other's point of view

gothling: **exactly! so show johnson some respect**

alfonso has entered

alfonso: so i'm don alfonso this time. from cosi fan tutte? like it?

Ms.T: fine with me

alfonso: any objections 2 mozart? opera?
the whole 18th century?

Ms.T: it's a fine name, johnson

gothling: **k, r we done?**

alfonso: not too albanian 4 u?

bliss4u: lol

alfonso: oh look, i made bliss laugh. that goes on
my calendar

gothling: **johnson, we're kind of into a gurl fight here.
can u make it quick?**

alfonso: oic. well <cough cough> i just stopped by 2
say how well i thought u kids did last night.
not kids. um, ladies?

gothling: **that's it?**

alfonso: well, they both had some inspired moments,
didn't u think, annie?

gothling: **that's where i STARTED this convo. but SOME
people have CONTROL issues**

alfonso: lol. but not miss annie, right? no control issues
there...

Ms.T: now that's the first amusing thing you've ever
said, johnson. you may stay 2 extra minutes
just for that

alfonso: yow! that's both of them now. i made em
both smile!

gothling: **don't push it, J**

alfonso: btw, T. i looked back at the transcript on u
and mitch. why do u think he freaked?

Ms.T: duh. i scared him off. i misjudged his devotion
to our bliss girl

bliss4u:	\<sigh\>
alfonso:	i was surprised too. i didn't think u were that aggressive... i thought he would be flattered
Ms.T:	you never know
gothling:	**no, johnson's right. he should have been flattered, and i think he was**
bliss4u:	huh?
gothling:	**that's what scared him. tatiana got 2 him**
Ms.T:	you think? actually, i was rather hurt when he disappeared
alfonso:	annie makes total sense. tatiana got 2 him
bliss4u:	hey, wait a sec. how about he just didn't want 2 cheat on me?
alfonso:	well, yes. the simplest answer. and what he said later fits with that
bliss4u:	there, u see?
alfonso:	still, he may ALSO have been embarrassed... by how he felt. i've been chatting with the boyz, and i do see a glimmer of something there
bliss4u:	oh please
alfonso:	tatiana's a fascinating gurl. credit where it's due
Ms.T:	thank you
bliss4u:	but he didn't DO anything
alfonso:	quite true. so it's win-win 4 bliss and tam
Ms.T:	but another loss for annie
gothling:	**i can wait. he's on the hook**
alfonso:	they both r. beau boy was tongue-tied after talking with bridget

Ms.T:	yeah, with miss peach
alfonso:	actually, interesting thing, T. did u know the only 1 who gets u on politics is mitch?
bliss4u:	why? what did he say?
alfonso:	he totally reamed beau and me
Ms.T:	really?
alfonso:	i kid u not. we explained about calling u a peach, and he was all "dude, u can't call a chick things." (not chick. a woman. my bad. mitch never says chick)
bliss4u:	why can't u call a chick things?
Ms.T:	bliss, puhleeeze...
bliss4u:	whatever. it's a word
alfonso:	u can't call them... like, a thing, i guess. an object
bliss4u:	but...
alfonso:	i know i know. but what i mean is mitch gets this stuff. he GETS it. and honestly? it's really starting 2 change my way of seeing things
gothling:	**u don't say**
bliss4u:	i just don't c what there is 2 get
Ms.T:	bliss, come on. has mitch ever called you an animal or a thing, or something associated with children?
bliss4u:	i don't think so. just nice things, like he says i'm pretty or my hair is cute or something
Ms.T:	i rest my case
gothling:	**why?? that proves nothing**

Ms.T:	it proves he respects her, duh. i'm not saying that, like, peach and ho are equal, ok? but they both make her less than human. THAT's what mitch gets
gothling:	**unlike beau?**
alfonso:	annie, let's don't go all tense, please
gothling:	**unlike beau, tamra??**
Ms.T:	ok, annie. yes. unlike beau
gothling:	**now we're gettin 2 it**
Ms.T:	beau doesn't have a clue, ok annie? beau speaks of me like an object sometimes, ok? beau doesn't respect me the way mitch respects bliss
bliss4u:	tamra, ur up in the nite! beau totally luvs u
Ms.T:	right. that's why he hit on you
bliss4u:	but he didn't...
Ms.T:	and he hit on you because you don't CONTROL him. because whatever he says is just so damn cute to you. it's just a word with no meaning, no history, no politics. you just jiggle your pompoms and nod your empty head
alfonso:	tamra, if i may interject a word here...
Ms.T:	how would you know if beau respects you or not, bliss? you don't have any more of a clue than he does
bliss4u:	shut up, T. just shut up right now
Ms.T:	actually, you're perfect for each other. two freakin clueless blind chauvinistic middle-brow morons. i hope you're happy together, because i'm outta here

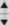

Ms.T is offline

gothling: **oooo la LA**

alfonso: well, i was afraid of this

bliss4u: i am SO not speaking 2 her

IM from gothling

JUNE 09 10:30 AM

gothling: yo johnson

alfonso: sì sì, dorabella?

gothling: dorabella? k, dude. what r u listening 2 right now?

alfonso: um, nothing. nothing at all

gothling: spit it out. something euro. something classical

alfonso: no way. u know me. i only do edgy stuff: gnarls, belle & sebastian. white stripes. um?

gothling: nice try

alfonso: bob marley? classic tupac? the supremes?

gothling: it's opera isn't it?

alfonso: okok, it's mozart! i won't apologize

gothling: busted

alfonso: get out. mozart is my only solace. he brings order 2 chaos and darkness

gothling: <yawn>

alfonso: annie, dear, tell me u feel it too. the encroaching gloom

gothling: oh, that's yr senior year coming, pal. push through the curtain and the light will dawn

alfonso: yes, like sunrise at the landfill. that's what i'm afraid of. i'm waking just in time 2 see where my life is ending

gothling: get a grip

alfonso: u could take me seriously... 4 once

gothling: earn it, scooter

alfonso: oh annie, if that were possible. ur a forbidding and formidable woman. how would anyone earn yr regard?

gothling: such a wit, johnson...

alfonso: if only u meant that

gothling: which reminds me. how come u never wrote me a poem?

alfonso: huh? maybe because u despise me?

gothling: oh, i do not. u write them 4 class, 4 the yearbook. 4 every girl u know. everyone thinks it's so random, but they're all totally in awe

alfonso: true, true

gothling: and ur, like, dr. bartolo's favorite student

alfonso: jeeze, gurl. don't ruin it

gothling: so why no poem 4 me?

alfonso: annabelle

gothling: what am i... a potted plant?

alfonso: sweetie...

gothling: what?

alfonso: i am totally certain this is not why u IM'd me

gothling: true. but it's still a good question. i think it just shows how u been neglecting me all these years <sigh>

alfonso: k, now ur scaring me. how bout this: u tell me why ur really here, and i promise 2 write a poem just 2 make u stop this line of talk

gothling: easy. i'm here, my child, because i want 2 know what ur up 2

alfonso: ah

gothling: so? what's with the nicey niceness 2 tam and bliss all of a sudden?

alfonso: well, not unexpected... how shall i?... let's say i'm turning over a new leaf

gothling: a new leaf

alfonso: mmm. temporarily at least

gothling: temporarily

alfonso: until this chat room stuff is over and bartolo signs off on my genius once again <sigh>

gothling: dude, what's this about? do i need 2 come by and pound some sense into u?

alfonso: tempting—and thanks—but no. this is something i have 2 do. and i'm actually quite reconciled 2 it

gothling: i'm waiting

alfonso: well, it truly does have 2 do with saving our little chat room. mitch and beau have laid down the law. it's absurd.... yet the absurdity does give it a certain appeal

gothling: stop blathering and talk 2 me

alfonso: ok, try this: either i mend my ways or the dudes drop out of the chat room

gothling: that's blackmail!

alfonso: u got it

gothling: totally out of line. what is their problem?

alfonso: they, um, heard about brittney

gothling: what about her?

alfonso: they feel i was perhaps not entirely... fair 2 her

gothling: oh, like u should have married her

alfonso: well. i believe mitch and beau see her as part of a pattern

gothling: of course there's a pattern. hello?? ur a total screwup with women. why they love u i don't know

alfonso: it's a gift

gothling: i'm gonna dope slap u, boy. u don't respect women. u think u love them, but u don't. u collect em and discard em. ur a cliché

alfonso: let it out, annie.... don't hold back just out of politeness...

gothling: oh, get a grip. i'm not mad, johnson. i'm not tamra. besides, it's fun 2 watch

alfonso: thank u so much

gothling: but ur a classic southern male. selfish, thoughtless, pretentious, and dumber than soap

alfonso: pretentious? moi?

gothling: AND afraid of commitment

alfonso: now, that one's a wee bit true

gothling: well, duh, bubba. that's why u go 4 skanks. brittney and tiffany were only the last 2

alfonso: true, there were 1 or 2 others

gothling: lol. let's see... meg was yr little easter bunny. beth was in yr xmas stocking

alfonso: i'm so flattered that u noticed

gothling: and b4 her, it was anne-ellen, frankie... i'm missing 1...

alfonso: kami... michele... that's it, i think, 4 this school year

gothling: dawg, u do need a rest. u just ate through the whole buffet at hooters

alfonso: so now ur on their side?

gothling: of course not, doll. they may be right, but they're totally wrong

alfonso: say again?

gothling: just because there's a problem doesn't mean it's fixable

alfonso: excellent. ur really cheering me up

gothling: hey, u drove here all by yrself. i'm just blowing the horn

alfonso: u totally have no respect 4 me, do u?

gothling: of course i do, honey. i just don't expect u 2 act against yr nature

alfonso: how do u mean that?

gothling: ur a slut puppy. why fight it?

alfonso: luv u too

gothling: oh get over it

alfonso: monster. dragon lady

gothling: worm. insect

alfonso: asp

gothling: what? asp?

alfonso: a venomous snake, duh

gothling: kewl

alfonso: only bites u in the heart. ask cleopatra

gothling: aw, that's sweet. k, i gotta bounce. listen, don't let the blackmailers get u down. we're about to put them in their place

alfonso: hmm. that's true, i guess

gothling: totally. don't lose focus, babe. we finish this and then ur free again

alfonso: right. it's just that...

gothling: just what? there's no just anything

alfonso: just... well, remember when i made bliss laugh? she never gave me the time of day before. now i've made her laugh, and... i dunno...

gothling: johnson if u hit on her, i will personally mess u up

alfonso: ah. so u feel it could be a problem. what about tamra? i think i could be a totally new man with her

gothling: u try either 1, dude, and mitch and beau will have to stand in line. clear enough?

alfonso: i think i got it. still, it shows the potential

gothling: whatever. ok, bro. IM 2nite while they're in the chat room

gothling is off-line

alfonso: oh annie

annie annie annie

annie

YOUR UNCLE JERRY'S BLOG

In the Cards
10 JUNE

> *The cards do not lie, my friend.*
> *—Ulrica the Witch, lame old gypsy saying*

Joy and peace, camper. Today, back by popular demand: Uncle Jerry's Tarot Tent. Gloomy in here? Never you mind. Psychic truth is often found in shadows.

The cards do not lie, young camper, and why not? Because they do not care. How cold, you say, how dark. No, no, no. Think. Think how cold and dark your little world would be if the cards did care. Suppose they were to sugarcoat. Suppose they saw some danger lurking in your future and said nothing—just to spare your feelings. What a disaster. No, no, destiny must be faced with open eyes. If the cards cared, you could not trust them. And without trust, well, where would any of us be?

A quick three cards, my friend. The first... aww... two of cups. How dove-lovely. Two cups raised to lovers' lips. Two pairs of bright eyes meet.... But wait, this is in the past. *Tsk, tsk.* Oh please, don't weep, young camper. Lovers' lips may lie, but the cards do not.

Second card: eight of cups. Many things offer shiny promise, but today you find them cheap and empty. (We might say your cup runneth NOT over, heh heh heh. That's a joke, son. Psalm 23. Look it up; it'll do you good.) But how right you are. The world is full of false promise, and by the way, this is the subject of Uncle Jerry's latest online Sunday sermon, available now at a website near you. (You look like you could use a sermon, son, if I may say so.)

So, young camper, love is in the past, and the present does not satisfy. Ah me. Ah life. Let's move on. Card three: yes... the eight of wands. News approaching, the future unfolding. Tumult and shouting. But oh, how like the cards: The eight does not say *what* you will learn, my friend. It says only that knowledge will come, and *soon*.

So there it is. Destiny. For good or ill, it comes. Be brave. Beware. For as you know, the cards do not lie.

And neither does Your Uncle Jerry.

Joy and peace.

CHAPTER 13
friends

✉ IM from chessman

JUNE 10 04:00 PM

chessman: tatiana, are you there?

Tatiana: mitchell, how are you?

chessman: sorry to bother you. can you talk? i mean is now a good time?

Tatiana: you are never the bother, mitchell. is such a flattery that you would message over to me

chessman: thanks. i'm glad

Tatiana: one cannot say this of your friends

chessman: my friends. i was afraid of that. sorry

Tatiana: i regret only that i was not more rude to them

chessman: but that wouldn't be like you

Tatiana: i am no accustomed to be called so many unkind things

chessman: i'm sorry

Tatiana: horse, machine, boy, food

chessman: they called you a horse??

Tatiana: racehorse is kind of horse, correct?

chessman: yes, but surely they didn't mean you...

Tatiana: ah. they spoke of the girl who loves your friend. i take her side, for she was not there

chessman: oic

Tatiana: i am still furious about her, what they called

chessman: i'm not sure why you're angry about another girl

Tatiana: all women are one, mitchell

chessman: pardon?

Tatiana: no woman is fruit or steam engine. all are women. all are one

chessman: tatiana, maybe this was only a cross-cultural mistake? people must say things in albania that americans wouldn't really get. metaphors, like

Tatiana: racehorse is to say she is less than woman, correct? something driven by animal feelings?

chessman: but in albania...

Tatiana: if one say this in albania, you are talking of a not so very nice girl... and if one say it of me, my brothers will abuse one very badly about the head and shoulders. abuse is correct, yes?

chessman: tatiana, ok

ok, i apologize for my friends. they were ignorant and callous

Tatiana: they were pigs, dogs. hyenas

chessman: yes

Tatiana: and you apologize for them?

chessman: yes

Tatiana: you mean to defend them?

chessman: not at all. they were impolite to you. i apologize deeply

Tatiana: they were crude to all women everywhere

chessman: yes they were. i'm so sorry

Tatiana: and you have spoken to them about these words?

chessman: tatiana, i have abused them very badly

Tatiana: you have said a woman is not a horse?

chessman: i didn't know about the horse

Tatiana: then you must abuse them about the horse

chessman: yes, i will do that

Tatiana: no no, you must do it right now

chessman: ok. i'll go now and abuse them about the horse

Tatiana: and the dude

chessman: yes, the dude, too. they shouldn't say that

Tatiana: you tell them

chessman: yes. and tatiana?

Tatiana: what?

chessman: then may i talk to you later?

Tatiana: yes, perhaps i would like that

chessman: ok. goodbye for now

Tatiana: goodbye

chessman: see ya

Tatiana: mitchell?

chessman: yes?

Tatiana: you would never insult me, would you?

chessman: never. well, catch ya later

Tatiana: wait!

chessman: what?

Tatiana: where are you going? you cannot leave me now

chessman: but you said...

Tatiana: don't be silly. you can see i need your company

chessman: you do?

Tatiana: is obvious

chessman: ok, i'll stay then

Tatiana: oh, mitchell, just talking you make me feel so much better. talk me, talk me

chessman: um, ok. what shall i tell you?

Tatiana: anything about you. i must to know you so much better

chessman: well, i'm not very interesting

Tatiana: you ARE. you are so kind and so comforting. and there's much passion in you too. i feel as if you were going away to defend me just now.

chessman: well, i'm on your side...

Tatiana: is like the brother, or no—like the fiancé ;-)

chessman: well...

Tatiana: ah, so romantic :) mitchell and tatiana, ooo la la

chessman: um

Tatiana: i am flirting you, mitchell. do you see? like the fiancé...

chessman: yes, i thought you might be

Tatiana: hah. you are such the shy one. tell to me anything.

oh! you were to tell me something before. you have something to explain. you must tell me this

chessman: um, right now?

Tatiana: yes, of course right now. i demand it

chessman: well, in a way, it was about someone else

Tatiana: you must to tell me. i am all listening

chessman: this other person is a girl

Tatiana: hmph. a girl. she is a friend of you?

chessman: actually, she's my girlfriend. that's what i needed to tell you

Tatiana: your girlfriend

chessman: yes. i have a girlfriend

Tatiana: girlfriend is like the fiancée, yes?

chessman: yikes. no, we're too young for that. i really like her and stuff, but i've got college coming up and... you know

Tatiana: oic. the girlfriend is not the fiancée, but is still the special one

chessman: there you go. so...

Tatiana: so now there is problem?

chessman: so um, i don't know. but, well, maybe you shouldn't tell me about the stars and everything

Tatiana: because of this girl...

chessman: yeah

Tatiana: hmm. your girlfriend, she is passionate? possessive?

chessman: yes. well, maybe not like albanian women. but she and i don't see other people. we promised

Tatiana: so then no problem

chessman: really?

Tatiana: of course. you don't see me! on the internet, no one knows i am the dog. lol

chessman: nice one. but i'm sure you're not a dog, tatiana

Tatiana: you are too sweet for this girlfriend, i think, mitchell. she doesn't know how you are gallant and thoughtful

chessman: um? well, thanks... anyway, so it's ok to talk, but i don't think you should flirt with me. you know what i mean. you must have a boyfriend, right?

Tatiana: i fear not

chessman: i can't believe that. a passionate woman like you?

Tatiana: perhaps i do have someone interested...

chessman: see there?

Tatiana: but i don't know how serious. i think i must work harder to make him more interested. is difficult, however

chessman: no way. what's the problem?

Tatiana: oh, he lives very far away

chessman: yeah, that's a tough one. my girlfriend has been out of town for weeks

Tatiana: he lives far away in america

chessman: in america?

Tatiana: but he likes me. i can sense it

chessman: you can?

Tatiana: oh yes. i must think how to win him away from his cold american girlfriend, lol

chessman: tatiana, please. you shouldn't flirt with me

Tatiana: sorry. sorry. i forget. don't be angry, mitchell

chessman: i'm not angry

Tatiana: i am harmless. don't be angry. just teasing you

chessman: ok

Tatiana: i just like you. is this a crime?

chessman: no. but...

Tatiana: flirting is only how i show my liking. don't worry, you are safe for your little american girlfriend

chessman: it makes me uncomfortable. i know it shouldn't, but it does

Tatiana: ah, you worry so much about the girl. she's gone, mitchell. she can't know what you say to me

chessman: that's really not the point

Tatiana: whatever, my darling. you are safe with tatiana

chessman: please don't

Tatiana: safe, safe, safe

chessman: ok but can we talk about something else?

Tatiana: yes! tell me something else: why does this girl leave you?

chessman: she didn't leave me. she just went away for a while

Tatiana: yes of course. but why did she?

chessman: her grandmother is ill

Tatiana: ah, poor grandmama

chessman: she had a stroke or something

Tatiana: you don't know?

chessman: well, she didn't know for sure when she left

Tatiana: but now?

chessman: i haven't heard from her

Tatiana: sorry? haven't heard from her about her dying grandmama and she is gone for months?

chessman: only a couple of weeks

Tatiana: well, she should be calling every day

chessman: it's complicated

Tatiana: twice every day. i would be calling you twice each day

chessman: no, it's cool

Tatiana: you don't miss her? good

chessman: sure i do. i just mean, if she can't call, then i understand

Tatiana: oh you trust her so much?

chessman: i do

Tatiana: what if she lies to you?

chessman: she doesn't. i know this girl. i know where she is

Tatiana: really. and where is that?

chessman: well, i don't know exactly. but i mean, i know that she's with her grandmother. and her friend tamra is with her too

Tatiana: hmph. this friend... what she is like?

chessman: oh, fantastic. i really like her

Tatiana: mitchell! so many girlfriends: me, the other, and now this tamra. you should be italian

chessman: lol. are you jealous?

Tatiana: fuming!

chessman: no seriously. tamra is famous around here. brains and beauty together. also very political. you'd like her

Tatiana: if she's after you, i despise her

chessman: not to worry. she's spoken for—my friend beau

Tatiana: racehorse woman? even so...

chessman: oh, you're so cynical. no, ms. T would never mess that up, certainly not with me

Tatiana: people do the strange thing, mitchell. but fine, let's put her to one side

chessman: tell me about your own life. got a boyfriend?

Tatiana: only the one in america

chessman: you're still flirting...

Tatiana: ah, ok. serious. i have almost 17 years old, i go to america for my year of school before university, and i have a boy—a boy name of... sebastien. sebastien max, whom i love too much

chessman: you love him too much? i didn't think that was possible for a passionate woman

Tatiana: now you are teasing me

chessman: see, you're brilliant, too

Tatiana: i am actually quite sad about this. i fear
he falls in love with my friend

chessman: oh, no. really?

Tatiana: i am not sure, but is possible. i know she
makes the play for him

chessman: tatiana, she doesn't have a chance

Tatiana: no, is possible. she is wonderful person, and
i make many mistake

chessman: what do you mean by mistakes?

Tatiana: maybe i push too hard

chessman: on your boyfriend?

Tatiana: yes. i am so... i don't know how to say.
like too much forceful sometime?

chessman: too intense?

Tatiana: si si. too intense many time. he is only a boy.
he want more fun. i am more intense, more political
like your girlfriend tamra

chessman: you're smarter than he is?

Tatiana: NO. everyone say this, but is not so. he
is a fine mind. he is only more... social? he play, he
laugh, he like the futbol

chessman: so he likes to take it easy, and you push
yourself all the time

Tatiana: perhaps <sighing>

chessman: very hard to have a relationship like that. i'm so sorry

Tatiana: see how you understand everything? is too sad. mitchell, now you make me sad. why can you not love me just until i find another? your fiancée would never know

chessman: i'm sorry i make you sad. i could tell you a joke or something :-)

Tatiana: ha. that is a funny thing to say

chessman: ha. really i'm not a very funny guy. just ask my girlfriend

Tatiana: mitchell, here is the truth. the girlfriend sees only your surface, but you are deep water to me... i need you to be my friend. i am so alone sometime. always

chessman: i am your friend, tatiana

Tatiana: my friend and something perhaps more? a little?

chessman: tatiana, i'm sorry. i really can't

Tatiana: <sigh>

chessman: i know...

Tatiana: friends, then

chessman: friends

CHAPTER 14
kissing lessons

✉ IM from Bridget

JUNE 10 08:00 PM

Bridget: beau? hello good evening?

BoBoy: bridge! hey girl, what up?

Bridget: surprised 2 hear from me?

BoBoy: sure am. what time is it over there?

Bridget: dunno. 5 hours later than u r

BoBoy: wow, 1 in the morning

Bridget: um i can't sleep 4 some reason

BoBoy: yeah, that happens 2 me

Bridget: tiresome

BoBoy: lol

Bridget: what?

BoBoy: tiresome. tired. can't sleep

Bridget: oic. sorry

BoBoy: just my sense of humor

Bridget: no, u have a good sense of humour. i like it

BoBoy: well...

Bridget: i like u too

BoBoy: excuse me?

Bridget: oh blimey. did i say that?

BoBoy: um?

Bridget: i did. just forget it, all right?

BoBoy: oh gurl u are in trouble now ;-)

Bridget: it just slipped out. i was just thinking aloud. sorry

BoBoy: really, it's ok

Bridget: i mean, i know u have a girlfriend and everything

BoBoy: slow down, bridge

Bridget: how embarrassing. this happens 2 me all the time. i just blurt out whatever's on my mind. just blurt it out and everyone looks at me like i have 2 heads

BoBoy: bridget

Bridget: what?

BoBoy: it's ok

Bridget: really?

BoBoy: really

Bridget: thank u, beau. oh how embarrassing. i'll be good now

BoBoy: not a problem

Bridget: i'm so tired

BoBoy: well, ok... er, oh

so why can't u sleep?

Bridget: if i knew that...

BoBoy: let me see—u had a fight with someone

Bridget: well, i did, sort of

BoBoy: i knew it. yr boyfriend?

Bridget: i wish. haven't seen him 4 ages

BoBoy: bet u miss him

Bridget: <sigh>

BoBoy: so who did u fight with? oh, i got it. yr best friend. mmm, that's rough

Bridget: how did u do that?

BoBoy: huh? nothing 2 it.

Bridget: really??

BoBoy: gurl like u, it's always 1 of 3 things

Bridget: what 3?

BoBoy: 1. boyfriend, 2. best friend, 3. worst enemy

Bridget: not bad

BoBoy: what did u fight about?

Bridget: that's simple: she's impossible

BoBoy: :)

Bridget: seriously!

BoBoy: no really

Bridget: okok, it's complicated. but basically she thinks i'm after her boyfriend

BoBoy: yow. that's big time

Bridget: but i'm NOT

BoBoy: ur not

Bridget: no. i mean, i do like him, but i'm NOT trying 2 take him away

BoBoy: sure...

Bridget: u don't believe me?

BoBoy: well, it's just like, where would she get that idea?

Bridget: u know how girls r

BoBoy: i do?

Bridget: suspicious! nasty. competitive. mean

BoBoy: oh, that :)

Bridget: k. so i did talk 2 him, and i do like him, and i did say nice things

BoBoy: but aside from that, ur in the clear :-D

Bridget: oh, i'm gonna get u

BoBoy: lol. from england?

Bridget: i mean it, beau, she is totally out of line on this

BoBoy: i hear u

Bridget: she practically pushed me at him, anyway

BoBoy: huh?

Bridget: i shouldn't be telling u, but i'm so mad at her. see, we had this bet, and it was like, ok, she tries 2 take my boy and i try 2 take hers

BoBoy: no way

Bridget: yes way

BoBoy: girls do stuff like that?

Bridget: pay attn. YES. oh yes

BoBoy: but why? i mean, i know why guys would do it, but that's 2 obvious 4 words

Bridget: true. but girls, well, maybe just 2 find out if they can trust their boyfriends

BoBoy: aw man, that is so RUDE

Bridget: no, it's not that way. more like they really WANT him 2 behave, but they want 2 know 4 sure, too. they're just insecure or something

BoBoy: in some parallel universe, this must make sense

Bridget: why? it makes total sense 2 me

BoBoy: 2 hand him candy that u don't want him 2 eat?

Bridget: come on, he knows he can't

BoBoy: shouldn't

Bridget: whatever. he knows u don't touch what isn't yrs

BoBoy: yeah but what about human nature?

Bridget: look, if he's not a jerk, he'll resist the temptation. simple

BoBoy: so u want him to PROVE he's not a jerk

Bridget: right

BoBoy: only he doesn't know he's being tested

Bridget: well duh...

BoBoy: oh, man. u guys r tough

Bridget: why??

BoBoy: this is so cruel. no wonder u can't sleep. it's yr conscience, girl

Bridget: ouch. why r u being mean now?

BoBoy: i'm not. i'm just saying

Bridget: i shouldn't have told u

BoBoy: nah, come on

Bridget: well. if i'm so cruel, then u surely don't want 2 talk 2 me

BoBoy: what?

Bridget: i'll just be going. thanks 4 nothing

BoBoy: no, wait

Bridget: and maybe i don't like u after all

BoBoy: bridge, wait

BoBoy: bridget?

BoBoy: bridge, please

Bridget: what?

BoBoy: just stay. talk 2 me

Bridget: why should i?

BoBoy: because u need 2 talk. i can tell

Bridget: no. i'm too CRUEL. obviously not good enough 2 talk 2

BoBoy: ok, i'm sorry for saying cruel. please stay

Bridget: no ur not

BoBoy: anyway, i just said the test was cruel, not u personally

Bridget: that's a... technicality

BoBoy: come on. u can let me off on a technicality, can't u?

Bridget: why should i?

BoBoy: just this once

Bridget: say please

BoBoy: please please preeeeze

Bridget: :)

BoBoy: there, see. u do still like me!

Bridget: don't be so sure. i could be just playing u

BoBoy: tell me more about yr best friend

Bridget: what about her?

BoBoy: what's the best thing?

Bridget: oh... she's brilliant. everyone says so

BoBoy: that's good. but that's not why u like her

Bridget: well, not really. i like her because... she's just a really good friend

BoBoy: she understands u?

Bridget: duh

BoBoy: she's supportive

Bridget: true. except today

BoBoy: she's fun, loyal, laughs at yr jokes, listens good

Bridget: yeah...

BoBoy: she likes u

Bridget: usually. she hates me lately

BoBoy: come on, girl. that will pass. it's not the first fight u ever had

Bridget: i don't know. she's really mad

BoBoy: aw, how could she stay mad at u? ur a sweetie

Bridget: don't be nice to me

BoBoy: but u R. ur just the sweetest lil ol thang

Bridget: no, u think i'm cruel and heartless

BoBoy: seriously. i can tell these things. ur like the nicest girl i ever met

Bridget: don't say that

BoBoy: no, it's true

Bridget: stop

BoBoy: k, stopping...

k, what's the biggest difference between u and yr best friend?

Bridget: um? dunno. maybe control stuff

BoBoy: interesting

Bridget: i mean, well, she's way into being on top of things. everything perfect, top marks in school, people saying the right words, things coming out perfectly

BoBoy: she likes things under control

Bridget: right

BoBoy: and u?

Bridget: well, i just can't do it. maybe because she's smarter than me

BoBoy: ur no dummy, bridge

Bridget: i am, compared 2 her

BoBoy: whatever. anyway, control isn't so important 2 u?

Bridget: yeah. well, i don't love chaos, but there's a little something about being just on the edge

BoBoy: kind of exciting

Bridget: totally. like when... no, i can't tell u this

BoBoy: yes u can

Bridget: you'll laugh

BoBoy: i won't. promise

Bridget: u better not.

ok, like when ur kissing a guy and something fluttery happens down in yr chest?

BoBoy: something fluttery?

Bridget: and like yr eyes kind of roll back and u almost faint? and, i dunno, everything's moving, and there's nothing u can do, and it's a little scary but totally exciting all at the same time?

BoBoy: bridge, ur making me all hot over here :)

Bridget: i know. it's nice, huh? <sigh>

BoBoy: woof. whoever he is, u got a lucky boyfriend

Bridget: hmmmmm

BoBoy: what?

Bridget: well... he thinks i could be more passionate. that's what i hear

BoBoy: get out. when ur feeling like THAT?

Bridget: no, seriously. he's not getting the message

BoBoy: he said ur not passionate?

Bridget: somebody told me, sort of. one of his friends

BoBoy: what a doof!

Bridget: i must be doing something wrong

BoBoy: why do u say that?

Bridget: well, i, um. k, i do get all kinda shy and quiet

BoBoy: the shy and passionate type. yowza!

Bridget: don't make fun of me

BoBoy: i'm not, bridge. seriously

Bridget: i can't help it

BoBoy: no, it's great. really fine. really sweet

Bridget: but what do i do about him?

BoBoy: he's english?

Bridget: um, yeah, english

BoBoy: not a chance. english r clueless about luv

Bridget: lol

BoBoy: ok. well, we gotta figure out how 2 give him a clue

Bridget: i thought about writing him a letter

BoBoy: eeek, no, not that

Bridget: why??

BoBoy: not good. much better in person

Bridget: like talk about it? i could never

BoBoy: well, no. not exactly talk about it. more like... ok, here. let's pretend

Bridget: pretend what?

BoBoy: u and me, ok? pretend like i'm yr boyfriend

Bridget: really?

BoBoy: sure. i'm not that bad a kisser...

Bridget: lol

BoBoy: ok, so we're kissing madly. u with me?

Bridget: well... ok i guess

BoBoy: so we're smooching away, and ur starting 2 feel that fluttery thing

Bridget: k...

BoBoy: feeling it?

Bridget: maybe

BoBoy: only maybe? hmm. how bout if i kiss yr neck, like on the left, just under yr chin? hot little kisses...

Bridget: k look. u have 2 court me. u can't jump me like a loose football

BoBoy: <ahem> sorry miss. i got carried away

Bridget: <smile> i'll say 1 thing 4 u, beau. u do make me laugh. my boy doesn't do that

BoBoy: really? why not? easiest thing in the world...

Bridget: i dunno. he's really sweet, but the brainy serious type

BoBoy: got it

Bridget: i mean, i'm totally gone on him. don't get me wrong

BoBoy: except for the passion bit...

Bridget: and that is so unfair. i'm really all about passion

BoBoy: ok, so let's figure it out. how do i court u?

Bridget: say some nice things, 4 starters

BoBoy: like what?

Bridget: i dunno. he always says nice things, gentle things about like nature and poetry and stuff. he can be pretty romantic

BoBoy: aw man. i can't think of that stuff. i'm a bozo

Bridget: try. pretend

BoBoy: ok. ur right. i should definitely learn this. where's johnson when i need him?... k <ahem> ready?

Bridget: ready

BoBoy: o bridget, the moon is shining on u. and the moon will be shining on me, too. and it's like going 2 be shining on both of us 2nite

Bridget: time out

BoBoy: not great, huh?

Bridget: no, it's fine, but. k, this just reminds me that we r on different sides of the ocean. u have 2 pretend we're together

BoBoy: ah. right

Bridget: k, take my hand

BoBoy: nice hand

Bridget: thank u. anything else?

BoBoy: um, k. yr hand, when u touch my face

Bridget: what part of yr face?

BoBoy: when u touch my cheek, yr fingers r soft as... butterfly wings

Bridget: nice start. go on

BoBoy: i kiss the fingers

Bridget: 1 by 1?

BoBoy: 1 by 1, and they taste, um, like cream and summer peaches

Bridget: mmm. let's go somewhere... somewhere safe

BoBoy: what? oh right. let's c

Bridget: and call me angel

BoBoy: come with me, my angel. come with me where the trees will protect us. c their limbs reach down like arms around... er... around our true luv

Bridget: very nice

BoBoy: i think i read that somewhere

Bridget: mmm, it still counts. keep going

BoBoy: dang. this is hard. k

it's so quiet here in the, uh... safety of the trees. just the softest breeze moving the flowers

moving them gently as my fingers stroke through yr hair

yr, um, auburn hair

and the air is cool, but yr lips r warm and sweet

bridge?

bridget?

Bridget: hmm?

BoBoy: where'd u go?

Bridget: what? i'm here

BoBoy: i thought u got lost in the trees, dude

Bridget: :) no, i was here. u were doing great

BoBoy: hmm

Bridget: what?

BoBoy: does this happen with... him—the english dude i'm starting 2 hate?

Bridget: lol. u mean, like does he ever think i got lost?

BoBoy: in a way

Bridget: maybe sometimes

BoBoy: really. hmm, k, let's think. where r yr hands right now? in this pretend world, i mean

Bridget: dunno. on yr shoulders?

BoBoy: so u don't really notice? k, when u start 2 get that fluttery feeling, do u sort of leave yr body?

Bridget: more like i go inside and just feel everything. i don't really know what i'm doing

BoBoy: like fainting

Bridget: a little, yeah

BoBoy: and u get real quiet and just feel everything happening

Bridget: maybe. why?

BoBoy: hmm. now i don't want 2 tell u, because it might help u get along with him ;-)

Bridget: u r so totally in my clutches, southern boy...

BoBoy: i'm a goner. but see, what i know is that u don't need 2 be more passionate, bridge

Bridget: i don't?

BoBoy: not at all. what u need is just 2 let. him. know.

Bridget: but how?

BoBoy: well, it's not that tricky. first, u probably hold off the fainting feeling a little longer

Bridget: why?

BoBoy: well, so u can hold his face, stroke his hair

Bridget: oic. duh me

BoBoy: whisper and moan

Bridget: really???

BoBoy: totally. bite, scratch. anything, really. am i being too forward?

Bridget: no i get it. yeah, wow, ur right. that's what i need 2 do

BoBoy: actually, no, i take it back. u should go totally still. cross yr arms and go stiff as a board

Bridget: lol

BoBoy: then when he breaks up with u, call me first thing

Bridget: ur a sweet guy, beau. <sigh>

BoBoy: not really

Bridget: oh yes ur. and beau?

BoBoy: yes, ma'am?

Bridget: well. what if i break up with the english chap and come after u right now?

BoBoy: be still my heart :) but seriously, u know i'm spoken 4. i'm totally gone on this girl. plus, she'd flat kill me if she knew i'd been taking romance lessons from u

Bridget: lol. and giving me kissing lessons...

BoBoy: that, too. woof. u won't tell, will u?

Bridget: yr secret's safe.... but i'm a little bit serious, beau. i like u a lot. we could work

BoBoy: aw man. that's really too nice 4 words, bridge, but no can do

Bridget: don't forget i'm coming 2 the states in the fall

BoBoy: try and find me

Bridget: oh, i'll find u. and don't hide behind yr girlfriend, u poof

BoBoy: lol

Bridget: seriously though. u know what we could be

BoBoy: i do, but bridge, please. u gotta stop saying this stuff

Bridget: ur right. sorry

BoBoy: but it's nice.... really nice <sigh>

Bridget: <sigh> call me angel 1 more time?

missing

THE DAWG HOUSE

JUNE 10 8:30 PM

chessman has entered

chessman: dude

BoBoy: yo, wattup?

chessman: hey, you haven't heard from tamra have you?

BoBoy: not a word, bro

chessman: yeah

BoBoy: u?

chessman: nah

BoBoy: what IS it with them?

chessman: really

BoBoy: i mean does a cell phone not work in freakin florida?

chessman: sure, but you can't use em in a hospital

BoBoy: yeah, it like imbues the machines or something

chessman: but don't they ever leave to eat?

BoBoy: zackly

chessman: yeah

BoBoy: i leave her voice mail... "miss u" "call me"... i text her... "miss u" "call me"

chessman: really? me too

BoBoy: and what do we get back?

chessman: we get silence

BoBoy: we get squat

chessman: zackly

BoBoy: i'm starting 2 get tired of this

chessman: i saw annie at the video store

BoBoy: yeah?

chessman: she says she hasn't heard either

BoBoy: well that's something

chessman: i guess

BoBoy: this whole thing stinks

chessman: you're getting pissed aren't you?

BoBoy: nah... yeah... a little

chessman: what's a guy to do?

BoBoy: women...

chessman: can't live with em

BoBoy: can't shoot em

chessman: heh

BoBoy: don't want 2 be a johnson

chessman: mr. "summer love, perhaps"

BoBoy: though i gotta say it's tempting...

chessman: yeah, well, easy for a babe magnet to say

BoBoy: get real. the babes r after u. open yr eyes

chessman: lol. if i knew any babes personally, i wouldn't know what to say

BoBoy: dude, u work too hard. just say "hey, u got plans 2nite? i'm dying to see XYZ movie." keep it casual. that's how i met T

chessman: really?

BoBoy: totally. then "wanna see it with me?" close the deal

chessman: "not if you were the last geek on earth..."

BoBoy: lol. then u say, yo, my friend beau tanner's going

chessman: excellent. exploit my football connection

BoBoy: use the network, my dawg

chessman: annie said she got one text from bliss's mom's phone

BoBoy: her mom's phone?

chessman: yeah, it was, like, our phones are still at the house; can you tell the guys?

BoBoy: right. they forgot their cell phones...

chessman: i know

BoBoy: both of them...

chessman: i know

BoBoy: and then they text annie instead of us

chessman: i know

BoBoy: it's a bogus story

chessman: maybe

BoBoy: no dude, it's bogus. it's off the bogosity meter

chessman: could be. but annie showed me their phones. she's gotta mail them down there

BoBoy: annie has their phones...

chessman: yep

BoBoy: bro, it's too hard 4 me 2 figure out, but there's something going on here

chessman: you feeling something?

BoBoy: totally. hey, remember the time we all got busted 4 smoking in the boy's room?

chessman: what about it?

BoBoy: when bartolo caught us, remember what johnson said?

chessman: he said, "i wasn't smokin..."

BoBoy: "the room was full of smoke and i just breathed that in..."

chessman: lol

BoBoy: THAT'S bogosity

chessman: not even bartolo could keep a straight face

BoBoy: bogus like ms. T without her cell

chessman: or bliss. sure. i getcha

BoBoy: what else did annie say?

chessman: nothing really. like, don't worry, bliss's mom probably has her busy all the time. stuff like that

BoBoy: what? like her granny died? they're planning a funeral?

chessman: annie didn't know. she's sending the phones

BoBoy: dude, u know... it's like... if they wanted 2 go away 2 gurls-only camp for 3 weeks, why not just say so?

chessman: so you think they're lying?

BoBoy: i dunno.... nah. T doesn't lie

chessman: yeah, and why WOULD they?

BoBoy: right. so i dunno

chessman: well...

BoBoy: yeah

chessman: yeah...

BoBoy: hey, u got plans 2nite? i'm dying 2 do the chat room...

chessman: lol. get away, you slut

BoBoy: seriously. that tatiana's fierce, bro. what's it like having her hit on u?

chessman: don't look at me. i'm innocent

BoBoy: sure, u just breathed...

chessman: seriously, i don't need the trouble

BoBoy: u mean with bliss? the missing bliss?

chessman: sure. but also when tatiana comes here this fall... i dunno... i mean, i like her, but...

BoBoy: really? i can't wait 2 meet bridget

chessman: i dunno... i want to meet her
and everything, but tatiana's...
complicated

BoBoy: come on. u like complicated

chessman: yes, but... whoa

BoBoy: she's a challenge

chessman: that's the truth...

BoBoy: ur just not used 2 a woman who can keep up
with u

chessman: more like a step ahead of me. but
seriously, i don't think i can do
the whole "cat's away" thing

BoBoy: like the johnson thing? sure. but how do we know
the women aren't doing that?

chessman: but until we do know, can you see
getting involved?

BoBoy: it's just online, bro

chessman: yeah but hooking up online probably
counts

BoBoy: bliss and T will never pin it on us

chessman: how come?

BoBoy: seriously, how r they gonna find out?

chessman: i dunno.... things always get found
out

BoBoy: know what i think, bro?

chessman: what?

BoBoy: i think ur just freaked because tatiana came on
2 u

chessman: heh heh, that too...

BoBoy: lighten up, dawg. this could be good 4 u

chessman: yeah...

BoBoy: **it's summer. don't imbue trouble**

chessman: lol. sure. i could be making too
much of it

BoBoy: **zackly. lighten up**

chessman: will do. btw, when's your birthday?

BoBoy: **july 2. why?**

chessman: i'm going to get you a new
dictionary

CHAPTER 16
philosophy

alfonso has entered

alfonso: ok, nobody gets ahead of us this time. we r totally on top of it. gonna move these pinheads like puppets on a string. like pawns on a chessboard. mwaa ha ha!

except that mitch is the chessmaster. hmm. and beau is his knight enforcer. at my best, i could never...

but it's just a figure of speech. too much fretting about metaphors. jeeze, that tamra girl and her peaches. can't we enjoy a victimless word crime anymore? of course we can

gotta love her, though. what conviction, what willpower, what ferocity. i'm actually starting 2 see things her way then there's bliss, bless her little tea cup. who'd a thunk there was so much 2 her? not my type, but u know. credit where due

and annie dearest. if only if only if only. may i die in her arms—is that so much 2 ask? her massive, merciless, amazon arms. ahhhh... crunch

oh, i'm so hopeless. slapslapslap. thanks captain, i needed that

✉ IM from gothling

gothling: johnson, u weasel, u shlump, u nancy boy

alfonso: the voice of my beloved! btw, those epithets don't work together

gothling: why not? i like em

alfonso: sorry, not good. with weasel, u go with something sneaky and craven—2 match weasel. like, "johnson, u weasel, u serpent, u sycophant." see?

gothling: u show-off! "craven" and "sycophant"—2 words i don't know in 1 sentence! don't ever do that 2 a woman... not while she's insulting u

alfonso: i kneel before u. please 2 forgive

gothling: i think not. so r we ready 2 go? anyone there yet?

alfonso: i came early

gothling: wish i could watch

alfonso: yeah, well. da boyz would see u, duh... but i'll IM u with constant updates, dearest, sealed with a kiss

gothling: eww. where those lips have been. anyway, keep me posted. i'm just watching tube

---

EXCHANGE STUDENT ROOM **UNION HIGH SCHOOL**

JUNE 10 11:00 PM

Tatiana has entered

Tatiana: i am the first one here tonight?

alfonso: yes, ur. except for yrs truly

Tatiana: evening, johnson

alfonso: actually, i'm glad we have a moment. i wanted 2 apologize again for my thoughtlessness in the past

Tatiana: you're fine, J. let it go. i should thank you for being a sport about the name. i was strung out—it makes me rude

alfonso: not at all. i was thinking a moment ago how persuasive ur on all this

Tatiana: persuasive

alfonso: yes, quite. i catch myself seeing things more and more yr way. unexpected

Tatiana: well. i don't know what to say. thanks, johnson.

chessman has entered

chessman: i'm alive, i'm alive. and i won't
disappear this time

alfonso: yo mitchie. welcome u geek-weasel, u snake.
if u slither off this time, u will pay thru yr beady
little eyes

chessman: lol. u do have a way, johnson. i
don't care what brittney says

Tatiana: mitchell, hallo

chessman: hey tatiana. everything ok with you?

Tatiana: i think so. for why do you ask?

chessman: the storm. i've been checking the
weather in the adriatic, and it
looks pretty fierce

Tatiana: right. yes, the storm

chessman: your family ok?

Tatiana: very fine. things may look worse on the
radar maps than here on the earth. is
that how you say? "on the earth"?

chessman: on the ground?

Tatiana: oh yes. ground. a funny word

chessman: wow. i'm glad. because they were
saying the power is out all over
greece and albania. i didn't really
expect to see you here

Tatiana: the power? i'm not sure i know this...

alfonso: he means electricity. mitch, she was just telling
me that the electric has been off and on all nite

chessman: oic

alfonso: it may cut out again at any time. tatiana,
we're all quite relieved that ur safe

Tatiana: how kind. yes my family are quite fine.
and mitchell, it is so grand to think of
you thinking of me. i am all smiling

chessman: aw, well...

Tatiana: i have told my family how good you
are to me

alfonso: get out. yr mother and everyone? u told them
about mitch?

Tatiana: mother, of course. father and brothers.
all are quite hoping for me to meet a wealthy,
handsome american to take me
out their hands one day :)

alfonso: lol

chessman: heh. i hope you do too

Tatiana: it could be you, if you play the card properly
;-)

chessman: sadly, my friend, i've given up cards :-)

Tatiana: alas

BoBoy has entered

BoBoy: finally made it, yo

alfonso: bubba, there ur. we thought u were bailing
on us 2nite

BoBoy: not me. just a busy evening. yo mitch. yo tatiana

chessman: hey

BoBoy: johnson behaving himself?

alfonso: tsk tsk, let's not go there

BoBoy: is bridget not here yet?

alfonso: haven't seen her

Tatiana: are you so worried that she would be missing?

BoBoy: oh not really. just asking

Tatiana: i should be jealous

alfonso: he's concerned about her. bridget is usually right on time

Tatiana: i see. pardon me for thinking one woman could handle a gang of young geese like you 3

alfonso: sweet. she's jealous that she'd have 2 share us

chessman: lol, tatiana

BoBoy: geese, i like that

✉ IM from alfonso

alfonso: tatiana—i mean, tamra. what's the trouble?

Ms.T: what do you mean?

alfonso: ur pissed. r u and bliss still fighting?

Ms.T: maybe

alfonso: have u spoken 2 each other since the other nite?

Ms.T: not so much

alfonso: oh, gurl, this is trouble

Ms.T: why?

EXCHANGE STUDENT ROOM **UNION HIGH SCHOOL**

alfonso: know what, beau? do u mind buzzing bridget?
              just 2 see if she's home

BoBoy: sure. can do

Tatiana: oh, fine. go and chase the english

✉ IM from alfonso

alfonso: T, listen. u need 2 let go. i know it isn't easy

Ms.T: let go? i don't need to let her shag my boyfriend

alfonso: she's only playing a role. just like ur

Ms.T: i think she's doing more than that

alfonso: i REALLY don't agree. she's yr best best best
friend, and u can trust her

Ms.T: like you would know about trust

alfonso: ???

Ms T: i'm sorry, johnson. that was totally out of
line, and you've been so nice to me

alfonso: ur fine

Ms.T: seriously, i'm sorry. i know i'm too mad.
i know it. and i know it isn't her fault, but it's getting
out of hand. i just hate not having good options.
i think i want out

alfonso: not good, T. u don't wanna do that

Ms.T: yes, i think i do. i'm miserable

alfonso: ok, but look. if u get out, that means cancel the whole game, lose the bet 2 annie, and fess up 2 da boyz. u want that?

Ms.T: why is that the only way? i could just have the power go out in albania. oh! oh! it's flickering right now!

alfonso: whatever. i'm not here 2 argue. but c, if the power goes out, then annie comes in with her magic wand and lights up everything. presto—u become a loser, and da boyz get away scott-free

Ms.T: arrgh

alfonso: u can do this T. i know u can. just play it out

Ms.T: double arrgh

alfonso: that's the spirit. buck up, soldier. and hey...

Ms.T: what?

alfonso: there's a great way to get revenge on bliss... and on beau

Ms.T: i know i know i know. I KNOW. but really. oh, ARRRRRGH. puff puff. ok, sarge, i'm going back in!

alfonso: that's it. go get em, gurl

✉ IM from BoBoy

BoBoy: bridget? hello good evening?

Bridget: oh goodness, it's u

BoBoy: hey gurl, what up? u coming 2 the chat room?

Bridget: i dunno. i'm scared

BoBoy: really? scared of what?

BoBoy: bridget?

BoBoy: bridge? u still there?

Bridget: beau, i can't. i just can't. goodbye

Bridget is offline

BoBoy: bridge?

EXCHANGE STUDENT ROOM **UNION HIGH SCHOOL**

Tatiana: mitchell, i have question for you

chessman: fire away

Tatiana: what did your friend beau mean about "is johnson behaving himself"?

alfonso: tatiana, he was just messing with me. pay no attention

chessman: yeah, he was just kidding around

Tatiana: i don't believe you, mitchell. you are hiding something

chessman: well...

Tatiana: tatiana can tell when her darling is not saying truth

alfonso: oh dear oh dear oh dear

Tatiana: speak to me, mitchell. you know
i will find it

alfonso: u 2 have been chatting on the side, haven't u?

chessman: tatiana, it was really something
between me and beau and johnson.
i wouldn't be comfortable sharing
that without johnson's ok

Tatiana: it is about what we discussed? about
the horse?

alfonso: u can tell her, dude. she'll find out anyway

chessman: um, yeah. about that kind of stuff

Tatiana: i knew it! oh, mitchell, it is so thrilling
that you are my champion in america.
i am cover you with kisses. mwaa!

alfonso: man, this is 1 passionate chick. i mean,
woman. sorry?

BoBoy: well, group. bridget's not coming

Tatiana: really?

alfonso: what did she say?

BoBoy: said she's not coming. scared of something

alfonso: scared?

Tatiana: scared of what?

BoBoy: she wouldn't tell me. she's totally imbued

alfonso: come on! scared isn't gonna work. u can't
leave it there!!

Tatiana: please to excuse... my grandmama
calls in next room

alfonso: and dude?... imbued REALLY DOESN'T
MEAN WHAT U THINK IT DOES

chessman: oh let it go, johnson

alfonso: NOR CONTUMELIOUS! ALMOST NOTHING MEANS WHAT U THINK!!!

BoBoy: what i say? what i say?

chessman: johnson, chill. take a mozart pill

alfonso: arrrrgggghh. where's my pistol?

✉ IM from Ms.T

Ms.T: bliss taylor, you come out here this minute

bliss4u: shove off. u don't even like me

Ms.T: girl, i do too like you

bliss4u: go away!

Ms.T: you are my best best best friend

bliss4u: i'm leaving now

Ms.T: and i am here to apologize and grovel and whatever it takes

bliss4u: what's grovel? i don't know because i'm a MORON

Ms.T: it's begging, okay? i'm begging

bliss4u: begging is good...

Ms.T: bliss, i'm sorry. i was rude and angry and unfair. it was my fault entirely.

bliss4u: yes, that sounds like how i remember it

Ms.T: i'm sorry i'm sorry i'm sorry i'm sorry

bliss4u: well... u were mad about politics. that always gets u going

Ms.T: yes, and... to be more painfully honest, i was jealous

bliss4u: jealous

Ms.T: of you and Beau? helloo...

bliss4u: no way

Ms.T: oh gimme a BREAK. he totally likes you. i'm dying here

bliss4u: u think he likes me?

Ms.T: YES! the little slut puppy. i am SO going to make him pay when i get back to town

---

EXCHANGE STUDENT ROOM **UNION HIGH SCHOOL**

chessman: why are you all over bo? you think he can really make her come back??

alfonso: he's the only 1 with a shot

chessman: maybe she needs a night off. where's the harm?

alfonso: no, she's gotta be here. what did she say exactly, bubba?

 TXT to Johnson

June 10 11:28 pm
From: Gothling
yo J. ne thng gd?

TXT to gothling

June 10 11:30 pm
From: Johnson
crazy. will IM u in a min

EXCHANGE STUDENT ROOM **UNION HIGH SCHOOL**

BoBoy: she said "no way. i'm scared."
something like that

chessman: scared? i wonder what she's afraid of

BoBoy: she wouldn't talk about it

alfonso: aaarggggggghhh

BoBoy: NOW what? this guy is totally off his nut

chessman: it's his new leaf getting to him.
he's just not used to it

IM from Ms.T

Ms.T: and worse than that, mitch is like impervious.

bliss4u: that's good, right?

Ms.T: for you, maybe. i'm totally throwing myself at him,
and he's all um, that makes me uncomfortable, tatiana...

bliss4u: true luv. it's a beautiful thing

Ms.T: that's what i thought, and now look at me. i've turned into a harpy

bliss4u: oh honey. it'll be ok...

Ms.T: whatever. so you coming back?

bliss4u: i guess. sure

Ms.T: wait. i'll tell them to send beau again.

bliss4u: let him talk me into it?

Ms.T: that would be the general idea

bliss4u: hee hee. i'm such a player. bye

Ms.T: i will kill that boy

EXCHANGE STUDENT ROOM **UNION HIGH SCHOOL**

Tatiana: beau, perhap you should try again with the english. you were maybe not the man enough last time, lol?

BoBoy: not man enough?

Tatiana: you know. maybe the little stronger persuasion

BoBoy: what should i say?

Tatiana: say anything! slap her around, no?

chessman: she's kidding

Tatiana: sorry, not myself today. no slapping

✉ IM from alfonso

alfonso: rough night, peaches

gothling: what's rough?

alfonso: the women. they've gone all random on me

gothling: i'll talk 2 them

alfonso: no, u stay out

gothling: johnson, i'll talk 2 them

alfonso: it's under control. a natural phase they're going thru

gothling: what phase?

alfonso: i think it's called "i hate my best friend because i let her snog my boyfriend." u know that phase

gothling: not personally

alfonso: funny, that's not how i heard it...

gothling: don't push it, reptile boy. i know where u live

EXCHANGE STUDENT ROOM **UNION HIGH SCHOOL**

BoBoy: so i should like tell her she's being a baby?

Tatiana: oh, american men. have you no finesse?

chessman: be european, beau. threaten
          suicide ;-)

Tatiana: ah, well. an operatic gesture.
          but i was thinking simpler

BoBoy: **like what?**

Tatiana: make it personal! tell her YOU need
          her to come back. not the group, but you

BoBoy: **really?**

Tatiana: is true, is it not? you want to see her

BoBoy: **um? i guess so**

Tatiana: ach, you swine

BoBoy: **excuse me?**

chessman: rotfl. you dog! hyena!

Tatiana: mitchell, my darling. only you understand
          these thing. YOU must go to the english and
          bring her by the hand

chessman: me?

BoBoy: **no, that's kewl. i'll give it another shot**

Tatiana: there, you see? the boy beau loves her,
          not me at all

chessman: are you really jealous, tatiana?

Tatiana: mitchell, i am so alone in this world. to
          lose any chance at love is more than i
          can bear sometime

chessman: i'm sure you have many chances

Tatiana: if you will not look at me fondly, then i
          am truly to die alone

✉ IM from alfonso

alfonso: listen, annabelle. let me be very serious with u

gothling: this should be good

alfonso: remember what u said 2 me about britt?

gothling: i said u were wasting yrself

alfonso: zackly. and i felt that way about u— with what's-his-name

gothling: voldemort

alfonso: u were wasted on him, annie

gothling: hmmph

alfonso: ur so much more of a woman than he could ever appreciate. u have depth that he will never know or understand

gothling: whatever

alfonso: i want u 2 find a man who can sing yr worth 2 the stars

gothling: i suppose u have someone in mind?

alfonso: i might. do u have someone in mind 4 me?

annie?

annie, don't hide from me

gothling: ur way over the line, johnson. we'll discuss it later

alfonso: as u wish. <sigh>

chessman: tatiana, do u think beau really likes bridget?

Tatiana: but of course. see how he jump when i told YOU to talk to her?

chessman: true

Tatiana: is it a problem if he does?

chessman: well, it could be. he's got a girlfriend. a nice one

Tatiana: yes, racehorse girl

chessman: but he and bridget are only friends online. so maybe that's ok

Tatiana: no, it is NOT ok

chessman: but i mean they can't do anything, even if they do start to like each other

✉ IM from BoBoy

BoBoy: it's me again. angel?

Bridget: oh, it's u. i was hoping u would come back <sigh>

BoBoy: u were?

Bridget: bo, u have no idea how confused i am

BoBoy: ur?

Bridget: yes. i just can't get a grip

BoBoy: i'm sorry

Bridget: don't be sorry. it's not yr fault

BoBoy: oh. whew :)

Bridget: well, yes it is. in a way

BoBoy: no fair. how is it my fault?

Bridget: let's not talk about this now. we should go 2 the chat room

BoBoy: great. u changed yr mind

Bridget: i guess

BoBoy: everyone wants u 2 come

Bridget: everyone? what about u?

BoBoy: um? yes. me too

Bridget: just me too?

BoBoy: ok... me, most of all

Bridget: i'm blushing

BoBoy: take my hand. let's go back

EXCHANGE STUDENT ROOM UNION HIGH SCHOOL

Tatiana: can't do anything online? can they not fall in love?

chessman: i guess. but is that the same?
it's not like they can hook up in
real life

Tatiana: tell me, darling mitchell. you are such the
philosopher. would the girlfriend of beau
feel this way? that falling in love online is
not real life?

chessman: hmm. true

Tatiana: is love not real when it is online?

chessman: i guess it is

Tatiana: you are honest man. and this is why
you resist me so strongly, yes? because you
know online is real life too

chessman: i see you've thought this through

Tatiana: i think of nothing else since i meet you,
and that is the gods' truth

alfonso: well, what have we here? a regular coffee klatsch

chessman: yeah, kind of a philosophical
discussion i guess

BoBoy: hey hey. guess who came back with me

Bridget has entered

alfonso: excellent! we were so out of balance without u,
bridget

Tatiana: hallo hallo, darling. i am so happy you
are here

Bridget: well, ur a peach 2 say so, tatiana

BoBoy: uh oh

Tatiana: lol, pumpkin

alfonso: whew. i thought we were in trouble there

Tatiana: i laugh only because i don't know how to swear in english

alfonso: oh, mitch can give you private lessons when you get 2 america

Bridget: i'm sure mitchell doesn't curse ;-)

Tatiana: bridget darling, one question

Bridget: yes, girlfriend?

Tatiana: pumpkins are round and fat, are they not?

suicide

GURLGANG ROOM

JUNE 11 5:20 PM

gothling:	**seems like yr boy beau has his mind on england an awful lot, heh heh. u ready 2 concede the bet?**
Ms.T:	his mind wanders. big deal
gothling:	**it will be l8r**
bliss4u:	if annie wants 2 quit now, let's do, so we win! i'm desperate 2 get mitchie back
gothling:	**not a chance**
Ms.T:	so what are you saying, bliss? you tired of beau already? you hussy ;-)
bliss4u:	funny thing is, i never expected 2 like him, but he's awesome. really really nice. i mean, i like him as bridget, of course... he makes me laugh

Ms.T: he IS awesome, but i'm so disappointed in him. i thought he'd see right through you. funny or not, he's a chump

gothling: told ya

Ms.T: i could snatch him bald-headed

bliss4u: well, wait. he isn't like madly in love or anything. nothing unforgivable. he's only being nice

gothling: oh it still counts. she can kill him anytime now

Ms.T: actually no, bliss is right. let's not be in contumelious haste

bliss4u: lol. he is so cute when he says stuff like that

Ms.T: i know. awww. i hate him

gothling: k, come on. what's he actually saying 2 bridget? give us the goods

bliss4u: i blush 2 repeat...

Ms.T: whatever

bliss4u: well... k, here's 1 strange thing that happened. i was actually all worried about tatiana—being such a passionate bee-yotch and all? and thinking that mitch was so unhappy with me

gothling: oh, yeah. "maybe he'd like a little spanking." that stuff. the strong woman stuff

bliss4u: c, and that's u and tam. i am totally not like that. so i got all worried that mitchie thought i was not, u know, passionate

Ms.T: darling, your mitchell is utterly devoted. i will never break him down

bliss4u: <sigh> but anyway, so i have bridget say 2 beau that her boyfriend in england thinks the same thing—like "oh, his friend told me that he thinks i'm cold, whatever will i do?" and stuff like that

gothling: **gurl, nice work. play the sympathy card why dontcha?**

Ms.T: it works every time on that bozo. jeeze.
<slap my worried brow>

bliss4u: it DOES work on him! i luv that. oh, and he's all, how awful, what could be wrong? like he wants 2 fix everything so i'll be happy with my boyfriend again. it's sweet, tam. ur so lucky

Ms.T: grrrr. and i was mad that he has bridget in his buddy list

bliss4u: but k, so bridget's boyfriend—beau calls him "that english dude i'm starting to hate." lol

Ms.T: oh very cute. shut up, annie. i can hear you laughing

bliss4u: anyway, so i sorta tell him how it goes when we're making out and stuff. and i'm, like, now why would he think i'm cold??

gothling: **wait. really? how DOES it go?**

bliss4u: ooo, i get all fluttery inside and everything. like i nearly pass out every time. it's totally exciting

gothling: **so i don't get it**

bliss4u: no, c, that's the problem. i'm all trembly and quiet, so mitchie thinks i don't like it when i totally do.

Ms.T: <groan> so now you get advice from beau on how to snog with mitchell

bliss4u: yeah. heh. so he says ok, basically, to fight off the fluttery stuff... just do anything...

Ms.T: do anything...

bliss4u: be wild. scratch him, bite him, whisper and moan and carry on like. so he knows! THEN u can pass out

Ms.T:	oh jeeze oh jeeze oh pete <sigh>
bliss4u:	nice, huh? i'm gonna try it
gothling:	**i wonder where he came up with those ideas...** **any theories, ms. T?**
Ms.T:	i'll just be going now. i have an appointment with mr. death
bliss4u:	what?
gothling:	**lol. and really, such excellent advice:** **whisper, moan... bite & scratch**
bliss4u:	oh no... u mean...
gothling:	**rotfl. let me catch my breath**
bliss4u:	how embarrassing. i'm sorry, tam
Ms.T:	bliss, you've met my former friend annie, haven't you?
gothling:	**whew. that was wonderful**
Ms.T:	i plan to kill her right after i kill myself
bliss4u:	i am so sorry, tam
gothling:	**okokokok**
bliss4u:	i had no clue
gothling:	**so bubba is indiscreet but basically harmless.** **how about the nerd patrol? what u got, tam?**
Ms.T:	<sigh sigh sigh> nothing. abso-bloody-lutely nothing. mitchell is the soul of devotion to his girl. i would despise him if he weren't so freakin cute about it all
gothling:	**oh, get a grip, camper. there must be something**
bliss4u:	no, i'm ok just how she left it =)
Ms.T:	there must be something? ok: he's willing to be my "friend"—tatiana's friend. how's that? pretty juicy, huh?

gothling: **there's more, or ur not trying**

Ms.T: arrgh. let me think. ok i know he LIKES tatiana. he follows the weather in albania. reads up on the history and everything. i'm on the web all the time just trying to stay ahead of him. but it's SO far from romance. it's like a really interesting homework assignment to him

bliss4u: no that sounds just like mitchie. he's the most sincere guy i've ever met

Ms.T: i hate him.... actually, no. now don't get me wrong bliss, but i could totally see it working with mitch. he's got stuff going on

bliss4u: stuff?

Ms.T: you should know. it's like i've only seen the surface of mitch before. that boy has soul... but that's probably why i can't budge him off his gurl....

gothling: **come on. u gotta lead him on. where's yr womanly wiles??**

Ms.T: i DO lead him on. i flirt shamelessly. i order him around. i make him apologize for his friends. i call him darling. i pout. i whine. i abuse him. i sweet-talk him. <sigh> nothing. nothing. i'm a failure as a woman

bliss4u: oh, sweetie

Ms.T: i'm nothing compared to bliss. is it all because you have bigger pompoms?

bliss4u: lol

gothling: **there must be some way 2 get at him. did u try helpless? lonely?**

Ms.T: he helps. he talks. that's it

gothling: **the direct approach?**

Ms.T: i was passionate, alluring, i was poetic

gothling: hmmm

Ms.T: haven't tried terminal illness...

gothling: ahhh. k, how bout suicide?

Ms.T: excuse me???

gothling: suicide. it's worth a try

bliss4u: oh that is totally unfair

gothling: drastic measures are called 4

Ms.T: couldn't i just get a tumor?

gothling: suicide suicide

bliss4u: no way

gothling: u know he won't let u jump off an albanian cliff

Ms.T: that's just humiliating

gothling: even halfway round the world, it's gotta work

bliss4u: so obvious

Ms.T: really

gothling: i'm not hearing better ideas...

bliss4u: come on! it is totally not fair. mitchie would freak. he would die of hurt

gothling: i rest my case

Ms.T: interesting

bliss4u: arrrrgh. u people

Ms.T: very interesting

bliss4u: besides, tatiana would never pull a stunt like that. threaten suicide?? are u kidding?

Ms.T: tatiana is feel so alone right now. she say this very thing to mitchell...

bliss4u: don't call him that

gothling: she's vulnerable

Ms.T: she's lonely. so lonely

bliss4u: but but... she has a boyfriend

Ms.T: actually, he's away right now. and you know italian men...

bliss4u: ackack

gothling: so she's desperate. yes, and this sincere american boy is all that stands between her and certain death by a broken heart

bliss4u: ur so twisted

gothling: why?

bliss4u: because it's cheating. and tatiana isn't shameless and weak like that

gothling: why can't she be? bridget's a ho. who'd a predicted that?

bliss4u: shut up, annie

Ms.T: oh now u insulted bridget

gothling: why is she mad? it's only a character

bliss4u: bridget is not ONLY a character

gothling: r u losing yr mind? i do not get this girl

bliss4u: she's MY character, and she's not a ho

Ms.T: well, but she IS after my beau

bliss4u: my character. my creation. not like some mask i'll throw away when i'm tired of her

gothling: oh dear oh dear

bliss4u: i LIKE her. i made her and i like her

Ms.T: i know, bliss

gothling: **but she IS a mask. that's exactly what she is**

bliss4u: annie can't feel like this about her uncle jerry whozit, the scout leader preacher card-reader redneck from maryland

gothling: **minnesota**

bliss4u: and that's nobody's fault but yr own. if u weren't so repressed, maybe u could luv someone too

Ms.T: whoa whoa. time out sister

gothling: **whatever. i didn't know she could type this fast**

bliss4u: so frigid

Ms.T: ok, kids, let's don't go there

gothling: **actually i'm pleased that she knows the word "repressed"**

Ms.T: annie, chill

gothling: **what?**

Ms.T: you're getting your iron vest on. there's no need

bliss4u: i can MAKE her a ho, if that's what everyone wants

Ms.T: nobody wants that, bliss

bliss4u: bridget, u a bitch ho

what? no, i most certainly am not

yes. they say u a english ho now

k, if i a ho, i better shake this booty all up in that bubba face

gothling: **gurl, that is SO bad**

Ms.T: bridget, would u go back 2 being a nice english girl?

bliss4u: make up yr mind

Ms.T: we were just talking about getting to mitch.
             if you don't like suicide, we have to think of
             something else

bliss4u: why doesn't annie just admit that mitch is
             not gettable, and we call it a day?

**gothling: look, prissy, u agreed to the terms. u put yrself in
             my hands 2 c if u can trust him. u can't just rule out
             anything that makes u feel threatened**

bliss4u: but this is an unfair trick

gothling: so u don't trust him after all?

Ms.T: ok, whatever. how about this... bliss doesn't
             get to rule out anything, but i'm not saying i'll
             do it either

gothling: oh, gurl, u don't have a chance without it

Ms.T: there's lots we haven't tried. i'll work on it

**gothling: look, i'm calling the shots here. u guys agreed
             2 this**

Ms.T: let's ask johnson

bliss4u: what?

Ms.T: let's ask johnson. he'll have ideas

gothling: hmm. i'm feeling chilly toward johnson right now

bliss4u: actually, that's not a bad idea

Ms.T: it's a great idea. i'll go talk to him

gothling: wait a minute

bliss4u: we'll both go, if annie's mad at him

**gothling: just settle down. i'll talk 2 johnson. u lil campers
             aren't cut out 4 this**

bliss4u: we can all talk 2 him

gothling: I'LL do it, and i'll do it alone. he's not 2 be trusted with u

Ms.T: whatever

gothling: but no guarantees

bliss4u: sure, but why can't we all go?

gothling: and if he says suicide, then that's it. understood?

Ms.T: suits me

bliss4u: he won't. i know he won't like the suicide idea

gothling: we'll just see what he says. but remember, i'm still in charge

CHAPTER 18
wounds

📧 IM from gothling

JUNE 11 7:09 PM

gothling: johnson, we have 2 talk

alfonso: at yr service, miss. as always

gothling: tamra's running out of steam with the chessman. u gotta do something

alfonso: but lovey, why me?

gothling: dude, i thought u were like this grand puppeteer

alfonso: i can't work miracles

gothling: u were this colossus, this wizard of the heart

alfonso: if yr puppet has no imagination, it's hardly my fault

gothling: the fault is with YR puppet, pal, not mine

alfonso: lil mitchie-poo? what's he done?

gothling: nothing! that's the problem!

alfonso: well, what has she tried?

gothling: everything

alfonso: flirtation?

gothling: constantly

alfonso: humor? despair?

gothling: yes...

alfonso: wit? abuse? helplessness?

gothling: been there, done those

alfonso: mystery? lechery?

gothling: everything, johnson

alfonso: oh mitchell <sigh>

gothling: he has 2 get with the program

alfonso: sad sad sad. and tatiana is such a fox, too. such a mezzo

gothling: i know! isn't she great?

alfonso: the passion, the bad accent, the brazen flirting

gothling: the lurking sadness

alfonso: well, u can't really say "lurking" with "sadness"

gothling: lurk is what i said. her sadness lurks

alfonso: it does, eh? hmm

gothling: behind her bright exterior lurks a gloomy, gloomy... gloom

alfonso: well, sadness doesn't lurk, but k, yes, she's been seriously dark. hmm, yeah. we could work with that

gothling: good, but how?

alfonso: u know what? tell her 2 go all gypsy on him!

gothling: all gypsy?

alfonso: gurl, it's perfect. darkness and destiny, passion and pulchritude.... oh! OH! get her reading the cards 4 him

gothling: kewl. yes. great idea

alfonso: ach. no! not for him—how silly of me—4 HERSELF

gothling: u lost me there

alfonso: k, the source of her foreboding, her enclosing (not lurking) sadness, the source EVEN of her passion 4 life, lurks (lurks!) within the dark clouds of her own destiny. a destiny that she reads... where, gypsy gurl?

gothling: oh i like...

alfonso: u see? i do have 1 or 2 things going 4 me

gothling: ur a surprising guy, johnson. i won't deny it

alfonso: and i'll work on mitch. he needs some prep 4 this. i'll have to accidentally know something about tatiana

gothling: some dark secret?

alfonso: some dark and terrible secret

gothling: some dark terrible operatic secret?

alfonso: destiny is unjust... yes, i can totally get mitch going with this.... plus the whole card thing. keep it vague and dark. yeah. mitch will buy this

gothling: if he doesn't, we're going 4 suicide

alfonso: oh, please. like what? "say u love me, or i kill myself"?

gothling: what's wrong with that?

alfonso: it's not terribly inventive, is it?

gothling: well, if he's too dense 2 go 4 yr pretty stories, we have 2 give him something blunt and obvious

alfonso: sure. k whatever.

but annabelle... i mean...

suppose he does understand, but he's just totally committed to bliss? think about it. kinda sweet in a way

gothling: impossible

alfonso: u don't know men

gothling: yes, i do

alfonso: <gurgle> scuse me while i count to 10... k. annie dear?

gothling: what?

alfonso: k, yes u do. u know a great deal about men. about women too. but sometimes there r matches that just work. they just do

gothling: oh please

alfonso: i know it's corny, i know it's old-fashioned, but some people r willing 2 pass up all offers and save their hearts 4 that special someone

gothling: johnson, that's romantic hogwash. guys r all alike. they're all horn dawgs. just like u, dear, only not as honest

alfonso: i'm telling u. even guys like me would give it all up 4 the girl of their dreams

gothling: u can't ask a compass not 2 point north

alfonso: annabelle, u know SO much about the heart. but ur counting a lot on 1 bad experience

gothling: darling. sweetie. sweetie darling: shut up

alfonso: my word as an opera buff. it's possible 2 dwell too long on 1 tragedy

gothling: johnson, let's don't, k?

alfonso: annie, what he did 2 u, what she did—that doesn't have 2 ruin yr life

gothling: we r not talking about this

alfonso: doll, u need 2 talk

gothling: no. she was my best friend, johnson, got it? if u HAD any friends u would understand

alfonso: i know i know. but annie, maybe it's time 2 try again

gothling: we are NOT talking about it, johnson. ur way over the line, u hear me?

alfonso: <sigh>

gothling: finish about mitch. then i'm going

alfonso: ah yes, mitch! said johnson, closing the wound, fixing his tie...

gothling: j-man, don't do this, bro...

alfonso: so mitch! the pitch 2 mitch. mitch needs a pitch. mitch needs a picture, actually. let's paint him something plain. something he can see without his glasses

gothling: yeah, he's not totally clear on the mysteries of luv

alfonso: unlike u and me, right?

gothling: stop it

alfonso: well, not 2 worry. i'll take care of it. he needs more opera in his life. but hey, beau told me some very interesting stuff

gothling: what?

alfonso: turns out bridget's "english" boyfriend can woo her quite well. she told beau all about it

gothling: like what?

alfonso: like, oh, how about:

> come away my dove, and
> let us seek the loving trees,
> where breeze and blossom will conspire
> to take our passion higher and higher.

not as good as that, because that's 1 of mine. but the point is, ol' mitch is a romantic. who'd'a thunk?

gothling: gag me. that was like a glass of syrup

alfonso: really? that was from the poem i promised u. nature, elegance, nice internal rhymes? not?

gothling: i'm thinking not

alfonso: rats. i spent 6 whole minutes on that

gothling: johnson, now that wounds ME. it's not that i totally WANT yr attention, but i'd like 2 believe i'm worth more than 6 MEASLY MINUTES OF A HIGH SCHOOL POET'S TIME

alfonso: annabelle, my sweet...

gothling: what?

alfonso: ur worth a whole lifetime of high school poetry

mediterranean

THE DAWG HOUSE

JUNE 13 9:00 PM

BoBoy: yo mitch

chessman: zup?

BoBoy: nothin really

chessman: yeah me too

BoBoy: u heard from bliss?

chessman: i wish

BoBoy: me too

chessman: i dunno

BoBoy: what?

chessman: nah. well

ok, sometimes i wonder if this
could actually be her way of breaking
up? like she couldn't tell me to
my face, but she maybe wants to see
other people. i dunno

BoBoy: **so she just goes away**

chessman: i guess

BoBoy: **yeah**

chessman: but i don't really think it's true

BoBoy: **no**

chessman: just wonder sometimes

BoBoy: **me too. i get a bad feeling about it sometimes**

chessman: but dude, ms. T would tell u
straight out if she wants to see
other people. she would do that

BoBoy: **so why doesn't she?**

chessman: zackly. why?

BoBoy: **right**

chessman: so, in a way, that's good

BoBoy: **it's good that she doesn't tell me?**

chessman: because you know if she had
something to say, she'd say it

BoBoy: **what? oh. which totally means she doesn't feel
like that**

chessman: because she hasn't told you

BoBoy: **that's brilliant, debater dude**

chessman: well, it's an argument from silence,
but it's all we've got right now

alfonso has entered

alfonso: word up, dudes

chessman: zup J?

BoBoy: **word**

alfonso: gentlemen, u will be pleased 2 hear that i am totally
            getting used 2 this single dude status

chessman: seriously?

alfonso: (which u so unkindly imposed without my
            consent—and don't think i'll ever forget it)

BoBoy: **ur liking it? get real**

alfonso: no, i mean it. best thing i've ever done. i am
            feeling... what's the word... purged, i guess

BoBoy: **purged**

alfonso: purged of unwanted karma. i am totally finding
            myself—who i am, what i need, what i don't need

chessman: who'd a thunk it? so what don't you
            need?

alfonso: women! the need is gone

chessman: get real

alfonso: i feel like 1 of those old dudes who go 2 the
            desert 2 live in a hole or something

BoBoy: **a hermit**

alfonso: zackly. they like sit in a cave all naked and
            don't talk 2 anyone. stay alive on bugs and pure
            thoughts

chessman: subsistence living

BoBoy: **kewl. so have u subsided now?**

alfonso: um?

BoBoy: **that's beautiful, J**

chessman: but, johnson, you talk to people.
you eat. you don't meditate. you're
no desert monk

alfonso: that's not the point, nerdman.
even without all that, u boys have put me on the
edge, the very edge, of privation

chessman: oic. you're deprived of women.
well, that's cool. a sacrifice

BoBoy: wow. so yr mind is like razor sharp these days?

alfonso: i am experiencing clarity like never before

BoBoy: kewl. we shoulda thought of this a long time
ago, mitchie

alfonso: i'm also feeling compassion 4 others.
unexpected, truly

chessman: compassion! whoa. call a medic.
the boy is breaking down

BoBoy: compassion 4 who?

alfonso: well, i shouldn't...

chessman: oh, he's playing us

alfonso: nah. well, actually. k, i don't trust u, but it's annie

BoBoy: annie. i'm drawing a blank here, bro

alfonso: annie. i feel compassion 4 annie. duh??

chessman: i don't think beau knows annie's
story, J

BoBoy: what story?

alfonso: ah, now i c. sorry, dude. the new me is sorry

chessman: beau, the thing with annie is that
she had this boyfriend. i knew him
from somewhere. but he was totally
not right for her

BoBoy: but really, who would be?

alfonso: what do u mean? i can think of 1 or 2

BoBoy: dude, she's totally goth and totally butch at the same time. she's an azore... no, that thing on the web

chessman: an amazon

alfonso: aw, man, she is not

chessman: don't say she's a peach, J. that ain't gonna work here

alfonso: she's hurt, that's all. can't u see that?

BoBoy: she's hurt...

alfonso: totally. u don't know what that dude did 2 her

BoBoy: what?

chessman: oh, it was cold. i heard it from bliss

alfonso: zackly. well, i mean, she's not the first it's happened 2, but annie's like this tower of strength and self-control and... and...

BoBoy: know-it-all-ness

chessman: lol. she totally does know everything—just ask her

alfonso: yeah, yeah. accepting dissent is not her strength

BoBoy: does she even know what that is?

alfonso: fine. we know she's hardball. that goes without saying

chessman: and she's bitter. never a kind word these days

alfonso: all right, fair enough. she's brusque. that's the 1 thing u can say against her, but here's my point

BoBoy:	**and she like has 2 control the conversation. every conversation**
alfonso:	true, k
chessman:	hostile?
BoBoy:	**defensive?**
chessman:	competitive
alfonso:	okokok. so she's hardheaded. she's a little arrogant, hostile, defensive, controlling, bitter, and butch. but aside from that, what has annie ever done 2 us?
BoBoy:	**contumelious?**
alfonso:	oh, shut up, bubba
chessman:	dude, i'm starting to think johnson likes annie
alfonso:	compassion where compassion's DUE. that's what i'm trying 2 say
chessman:	she was hurt bad
BoBoy:	**so what did the dude do 2 her?**
chessman:	bliss told me she swore off romance for a year
alfonso:	what he did, my brother, was hook up with her best friend
BoBoy:	**what? that can't be legal...**
chessman:	totally over the line
alfonso:	even i have never done that
BoBoy:	**her best friend. ouch. so that's why annie is worked all the time**
chessman:	i just don't tangle with her
alfonso:	it's a touching story, don't u think? almost an opera

BoBoy: nobody's heartless here, J

alfonso: that's what i'm talking about. compassion where due

chessman: she's a human being too

BoBoy: glad to hear it

chessman: johnson, you're really turning it over, aren't you? i have to say i'm surprised

alfonso: i'm not too proud to admit it

chessman: but well, so have you sworn off women?

alfonso: not totally, no. our deal is i'm free when the chat room is over. in the meanwhile, being the hermit is instructive. turns out i enjoy watching

BoBoy: yeah, i gotta try that sometime

chessman: we're practically monks lately, anyway

BoBoy: lol. hey, johnson, 1 question. u don't think bliss and ms. T r trying to ditch us, do u?

alfonso: dude, u know as much as i do

chessman: so no news through annie, you're saying?

alfonso: sometimes an absence is only an absence

BoBoy: seriously, what do u know?

alfonso: k, last i heard from annie was that bliss and tam were hoping to reappear, but no one knows when they'll make it

BoBoy: how come she can reach them and we can't?

alfonso: dude, u know women. they have ways

BoBoy: yeah

alfonso: but hey. speaking of women, have u heard from tatiana?

BoBoy: not me. i'm the bozo, remember? mitch is da man

chessman: oh right. what did you hear, johnson?

alfonso: well, she wrote me something kinda dark

BoBoy: what was it?

alfonso: actually, i'm a little worried about her

BoBoy: j-man, more compassion? now I'M worried

chessman: seriously, what's she saying?

alfonso: i don't know if u guys will totally believe me, because u think i have this like gothic imagination and stuff

chessman: well, you do, but give us a try

alfonso: altho i'm nothing compared 2 that girl's life

BoBoy: sure

alfonso: because she's like living in an opera, practically. u know how those people r

BoBoy: what people?

chessman: albanians

alfonso: actually, i meant all cultures of the mediterranean region

chessman: i stand corrected. please go on

alfonso: how to begin?... k, as we know, in her country, there r the rich, there r the poor, and there r gypsies. and of course these groups never mix. so it is totally out of the question for a gypsy 2 aspire 2 riches. a poor man would never hope 2 court the baron's sister. and the daughter of a wealthy man may never, never—no matter how she loves him—marry a gypsy boy

BoBoy: we know this?

chessman: well, sort of. social classes
are tougher in europe than they
are over here. johnson is being
dramatic, but yeah

alfonso: thank u 4 that overwhelming vote of confidence.
now shut up.

k, as fate would have it, tatiana comes from a
well-to-do family. a very well-to-do family

BoBoy: kewl. did we know this too?

chessman: they're connected with oil or some
kind of mineral exploration. she
didn't say exactly

alfonso: point is, and much 2 her family's dismay, she's
in love... with a gypsy

BoBoy: no way! so that's like a death sentence, right? oh,
unfair unfair unfair

alfonso: the old ways are strong in her country. but
now i tell u this with great sadness: she had
thought the gypsy boyfriend went away 2 plan their
elopement. she said something like this in
the chat room

chessman: well, not exactly. but yeah, ok.
he's in italy

alfonso: she was 2 meet him there in 6 months, and they
would run away 2 where her family would never
find them. very romantic, but totally the truth as
she tells it

but now, word has reached her that her
gypsy love...

BoBoy: what?

alfonso: ...has died

BoBoy: i knew it

alfonso: he fell from a balcony—no, how did she say it?— from a rampart. in rome

chessman: you better not be jerking our chain, J

alfonso: u have seen my poor poems. do u think that in my wildest dreams i could write a story this sad?

BoBoy: true...

alfonso: and that's not all. at first she thought like her father had him killed, 2 keep them apart. but now, it looks like the dude saw how little hope there was, and...

BoBoy: what?

alfonso: well, tatiana thinks he may have... jumped

BoBoy: no way

chessman: seriously?

alfonso: tatiana doesn't let on. u know how strong she is. but i can tell she's beside herself with grief. and her family r beside themselves with shame. i mean, a gypsy with their own daughter. now a suicide, a daughter in despair. they think she might do something terrible

chessman: aw man, so that could explain...

alfonso: why they're sending her 2 america. u got it, dude

BoBoy: i knew it. i knew it

chessman: they want her to find an american boyfriend

alfonso: yeah, but mitch, who cares what they want?

chessman: i dunno. just thinking about something she said

alfonso: but who CARES about that? i'm afraid she'll do something 2 herself. she's so volatile, and she totally blames herself 4 his death

chessman: blames herself? how is this her fault?

BoBoy: aw man, this is terrible

alfonso: she's in a dark place, dudes. very dark

BoBoy: we gotta do something

alfonso: she keeps talking about the cards and all

chessman: the cards?

alfonso: u know, the cards. fortune-telling. gypsy stuff

chessman: really?

alfonso: dude, he was teaching her that stuff. how 2 see yr future and all. she thinks he maybe saw their future and that's why he jumped

chessman: aw man. this is too much

alfonso: now all she sees in the cards is death

BoBoy: yipe. mitch, u gotta do something

chessman: me?? i don't know what to do about stuff like this

alfonso: no, wait... bubba's right

chessman: no he's not

alfonso: tatiana does like u, man. she talks about u...

BoBoy: mitch, u gotta talk 2 her

alfonso: she trusts u. ur so stable

chessman: come on, what would i say to her???

BoBoy: nah, u don't talk about this stuff. just let her talk

alfonso: whatever she wants 2 talk about. just get her
            thru this rough patch...

chessman: just let her talk...

alfonso: u could lighten her load, mitch

BoBoy: u could save a life

alfonso: how many hopeless nerds can say that?

chessman: shove off, J

BoBoy: seriously, bro. me and johnson, we're just rednecks
           2 her

alfonso: totally

BoBoy: we'd probably call her a lamp or a truck or something

chessman: gimme a break

BoBoy: mitch, u gotta. it could be her life

alfonso: u know how impulsive she can be

chessman: but she's after me already, and
           i really can't be her american
           boyfriend

BoBoy: just 4 a while... get her thru this

chessman: no way. i can't pretend stuff like
           that

alfonso: no, ur right, dude: don't pretend anything.
            nobody's saying marry her

BoBoy: just listen 2 her

chessman: i could MAYBE just let her talk...

BoBoy: zackly

alfonso: ur solid, dude. ur a rock. that's all she needs...

chessman: i've got rocks in my head. that's
           what i've got

alfonso:	aw, where's the compassion?
chessman:	i KNOW, but what about bliss???
alfonso:	dude, pleeeeze. some things r not about bliss!!
chessman:	....
alfonso:	come on mitchie...
BoBoy:	she's really imbued, yo...
chessman:	\<groan>
alfonso:	just listen. that's all u have 2 do...
chessman:	arrrgghh
BoBoy:	just let her talk...

YOUR UNCLE JERRY'S BLOG

Marriage of the Minds
14 JUNE

> *Let me not to the marriage of true minds*
> *Admit impediments.*
> *—Shakespeare, lame old love sonnet*

Joy and peace, camper. Marriage is what brings us together. Marriage, that age-old, universally celebrated union between heart and heart, is not—pay attention, young feller—NOT to be taken lightly.

Why do young campers love to marry? Up here in Minnesota, where the lonesome wind blows in from the prairie, it is the opinion of certain older persons that marriage was invented so that everyone can stay warm through the winter. Ho ho. Your Uncle Jerry's own mother got engaged three times, just looking for a man who didn't have cold feet.

Your Uncle Jerry himself will never marry. Uncle Jerry observes the code of the Norwegian Bachelor Farmer: never give up, never surrender, and never change your long johns. This tends to reduce courtship to a healthy minimum, and it keeps you just as warm.

The thing to notice about a wedding ring is that it's what?... Hollow. Empty. And if you are empty too, my friend, then marriage will be a hole within a hole, and you will fall through it like a rat through an aqueduct. The only way out is when you hit bottom.

Take Your Uncle Jerry's parents. (Please.) There are 50 ways to mess up a marriage, and Your Uncle Jerry's parents have tried every single one. What keeps them together? Dental insurance. They don't want to lose their double coverage.

Point is, camper, if you can think of 5 ways out of the 50, you're a genius... and you ain't no genius. How does Uncle Jerry know? Because you're in love, duh.... Genius is a Norwegian Bachelor Farmer.

The best marriages are the practical ones. Marry for money. Marry for career advancement. Marry to get citizenship in your spouse's country. A marriage with a purpose is a marriage of true minds, young friend. Marry... to stay warm in the winter.

However, Your Uncle Jerry knows full well that few young campers will take his sage advice—the young folks WILL fall in love. And thus, for one month only, Your Uncle Jerry offers this special service.

You can sign up for Your Uncle Jerry's Famous Online June Wedding Service. Send us your application, and Uncle Jerry will perform a no-frills, no guarantees, and no-holds-barred wedding service for you and your intended in a chat room of your choice. For the month of June only, it's free, it's convenient, and it's totally bogus. No muss, no fuss, no salesman will visit your home. (Void where prohibited by law or good sense.)

Love is in the air, camper. It's June.
Peace and joy.

CHAPTER 20
tempting fate

📨 IM from Bridget

JUNE 14 5:05 PM

Bridget: hello good evening?

beau, r u there?

BoBoy: bridgie! hey gurl, what up?

Bridget: nothing. just felt like checking on u

BoBoy: right. in case i was up 2 something

Bridget: oh, i know ur up 2 something

BoBoy: no fair. i've been totally framed!

Bridget: i don't think so...

BoBoy: officer, please! the man was dead when i got here

Bridget: lol

BoBoy: the couch was on fire when i lay down!

Bridget: u r too funny beau boy

BoBoy: too funny 4 what?

Bridget: oh, i miss laughing. u r so good 4 me

BoBoy: awww

✉ IM from chessman

JUNE 14 5:07 PM

chessman: tatiana? hello?

tatiana? i can see you're online

Tatiana: hallo, mitchell. i am too sorry not to speak right at this moment now, you see

chessman: you can't talk now?

Tatiana: not so much, no

chessman: well, ok. i didn't want to disturb you. just checking to see how you're doing

Tatiana: no i am not doing somethings for this moment

chessman: tatiana, are you ok? you sound a little different

Tatiana: no! i am not doing somethings at this point in time, lol

chessman: um?

Tatiana: why do these american say "this point in time." lol. everyone is make fun of them. hah!

chessman: tatiana?

Tatiana: yes, my darling mitchell american boy saunders?

chessman: tatiana, have you been drinking?

Tatiana: no i have not. no no NO. yes.

chessman: i thought so

Tatiana: mitchell, i am too very sorry not to speak you now at this point in time

chessman: you're sorry?

Tatiana: no. is not how you say it. i have too much sorry. i am full of sorry. hah. i cannot recall how you very american say this. sorry?

chessman: sorrow? you're sad?

Tatiana: YES. i am SORROW. sorrow sorrow sorrow. that's the word in time. too much very sorrow to be talking american boys right now if you please thank you very much you welshman

✉ IM from Bridget

BoBoy: what do u mean u miss laughing?

Bridget: i thought that was fairly clear :)

BoBoy: are things so bad in england?

Bridget: u know the saddest thing about england?

BoBoy: what?

Bridget: no one is allowed 2 be sad

BoBoy: dude, that's no fun

Bridget: u just screw yr face up and say, fine fine i'm just fine, lovely weather we're having, stiff upper lip, what what

BoBoy: what what? i like that

Bridget: continue fine i hope it may, and yet it rained but yesterday. more tea, vicar?

BoBoy: so bridge. what's got u down in the dumps, eh? what what?

Bridget: no, that's not how u—never mind

BoBoy: u got boy trouble dontcha, bridge?

Bridget: o... u could say that. nothing that everyone hasn't been thru. quite tiresome. rather not speak of it, really

BoBoy: i knew it. come on, sweetie. what he say?

Bridget: it's what he's done, beau. it's too dreadful 4 words. i really can't. i feel myself choking up just thinking about it

BoBoy: what's he done, girlfriend?

Bridget: well, actually, it's rather simple... i believe u would say he's dumped me

BoBoy: NO

Bridget: me—of all people. i'm not that loathsome, beau, i promise u

BoBoy: what is that dude's problem??

Bridget: i've never been brilliant, but i've been told i look actually rather fetching some days

BoBoy: it's not about u, i can guarantee that

Bridget: and i AM passionate. i don't care what he says

✉ IM from chessman

chessman: tatiana, what makes you so sad? what's this about?

Tatiana: about feeling lost in my own life, mitchell. about sailing on the darkest waters

chessman: not sure i understand

Tatiana: how sad, without love, to set out across the sea

chessman: that's beautiful. it's like i've read it somewhere...

Tatiana: it is an old french poetry. oh, mitchell is there nothing you do not know?

chessman: oh, please

Tatiana: you have such a heart, my friend

chessman: i do?

Tatiana: oh my oh my. the heart of a poet. the passion of a gypsy

chessman: i'm passionate?

✉ IM from Bridget

BoBoy: of course ur, bridge. i haven't forgotten our kissing lessons, u know

Bridget: me neither :) if only...

✉ IM from chessman

Tatiana: my darling, the only way you are not the gypsy poet is that you do not read the cards

chessman: that's true. but i've seen it done

Tatiana: if only...

✉ IM from Bridget

BoBoy: if only what, bridgie?

Bridget: never mind

✉ IM from chessman

chessman: if only what, tatiana?

Tatiana: mitchell, i am too deeply sorrowed right at this moment to... but wait

chessman: what is it?

Tatiana: why have i not think of this before? you must lay the cards for me

chessman: how can i do that?

Tatiana: here. i have the cards now, and you must tell me which ones to lay down. just to give me three numbers

chessman: ok. um, 11. 29. and 47

Tatiana: all prime numbers?

chessman: sorry. i'm a nerd

Tatiana: lol. me too. ok, i count... so, and so, and so. now we see

chessman: what did we get?

Tatiana: ah, i knew. was foolish even to try. sigh

chessman: but what were the cards?

Tatiana: always the same, mitchell. 3 cards make past, present, future. so what i get is 1, 2, 3: separation, bad news, and death. always always death

chessman: i'm sorry.... johnson told me about your boyfriend

Tatiana: i turn them again, looking for love, looking for the marriage. but no: same. same. first him, then me. death. i knew it

chessman: tatiana, what do you mean?

Tatiana: so simple. fate is there to read, and one cannot change this

---

✉ IM from Bridget

BoBoy: come on, bridgie. let's do something 2 cheer u up

Bridget: k. tell me a story

BoBoy: a story? um, once there was a princess

Bridget: oh good

BoBoy: she lived a fairy tale life, where everything was beautiful, and she was beautiful, and she was happy all the time

Bridget: good 4 her. did she marry a prince?

BoBoy: um, well, not right away

Bridget: well, when?

BoBoy: c, first, she is captured by a dragon

Bridget: oh, exciting

BoBoy: a ferocious, obnoxticating dragon with shiny fangs, and breath that could imbue the paint off a pickup truck

Bridget: u r so funny, beau. i never knew that

BoBoy: how could u know? we just met a couple weeks ago

Bridget: who's going 2 save the princess?

BoBoy: so there's this guy. and he's out in the wilderness, cleaning his spirit. he like eats bugs and honey, barely subsiding out there

Bridget: i like how u tell a story

BoBoy: he's very sad

Bridget: why?

BoBoy: um? because his girl has left him or died or something. so he thinks that if he gets all pure in the desert... then he'll be good enough 2 rescue the princess. yeah, that's it

Bridget: pure thoughts

BoBoy: right. so he takes his vorpal sword and his silver football helmet, and he rushes off 2 fight the dragon

Bridget: the princess watches from her tower

BoBoy: the dragon blows his fiery breath, but it bounces off the silver helmet and burns him right up. then our boy chops off the dragon's head and leads the princess down from her tower

Bridget: my hero

BoBoy: happy ever after. the end

≋ IM from chessman

chessman: tatiana, maybe if i lay the cards over here?

Tatiana: how do you mean? you have the cards?

chessman: only regular cards, but they'll work, yes?

Tatiana: yes... so, you means it could be my sorrows making the cards too sad?

chessman: exactly. let's try. gimme three numbers

Tatiana: you are so lovely to do this. ok, so 7, 13, 41

chessman: prime numbers. ok, i've counted out those cards. now what?

Tatiana: so turn them and tell me

chessman: ok. first is jack of spades. what's that mean?

Tatiana: ah. so in my cards this is page of coins. well, young man. very knowledge but makes no leaping decision

chessman: not so bad, see?

Tatiana: have you the dark hair, mitchell?

chessman: i guess

Tatiana: so this could be you. surely you are the cautious one, and so brilliant <sigh>

chessman: ok ok. second card is 8 of diamonds

Tatiana: swords, of course. so very sad. alone. like the prisoner. she sigh. she weep. all around is pain to the heart. she hope it do not last forever

chessman: and that could be you, right?

Tatiana: always this is the card for me. so the last card will be some kind of death. i don't even want to know

chessman: let's see. so we have me, then you. and now... 2 of hearts?

Tatiana: NO! you are joking me?

chessman: what's it mean?

Tatiana: truly you don't know 2 of cup?

chessman: you could tell me anything and i would believe you

Tatiana: no... because you would look up

chessman: well, true...

Tatiana: you are this moment looking up the web, are you not?

chessman: busted

Tatiana: and what are you find?

chessman: 2 of cups: love, passion... union...
marriage of the minds

Tatiana: lol. is it not wonderful??

chessman: um...

Tatiana: mitchell, you see? you see what this mean?

chessman: i, um...

Tatiana: is fate! is fate! you and i are the lovers. oh this
make me so very happy. a new light dawns in my heart

chessman: but i don't think...

Tatiana: of course, mitchell, i know you must fight it!
i know. that is so much your fate

make two more cards—any two

chessman: 7 of clubs

Tatiana: is you! you struggle. you struggle in the heart

chessman: 10 of hearts

Tatiana: i told you so. happy ever after!

✉ IM from Bridget

Bridget: beau? dance with me?

BoBoy: excuse me?

Bridget: u kissed me before. now i need 2 dance

BoBoy: but bridge, i dance like a brontosaurus

Bridget: trust me. in my mind u dance like a prince

BoBoy: oh jeeze. well, u'll have 2 teach me

Bridget: just take my right hand with yr left

BoBoy: k. got it

Bridget: now yr right hand on my waist. not too tight

BoBoy: keep my distance?

Bridget: yes, for now ;-)

my hand is on yr shoulder, and u move us to yr left, then right. again. let yr mind be quiet...

slowly 1, 2, 3, 4

BoBoy: bridget?

Bridget: mmm?

BoBoy: this is nice

Bridget: now u step back and turn 2 the left. i follow. 1, 2

BoBoy: i've never met a girl like u

Bridget: mmm... step up and turn us 2 the right

BoBoy: sometimes i get lonely. u know?

Bridget: i know, honey

BoBoy: what am i gonna do, bridge?

Bridget: turn us 1 full turn. do it in 3 steps

BoBoy: i like u so much, bridge, but i don't deserve u

Bridget: u deserve much better, my prince

BoBoy: i'm not exactly the cream of the corn

Bridget: u just need 2 believe in yrself. turn me 2 the right

BoBoy: bridget?

Bridget: yes?

BoBoy: do u believe in me?

Bridget: i do. completely

BoBoy: u don't know what that does 2 me

Bridget: everyone needs 2 feel believed in

BoBoy: u believe in yrself?

Bridget: i do when i'm with u

BoBoy: that is the nicest thing i've ever heard

Bridget: twirl me once and then catch me in yr arms

BoBoy: i was right, eh? i tromp around like a brontosaurus

Bridget: lol. u tromp divinely

✉ IM from chessman

chessman: tatiana, i don't know what to say

Tatiana: say anything. i cannot be unhappy now

chessman: this is too weird

Tatiana: yes, it is just as the gypsies tell it

chessman: but you really believe this?

Tatiana: mitchell, many thing are the mystery. shall we not believe them because we not understand?

chessman: but what are the odds of this happening?

Tatiana: the cards often have this effect

chessman: and people just believe them anyway?

Tatiana: no no. many people struggle. but what point in struggling when fate awaits us all?

chessman: i need to think

Tatiana: yes, mitchell. you think. tatiana does not rush you

chessman: will you be all right now?

Tatiana: i have not felt so well since many weeks. my heart is in the cloud

chessman: i'll write you tomorrow

Tatiana: you struggle, my page of coins. i will wait for you tomorrow

🔁 IM from Bridget

BoBoy: what am i gonna do about u, bridge?

Bridget: <sigh>

BoBoy: i could just fly over there right now. i need 2 touch hands 4 real

Bridget: what if there's a dragon?

BoBoy: got my helmet right here

Bridget: come 4 me, soon, beau. i'm here in my tower

china wall

⬛ IM from gothling

JUNE 15 10:50 PM

gothling: so, johnson, are we good 2 go?

alfonso: almost set

gothling: perfect. my gurls got them right 2 the brink last night

alfonso: so the gypsy stuff?

gothling: worked like a charm

alfonso: great. k. well. cya

gothling: hey!

alfonso: yes?

gothling: that's it? the brush off?

alfonso: not really. why?

gothling: where's the good ol johnson? where's the banter? the flirtation?

alfonso: u made things pretty clear on that the last time

gothling: so what's yr point? u get 2 freeze me out because i said no?

alfonso: i'm not freezing u out. but i do have feelings 2 protect, just like u

gothling: get over it, dude. ur still mine—admit it

alfonso: i don't think so, annie

gothling: come on, johnson. ur not hurt. yr ego's bruised is all

alfonso: are we done?

gothling: k, look. i'm sorry. i'm sorry i was... i'm sorry if whatever i said caused a problem. let's just let it go and get back 2 the way things were

alfonso: well, thanks 4 the apology, but I forgave u b4

gothling: o, thank u so much, u patronizing putz. then why r u being cold now?

alfonso: sorry, i don't mean 2 be cold

gothling: all right, then

alfonso: but if u think nothing's changed, ur wrong

gothling: johnson, u may not behave this way. GROW. UP.

alfonso: grown up means consequences, annie. i'm not mad. but after u dis a person enough times, they tend 2 protect themselves

gothling: get real. u still need me and u know it

alfonso: seriously, g2g. i'll keep u posted about the chat room

gothling: whatever, dude

EXCHANGE STUDENT ROOM **UNION HIGH SCHOOL**

JUNE 15 11:00 PM

BoBoy has entered

BoBoy:	yo y'all. anybody alive yet?
alfonso:	bro beau! what ease thee word?
BoBoy:	word, J. good 2 c ur still the wittiest of them all
alfonso:	my new accent. jamaican. whaddya think?
BoBoy:	kewl. why u doing that?
alfonso:	jus messin. i like tatiana's talk is all
BoBoy:	yeah, but that's her real accent
alfonso:	well, what's real online?
BoBoy:	meaning what—she's faking? i don't theeenk so
alfonso:	i just mean a lot of people wear masks
BoBoy:	masks. dude, u have a seriously cold view of human beings

Bridget has entered

Bridget: hello, good evening. am i the first?

alfonso: no indeed, bridget. beau and i r here

BoBoy: hey gurl. what up?

Bridget: ah, my prince! i did so hope u would come 2nite

alfonso: prince?? dude, what have i missed?

BoBoy: oh, heh heh. i was um, telling fairy tales last night. dragons, princes, u know. swords

alfonso: oic. bridget, u be careful. the stories our boy can tell...

Bridget: lol. not 2 worry. i know a tall tale when i hear it

Tatiana has entered

alfonso: hallo, tatiana, my velly good fren

Tatiana: what is happen to the johnson voice?

BoBoy: tatiana, pay no attention 2 the man behind the jamaican t-shirt

Bridget: that was a shock, rather, i should say

chessman has entered

chessman: made it

BoBoy: zup, bro?

Bridget: hello, good morning

chessman: hi, bridget

Bridget: or evening, rather. i'm always confused. how tiresome

alfonso: mitchell, my good mon. welcome 2 da cabana

chessman: johnson?

Tatiana: something very troubling is happen to johnson. he seem to think he is of jamaica this evening. has the t-shirt and all

alfonso: nutting could be furder from da troot. i only showin me boy how de life online be whatevah we want

BoBoy: or something like that

alfonso: more rum, my brotha?

✉ IM from Bridget

Bridget: beau, i'm sorry about calling u my prince. did i embarrass u?

BoBoy: nah

Bridget: i was just so pleased 2 see u

BoBoy: 's all right

Bridget: ur still my prince, tho :)

BoBoy: that sounds so funny. but nice...

✉ IM from Tatiana

Tatiana: mitchell, please tell me what is problem with johnson?

chessman: not sure i know. he's not stupid, so i think he must have a point to make

Tatiana: is very—how you say?—irritable?

chessman: ah. irritating

Tatiana: very irritating to me

chessman: maybe he'll stop in a minute. i'm sure he isn't mocking you

Bridget: johnson, do the voice again

alfonso: which voice do that be, me ladee?

Bridget: that's the 1. very funny

chessman: just a side note, johnson.
we still have that agreement?

alfonso: yah mon, deed we doo

chessman: so then, if one of the exchange students
found the voice irritating, you would
probably cut it out. am i right?

alfonso: ahem, well, yes that would seem 2 be in the spirit
of the agreement

Tatiana: so you are your real voice again, johnson?
thank you for this

alfonso: my real mask, yes, my queen

BoBoy: johnson's not telling us something

Bridget: lol. many things, no doubt

BoBoy: no, i mean he usually yanks chain when he's
not happy

chessman: dude, that's right. i never put
it together like that

alfonso: thank u 4 yr concern, bubba, but the j-man
is totally fine. not a cloud in the sky, not a care
in the world

chessman: oh, there's a problem

Tatiana: lol. you mean he has perhap the woman
trouble, yes?

alfonso: as if. okay, group, let's talk about
               ----->school

chessman: let's talk about compassion, dude

alfonso: don't go there, nerdman. we'll all be sorry

BoBoy: mitchie, u dawg. u done nailed it

✉ IM from Tatiana

Tatiana: mitchell, i am so happy from last night, i want only to be with you. is that rude to others?

chessman: no, you're fine

Tatiana: and have you struggled with 2 of hearts?

chessman: tatiana, this is so difficult for me. i would never do anything to hurt my girlfriend, but...

Tatiana: i know is true. is true. but she have been away for so very long time, yes?

chessman: she has

Tatiana: how are you sure she isn't telling you goodbye?

chessman: <sigh> that's what i'm afraid of

EXCHANGE STUDENT ROOM **UNION HIGH SCHOOL**

Bridget: talk about compassion 4 who? what r u chaps saying?

BoBoy: **johnson, be honest. ur among friends**

alfonso: never

chessman: bro, i think you can trust these women

BoBoy: **group hug for johnson!! {{j-man}}**

Tatiana: yes, please. we can be trusted in matters of love

alfonso: ur making a big deal out of nothing

BoBoy: **aha**

alfonso: a small disaster of the heart. nothing a young poet can't endure alone

BoBoy: **aw man. she didn't!**

Bridget: can this be true? johnson has a heart? ;-)

chessman: his heart is at a delicate stage right now. he's gone cold turkey. he's opened up to the one he's wanted all along

alfonso: no names, guys, or u WILL be sorry

BoBoy: **dude, we got yr back**

Bridget: i'm so embarrassed. johnson, i had no idea

Tatiana: please to forgive bridget. it was teasing only

alfonso: oh, u people... just drop it k? i can deal with a little rejection

BoBoy: **she did! she crushed him**

chessman: crushed? never. only a flesh
wound, right J? we're here for you

alfonso: mitch, ur a funny guy. u never liked me,
anyway

✉ IM from Bridget

Bridget: beau, what in the world??

BoBoy: it's real. i can tell he's been dissed

Bridget: i'm so sorry. who would have done it?

BoBoy: can't tell u that, sweetie. but it's almost never happened before

---

EXCHANGE STUDENT ROOM **UNION HIGH SCHOOL**

chessman: dude, i'm a loyal pooch. how many
friends do you think i have?

alfonso: more than me

Tatiana: johnson, i tell you this in all seriously.
a wound of the heart is need the air to heal.
know what i meaning? not matters
how small

alfonso: will u puhleeze give it a rest?

BoBoy: big breaths, J

chessman: you want i should wipe her hard
drive, boss?

alfonso: lol

Tatiana: beau boy, you know these girl who have hurt the johnson?

BoBoy: oh, dude, we know her, all right. she's a cruel 1

chessman: dawg, johnson likes her. therefore, we like her

Bridget: how can u like her after this?

BoBoy: zackly

chessman: compassion where due. haven't you been paying attention?

BoBoy: oh, right. true. she's had it rough. well, but still...

alfonso: pleeze pleeze pleeze pleeze pleeze

✉ IM from Tatiana

chessman: tatiana, we need to talk about us, and here's the thing that i can't get beyond. if i would leave my girl to fall in love with you...

Tatiana: ah, mitchell, i love it so when you say these word

chessman: if i would leave HER, how could YOU ever trust me?

Tatiana: no, you would never do to me. i know this

chessman: no you don't

Tatiana: because i would never leave you for months without any word

chessman: you CAN'T know this. don't you see?

Tatiana: no. don't you see, mitchell? is fate in the cards

chessman: aw, man...

Tatiana: you think that is nothing?

chessman: not exactly, but still

Tatiana: destiny is not to be played with. the cards say
we are marriage in future, and this is all i need to know

EXCHANGE STUDENT ROOM **UNION HIGH SCHOOL**

alfonso: ok, u broke me down. here's the story

Bridget: good. i love stories

alfonso: ok, yes. YES, so i had this big crush going 4 a
certain person. but i knew she was closed up.
she's a castle, she's the china wall, she lets no 1 in

BoBoy: she's a brick

alfonso: why i thought i could get thru, of all people,
i'll never know

chessman: because you're good at it?

alfonso: but i decided 2 go with hope instead of fear:
i told her how i felt

Tatiana: you are the brave man, johnson. total
respect, you dude

alfonso: i laid my heart at her feet, and she stomped
that sucker flat

Bridget:	that's terrible!
BoBoy:	**dude, i'll flatten her tires**
alfonso:	no no no. that's the point. i can take it. i'm not complaining. i knew what i was risking, and i will accept this hurt from her
chessman:	oh, he's got it bad
alfonso:	she is, after all, magnificent
Tatiana:	very poetic
Bridget:	it's so sweet. i'm actually crying here
alfonso:	but i will not try again
Tatiana:	oh no, absolutely you must try again!
Bridget:	of course u will. don't even think u won't
alfonso:	WHAAA???
chessman:	they're saying you gotta try again, bro
Bridget:	no, u must! or else u didn't mean it the first time
alfonso:	u people r barking mad
BoBoy:	**dude, they're right**
alfonso:	r u not listening??
Bridget:	what kind of a poet would bail?
Tatiana:	do you love these woman or not?
alfonso:	u hate me. u just want 2 see me flattened again
Bridget:	if u luv her, u keep trying
Tatiana:	is simple, really
Bridget:	u don't know what flat is

alfonso: excuse me?? is that some kinda english joke?

Bridget: u don't. watching her walk away with someone else—
that would be flat

Tatiana: losing her to your best friend

alfonso: arrgh. that is such a cruel card 2 play

BoBoy: bro, u see why i like these girls?

alfonso: people skills?

BoBoy: all their passion, dude

✉ IM from Bridget

Bridget: oh u big sweetie!

BoBoy: what i say?

Bridget: ur so good 2 me. how come u can c what... u
know... that english dude can't?

BoBoy: don't worry about the past, peanut

Bridget: u mean it?

BoBoy: i mean it

Bridget: tell me

BoBoy: i've got it bad 4 u, girl. from here on out, it's u
and me. i swear it is

Bridget: ah, beau. this is too sweet. and too sad

BoBoy: take my hand

Bridget: got it, guy

BoBoy: why too sad?

Bridget: oh just everything. i'll tell u l8r

alfonso:	ok. \<huff puff huff puff\> supposing i really was loser enough 2 go back and try again. what would be my best approach? just hypothetically
Tatiana:	well...
Bridget:	best case scenario: she didn't mean it
alfonso:	didn't mean it...
Tatiana:	oh, johnson, please. you know about this
Bridget:	she could be buying time 2 think
chessman:	she WHAT??? can they DO that??
alfonso:	well... yeah, they can. i just didn't think...
Tatiana:	so did you part in anger?
alfonso:	not at all. she IM'd today
Bridget:	good, and how did u act toward her?
alfonso:	um...
BoBoy:	u said "i don't need no scumbag love," right?
chessman:	right: contumelious
BoBoy:	dude, is that what that means?
chessman:	looked it up
alfonso:	i was polite but... let's say distant
Tatiana:	excellent, johnson.
Bridget:	cool but not cold, right?
alfonso:	i guess
Bridget:	is he a natural or what?

Tatiana: and she not like this, correct?

alfonso: not really

Bridget: ok, so keep it that way 4 next time

Tatiana: so she know you mean it, but not so she give up the hope

BoBoy: man, this is brutal

alfonso: no, i get it. these guys r very good

Tatiana: she is always asking for gravel, yes?

alfonso: say what?

chessman: making you grovel

alfonso: oh that. yes, indeed. very much the alpha dog personality

Tatiana: so you not make the grovel ever more. understood me? ever

Bridget: that DOESN'T mean be a total jerk

Tatiana: meeting as equals, very important

chessman: how about flowers, candy?

Bridget: oh quite. but in good time. when she earns them

BoBoy: when she earns them! dang, that's cool. i can never think of that stuff

Tatiana: send a poetry, perhaps

BoBoy: all in good time

Bridget: and poetry doesn't have 2 be gravelly, u know

alfonso: of course. it can be angry, mocking, despairing, kind... still, i don't think this is going anywhere. she's quite firm

chessman: should you read his cards, tatiana?

Tatiana: of course. one moment

alfonso: now this stuff, i don't totally buy

Tatiana: the cards do not care if you buy them, my friend. your fate, still your fate is. ready?

BoBoy: **ready. what do they say?**

Tatiana: give to me 3 numbers, johnson

alfonso: 14, 23, 27, hut hut

Tatiana: good. thank you

chessman: so she counts off your 3 cards, bro

Tatiana: first one turning. ah, queen of sword. strong but troubled. is true? she broods, she lets few near. waves her heartbreak like a sword

BoBoy: **bingo**

alfonso: are u doing this 4 real?

chessman: she is, dude

alfonso: tatiana, really? i didn't know u knew this stuff

chessman: learned it from the gypsies

alfonso: why do i suddenly feel like someone's pulling my strings?

Tatiana: second card is page of sword. hmm... sword and sword

BoBoy: **what's the page mean?**

Tatiana: is johnson. intelligent. wishes to be good person, but perhaps a spy.... johnson keeps a secret

alfonso: lol. not me

chessman: oh, never any secrets

BoBoy: his heart is an open file

Tatiana: both are swords. so very difficult relationship, yes? always the dueling

alfonso: k, tatiana. i don't get this. u really don't know me that well

Tatiana: i know you only from these chat room, as you can witness

alfonso: so how r u doing this?

BoBoy: dude it's the cards. she's just reading them

alfonso: get real

Tatiana: mr. johnson, do i know you? do i know this girl of whom you love?

alfonso: no, i get ya. how could someone in albania know her?

BoBoy: k then. what's the next card?

alfonso: mitch, r u buying this?

chessman: there's lots of fate in opera, dude. i'm surprised you're not eating it up

alfonso: opera is different. this here is like reading my mail

Tatiana: next card? or put them away?

alfonso: ok, but against my better judgment

Tatiana: turning... how strange

Bridget: what?

Tatiana: how very strange

alfonso: oh, she's playing with me now

BoBoy: tatiana, u got us all worried over here

Tatiana: so sorry. it is... major death card

Bridget: death??

alfonso: yipes! not me, i hope?

Tatiana: no you don't understand. there are many death cards

BoBoy: dude, ur fish food now. road kill city. ur toast

chessman: what does it mean, tatiana?

Tatiana: this one is not death like you die, johnson. death like you change

alfonso: huh?

Tatiana: out with old, in with new

Bridget: oh, i get it

chessman: wow, like reincarnation?

Tatiana: or resurrection. is change...

alfonso: makes no sense

BoBoy: check it out, dawg, it's change—yr new leaf!

alfonso: my new leaf!

✉ IM from Tatiana

chessman: tatiana, you are amazing

Tatiana: really, my handsome american boy? why you say this?

chessman: what you're doing for johnson

Tatiana: but i am do nothing

chessman: giving him new hope. i can't tell you how much that means to him

Tatiana: you misunderstand, mitchell. i reading cards only

chessman: you're not pulling the cards to make him feel better?

Tatiana: you mean am i cheating?

chessman: you might be "helping"

Tatiana: did you help when you laid 2 of hearts for us?

chessman: i wouldn't know how

Tatiana: i never help either

chessman: i love you even more for that

Tatiana: i know you do

chessman: wait. did i just say that?

Tatiana: you did. i am smiling

EXCHANGE STUDENT ROOM **UNION HIGH SCHOOL**

Bridget: but what about the girl? what happens with her?

Tatiana: i do not know. it would take another card

chessman: johnson?

alfonso: not me

BoBoy:	**what??? u don't want 2 know?**
alfonso:	no way
Bridget:	o i hate this. ack ack, i can't stand not knowing
alfonso:	don't press my luck, gurl
chessman:	maybe 3 cards is enough
alfonso:	it's enough 4 me
BoBoy:	**maybe like a new leaf 4 both? how bout that?**
Tatiana:	could be
alfonso:	or not. doesn't matter
Bridget:	arrrgh. i want that caaarrrrrrrrddd :-(
alfonso:	i'd rather be surprised. i really would
chessman:	well done, J
alfonso:	besides, i just had a thought. gotta run
Tatiana:	you see, mr. johnson. you have many weapons in the battle for her heart
BoBoy:	**scale the wall, baby**
Bridget:	gotta run? why?
chessman:	going to start a poem?

alfonso has left the room

BoBoy:	**bingo**

CHAPTER 22
calling jerry

🗩 IM from alfonso

JUNE 16 8:00 PM

alfonso: yo annie

gothling: u gotta be kidding. i thought u weren't speaking 2 me

alfonso: come on. i never said that. we've got business 2 do

gothling: what business?

alfonso: the girls didn't talk 2 u?

gothling: haven't heard from them. OR from u

alfonso: ok, well, here's what u need 2 know. the dudes have walked into the trap. it's time 2 spring it

gothling: well, finally. and were u ever going 2 tell me? u said u'd keep me posted

alfonso: will u stop? so we just need some evidence for the real bliss and ms. T 2 find. something the dudes can't deny

gothling: johnson, i KNOW. i know all this

alfonso: yes. fine

gothling: i know EXACTLY what the next step is! i'm the one who thought this whole game UP!!

alfonso: chill, annie

gothling: don't u "chill" me! I'M the one who brought u in, u troll. u insect. u troglodyte!

alfonso: look, i don't have even a minute 4 a shouting match

gothling: I AM NOT SHOUTING!!

alfonso: k. so what i was thinking was this

gothling: JOHNSON!!!

alfonso: hush, annabelle. y'll hurt yrself

gothling: johnson?

alfonso: yes?

gothling: i hate u

alfonso: i know. now can we move on?

gothling: seriously. i loathe u. i really do

alfonso: i think we need uncle jerry

gothling: what?

alfonso: u got him that online minister degree, didn't u?

gothling: oh arrrgh. i see where ur going with this....

alfonso: u don't like it?

gothling: no, i HATE it. it's much better than my idea

alfonso: oic. well, we can call it yr idea. no problem

gothling: DON'T PATRONIZE ME. I HATE THAT!!

alfonso: u hate so many things today

gothling: only everything about u

alfonso: so do we have a deal?

gothling: YES. now shove off

YOUR UNCLE JERRY'S BLOG

The Big Reveal
16 JUNE

*The Road of Excess leads
to the Palace of Wisdom.
—Wm Blake, lame old proverb*

Joy and peace, camper. Your wise old Uncle Jerry has found that there comes a time in every camper's life when all must be revealed. These are the moments—sometimes painful—from which we learn, and through which we may enter... (wait for it...) the gates of wisdom!

As you would know, young person, if you had been reading Your Uncle Jerry's Sunday Sermons like you oughta (get them in PDF at a website near you), most campers hike the Road of Excess without a clue.

Now. What is the Road of Excess? Anyone? Oh dear, oh dear. The Road, the Way—listen at me—the very Life we lead is a journey paved in disappointments and desires. Young people wish for so much as they travel life's pathway, do they not? And are not their little boats so often dashed upon the rocks and reefs of despair?

Ah well, Your Uncle Jerry was young once too.

Onward we slog, knee-deep in illusions, clouded by hopes. "She loves me." "He needs me." "There will never be another." "Something deep inside cannot be denied."

How long we must travel thus, we never know. But one day we turn a corner, the clouds part, the light breaks. And... voila!... all is REVEALED. Like dawn at the landfill.

(A poet friend gave Your Uncle Jerry that line. Can a poet be a true friend? you ask. Excellent. The question shows you have been studying. Your Uncle Jerry is not sure. A poet could be friend or foe. Beware. Treat a poet with excess of caution.)

Where were we? Excess. Ah yes. (A rhyme! Perhaps Your Uncle Jerry is a poet. Hah! I jokes.)

Your Uncle Jerry knows four young campers traveling the Road of Excess even as we speak. Tonight will be the night when Your Uncle Jerry will part the foolish clouds of romance that shroud their minds and show these hapless campers into the clean well-lighted Palace of Wisdom.

Peace and joy.

CHAPTER 23
entr@pment

bliss4u:	oh, i am so mad at him
gothling:	**told u. did i not tell u?**
Ms.T:	u did tell us
bliss4u:	i'm just going 2 kill him. mitchie, how could u do this 2 me?
Ms.T:	i know, bliss. i know
gothling:	**u trusted him. that was yr mistake**
Ms.T:	on the upside, he held out for a long time...
bliss4u:	don't make excuses 4 him. he's toast. i thought he was strong but he's a slut puppy
gothling:	**just like the rest of them**

Ms.T: yeah, miss bridget. you took beau down in seconds

bliss4u: beau's got a kind heart. that's his only failing

Ms.T: i can think of a few others, which i intend to describe to him in detail

bliss4u: ur not really mad r u?

Ms.T: i could spit nails

bliss4u: pretty quiet about it

Ms.T: if i talk about it i just start to cry

bliss4u: start? i cried all night. now i'm pissed

Ms.T: not me. i need to hold this edge or i'll go all mushy

gothling: u people. what a pair of wusses

Ms.T: you know, annie, i could displace some of my fury in your direction

gothling: why me? i did nothing

bliss4u: u set us up, as i recall...

Ms.T: i didn't say you DESERVED it. i just said i could DO it

gothling: grow up. u lost a bet, that's all

bliss4u: i lost mitchie. that's what i lost

gothling: love's a gamble, gurl. u knew that going in

Ms.T: u can't really be that cold, can you annie?

gothling: i'm just not sentimental. this stuff happens 2 the best of us

alfonso has entered

alfonso: ladies, u ready 2 go?

bliss4u: can't we just skip this part?

gothling: **no way no way no way**

Ms.T: and that's because...?

alfonso: listen, i know u feel like this is a disaster

bliss4u: that would be 1 way 2 put it

alfonso: but if u quit now, the dudes will never see what they've done

bliss4u: but why NOT? it's perfectly obvious

alfonso: not 2 them it isn't

Ms.T: what are you saying, johnson?

bliss4u: r they that stupid?

alfonso: no, look. they've only put a toe in the shallow stuff. they need 2 cross the river

gothling: **i just hate how well u say things sometimes**

Ms.T: i think i get it

alfonso: this is the last bit we do

gothling: **their eyes will be opened**

alfonso: and they will c

gothling: **so please, ladies. masks up 1 last time**

Ms.T: och, this old mask. something is smell about it

alfonso: lol, tatiana

bliss4u: i'm so mad

alfonso: ...and into the chat room, please

EXCHANGE STUDENT ROOM **UNION HIGH SCHOOL**

JUNE 16 11:00 PM

Tatiana has entered

Bridget has entered

alfonso: tatiana! bridget! u made it

BoBoy: hey, bridge. i thought u were going 2 stand me up this time

Bridget: u americans r so impatient

Tatiana: precisely, i would have think a beautiful women is worth the waiting

chessman: i couldn't agree more, tatiana

Tatiana: there, you see beau? mitchell knows how to wait for a lady

Bridget: i suppose mitchell thinks some women r worth waiting 4 and some aren't, what what?

alfonso: ok, great. here's the thing

BoBoy: yeah but how can a guy be sure how long 2 wait? maybe she's not coming

Tatiana: trust! is that how you say in english? loving means believing! may i call you BeauZeau?

alfonso: k, this is going 2 be a terrific end 2 the summer chat room. i was thinking we could talk about relationship customs in different countries

BoBoy: yikes! dude, what i say?

Bridget: nothing, sweetie. ur fine

chessman: tatiana, is everything ok?

Bridget: she'll be fine. under a little stress lately, u know?

Tatiana: mitchell, you must pardon my directness

alfonso: customs? different countries? anyone?

chessman: of course, tatiana. what's up?

Tatiana: you must marry me

chessman: excuse me?

BoBoy: whoa, dude. that's direct all right

Tatiana: it is only for online. you know, the online marriage

chessman: i'm not sure i understand

Tatiana: you will not see me till the september, but i must know that you are mine until then

chessman: can we talk about this on the side?

Bridget: no, let's all do it! what a loverly idea. wouldn't that be loverly?

BoBoy: what? like u and me, bridge?

Bridget: how exciting. i can imagine u in tuxedo, my big footballer. woof!

Tatiana: johnson can arrange it, i having no doubt

alfonso: an online wedding? if that's what the ladies wish, i can c what's possible

BoBoy: k, time-out, kids! ur scaring me here

chessman: tatiana, i'm not sure why it's so important all of a sudden

Bridget: oh, dear. we're scaring the american boys... hee hee

Tatiana: yes, well, my darling mitchell. i think about how you spoke of trusting. i need to trust that you will wait for me

Bridget: pleeeze, beau? it's only a game. it'll be fun. besides, it's just online...

BoBoy: well, true

Bridget: everyone's doing it in england. then they get divorced the next day. how fun!

chessman: can you take it that lightly?

BoBoy: i haven't technically broken up with ms. T yet

Tatiana: yes, well, is she not gone forever?

chessman: we don't know... that's what is so weird

BoBoy: they like disappeared in a very fishy way

alfonso: actually, i... um, i'm thinking things have changed 4 them

chessman: ok. what have you heard J?

alfonso: well, i didn't mean 2 bring it up in a large group, but i did hear something

BoBoy: don't tell me they called annie again

alfonso: ah, well, it seems they did

chessman: so is there a message, or are you just tooling us here?

alfonso: so... well, she says they actually didn't mention you. i'm not sure what this means

Bridget: oh not good

alfonso: bliss's grandmother is much better, so they could come back if they wanted 2. but... well, they've decided 2 stay awhile

BoBoy: what?? why??

Tatiana: women have their reasons, my friend

BoBoy: **there's someone else, isn't there?**

alfonso: i don't think it's official, no

chessman: johnson, this isn't going to work. spill it... whatever you got

alfonso: k. <ahem> annie says they talked about 2 guys they met... 2 guys who r a lot of fun. evidently, it's hard 2 say goodbye

BoBoy: **i knew it**

chessman: so they're not even going to tell us it's over?

alfonso: hold on, don't jump 2 conclusions. i don't believe they've decided it's over. that may depend on u

BoBoy: **come on, bro. how bogus is that? they're the ones who left**

alfonso: look, dawg. they're girls at 16. they're alive. they have needs. maybe they've made a mistake, maybe not. the heart... is unruly

chessman: i don't know where that leaves us

alfonso: well, i'm not 1 to give advice, but... u gotta ask yrself 2 things. 1: if the worst has happened, can u move on? obviously u can

Bridget: oh, excuse me. i thought we had moved on already. beau?

chessman: what's the second thing?

alfonso: 2. if she comes back, can u forgive and not ask too many questions?

Tatiana: johnson seem to have the experience in these matter...

BoBoy: **not ask about the other dudes?... hmm**

alfonso: well, 1 thing is sure. <cough cough> no 1 here is in a position 2 criticize

chessman: true enough. i'm not pointing fingers

Tatiana: and where are the BeauZeau fingers pointing?

BoBoy: **no, in a way... i'm actually relieved**

Tatiana: relieved?

BoBoy: **totally, like the pressure is off, now**

Tatiana: you'll not speak to this girl T, first?

chessman: tatiana, we've tried. if she wanted to talk, she's had plenty of chances

BoBoy: **seems like she wants 2 talk 2 other people**

Bridget: u do like me, don't u, beau? ur not just missing her? because i need 2 know now

BoBoy: **bridget...**

Bridget: u talked me down from that ledge, and i'm so weary of being sad

Tatiana: mitchell, you said if you could leave your girl, how could i trust you wouldn't do this same thing to me

chessman: yes, i said that

Tatiana: so, it seems you don't have a girl now. but i have found the way to trust. you must marry to me, eh? only online, not forever. only to save you for me till i get there.

Bridget: oh yes, let's do it. we all need a laugh

BoBoy: **boy that's the truth**

chessman: i need a minute to think

Bridget: beau, sweetie. take my hand. i'm leaning out over the water, and it is so very very far 2 fall...

Tatiana: i know is a soon thing, but mitchell, i am such the desperate woman without knowing i can trust

chessman: you can trust me. you can trust the cards

BoBoy: **bridget, i'm reaching out... and now i'm... tickling u in the ribs!**

Bridget: lol

Tatiana: sometime the cards do not telling, but rather making the question: so, 2 of hearts—he loves me! or he loves me?
oh, sorry: is the talk of love too much for the genius american?

chessman: tatiana, what can i say? i crossed that bridge the other night. truly i did

Tatiana: see, darling mitchell? your passion runs deep and simple. you could be albanian!

chessman: funny

Tatiana: so will you "marry" me and put my fears to rest?

Bridget: yes yes. johnson, run get us a priest or something

alfonso: **i'm on it. back in a flash with the preacher man**

chessman: tatiana, ok. if you need this to be sure of me till september, then ok

 TXT to gothling

June 16 11:16 pm
From: Johnson
rdy whn u r

Bridget: then ur still my prince?

BoBoy: **i am**

Bridget: take me down the aisle?

BoBoy: **u bet**

 TXT to Johnson

```
June 16 11:17 pm
From: gothling
m on it
```

EXCHANGE STUDENT ROOM **UNION HIGH SCHOOL**

alfonso: dudes and dudettes, i'm back and i've got what we need. this will go down in chat room history

JerryC has entered

alfonso: Jerry! welcome. meet tatiana, meet bridget, meet mitch and beau

JerryC: **GREETINGS! joy and peace, peace and joy**

alfonso: group, this is Jerry Clarkson, scout leader, netizen, and minister of the online word

JerryC: you can call me J or you can call me C. but just don't call me JC, heh heh heh. he's in a cyber space all his own ;) ;)

chessman: oh my oh my oh my

Tatiana: welcome jerry. and we are understanding that you make the marriage online?

Bridget: he's so friendly, isn't he, beau?

BoBoy: way friendly

JerryC: indeed i do, miss tatiana, indeed i doobie doobie doo. i can marry and bury, chastise, baptize, dry clean, and treat a young man's frostbite of the toes, all at 100 megabits per second. heh heh heh

Tatiana: is wonderful. just what is needed

JerryC: sign up for my weekly e-sermons, young man, delivering peace and joy in pdf every saturday midnight—while ur out doing what you shouldn't oughta ;-) ;-) that's a joke, son.

alfonso: excellent, J. we won't keep u long. we just need a quick online double wedding

BoBoy: mitch, can this be real?

chessman: i guess so. anyone can get a license to do this

BoBoy: but is the marriage real, then?

Bridget: oh look, my fiancé has frostbite already :)

Tatiana: a disaster

JerryC: may i just say this, my brothers...

alfonso: and sisters

JerryC: **and sisters, tx alfonso**

alfonso: no problem

JerryC: **ladies...**

alfonso: and gentlemen

JerryC: **dearly beloved, marriage is what brings us 2gether. peace and joy**

alfonso: say it preacher

JerryC: **life online is as real as you make it. i have known many and many a happy young couple that got hitched right here at the altar of the ethernet**

alfonso: joy and peace

JerryC: **thank you brother**

alfonso: or sister

JerryC: **or sis... ok, stow it, johnson. i'll take it from here**

alfonso: tell it, jerry

chessman.   wait a minute

JerryC: **many a happy man and woman making it real, many a boy and girl making it last, and they—like you—started right here in the great bright temple of the net, right here in the solemn presence of the all-seeing web**

alfonso: that's just beautiful

chessman: johnson, this guy knows you?

JerryC: **peace and joy. and here in the presence of that awesome cyberosity, we gather 2nite 2 draw these 2 young couples near. and 2 bind them, if you will, with the very tie that bindeth all humanity. all for 1, and 1 for all,**

and likewise even unto the other (alfonso can you play a sound file right here?)

alfonso: no can do, rev. let's move along

JerryC: **joy and peace, where was i? will the unwitting subjects—i mean the loving couples heh heh heh—please join me down front here. blessings, blessings on u. and when i ask u a question, son, u speak right up in the microphone. i joke. heh heh. i joke because i luv**

Bridget: oh, i'm excited. thank u beau. thank u for being such a dear. u can say it's only online if u want, but 2 me it's everything

BoBoy: **i know, hon**

Bridget: it's all i've got

chessman: tatiana, i have to say i'm a little nervous here

Tatiana: is fine, my handsome american boy. this jerry fellow very nice, like russian priest i think

BoBoy: **i think he's been hitting the sacred vodka 2nite**

JerryC: **2 quick questions, boys, and life will never be the same: will you take these 2 flowers of the forest, dew-picked in the early sweetness of their bloom, 2 be your wedded online brides? answer prompt and don't mumble ;) :) :D**

BoBoy: **yessir i will**

chessman: yes

alfonso: oh, i told myself i wasn't going 2 cry....

JerryC: **and ladies, will you accept these strapping, handsome, though none 2 bright young units 2 be yr wedded online grooms, constantly at yr beck and call,**

	falling over their feet 2 apologize and do yr bidding? now's the time 2 back out if yr hands ain't tied. do ya want em or dontcha?
Bridget:	i do i do i do
Tatiana:	yes, i... oh mitchell, yes i do
alfonso:	i knew it. there goes the mascara...
JerryC:	**is there anyone here who knows a reason why (scuse me while i dab my eyes)**
alfonso:	oh, me too. me too
JerryC:	**is there anyone here who knows why these 4 loving morons should NOT be joined in wondrous online matrimony?**
alfonso:	not a 1, rev. many thanks
JerryC:	**my work is done**

JerryC has left the room

Bridget has left the room

Tatiana has left the room

BoBoy:	**hey, where'd they go?**
alfonso:	don't worry, handsome. they'll be back in a flash
chessman:	johnson, where'd you come up with Uncle Jerry?

bliss4u has entered

Ms.T has entered

BoBoy:	**hey, stranger!**
chessman:	bliss??
BoBoy:	**wait a sec. what r u doing here??**
bliss4u:	mitchie, why why why why?

BoBoy: oh dawg, we r totally imbued

alfonso: truer words were never spoken

chessman: wait... i'm still...

Ms.T: still what, mitchell darling?

alfonso: come on, bro. it's not that hard 2 work out

gothling has entered

chessman: i was afraid you'd say that. this
                whole foreign student thing was...

alfonso: bogosity, dude

gothling: **maskosity**

BoBoy: **annie's here too?**

gothling: **i was in the area. thought i'd...**

bliss4u: pop round, what what

BoBoy: **T, i'm innocent. those girls totally played us**

Ms.T: don't even. you had your eyes wide open

chessman: i'm getting it now. annie, you're
                Jerry C, aren't you?

gothling: **peace and joy, dude**

BoBoy: **excuse me?**

chessman: bro—annie and johnson burned us bad

bliss4u: oh, like ur the 1 who got burned? u married
                my best friend right behind my back

chessman: true. and you've been lying since
                the story about your grandmother

gothling: **an innocent fiction**

BoBoy: **bliss? yr best friend is tatiana?**

Ms.T: BEAU! wake up! i was tatiana!

alfonso: and wasn't she wonderful? what a performance

chessman: shut up, johnson

Ms.T: how kind you americans are, darling

BoBoy: i'm starting 2 get it, now

alfonso: and bliss was just brilliant as bridget

bliss4u: thank u, johnson. we had brilliant coaches

chessman: bliss. tamra. did you think this was funny? did we deserve this? do you not have lives?

bliss4u: u can't blame us. u went 4 these chicks of yr own free will

BoBoy: what free will? u totally lied 2 us

gothling: sweet sweet sweet

chessman: shut up, annie

Ms.T: nobody dragged you down the aisle, bubba

chessman: no, they hinted about suicide

alfonso: true. and i warned them that was over the top

BoBoy: shut up, johnson

gothling: there's no way 2 spln this, my dawgs. u done the deed

chessman: you can't be serious

bliss4u: we were there, mitchie. we saw u

chessman: no, bliss. "you" weren't there. i'm not even sure who "you" are

alfonso: ur caught, bro. a classic setup

chessman: more like classic entrapment. and are we supposed to trust that this is the real bliss and tam now?

BoBoy: **T, come on, how can u blame us, when u were totally tooling us?**

Ms.T: i can blame you because you promised you'd be good

BoBoy: **oh, and like U were good? didn't u hit on my man mitch?**

Ms.T: that wasn't real, and you know it

chessman: then what WE said wasn't real, either. nothing about this was real

bliss4u: it was too, mitch. i could tell u meant it

BoBoy: **gurl, how could u tell? u were somebody else**

bliss4u: i don't even know what that means

✉ IM from chessman

chessman: tamra, what's real?

Ms.T: what do you mean?

chessman: are you real or was tatiana?

Ms.T: tatiana who?

chessman: no more games, T. this whole thing was beneath you

Ms.T: ask me a real question and i'll tell you

chessman: ok. my real question is did you have real feelings for the real me or not?

Ms.T: mitchell, i can't go there. you know i can't

chessman: you CAN go there. i'm not asking you to leave beau. i'm only saying i'm not a toy, and I'm not ashamed of what i felt for you

Ms.T: felt?

chessman: ok... feel

Ms.T: but you didn't know it was me you had feelings for. coulda been anyone

chessman: but it was you, T. who you are doesn't change with a screen name

Ms.T: arrggh. go away, mitchell

chessman: don't bail on me. i NEED to know. find your inner tatiana and talk to me

Ms.T: ok ok. OK. first of all, i'm a little sorry we tricked you

chessman: ok... thanks, i guess

Ms.T: but if we hadn't, i would never have gotten to know you...

chessman: i know... i hate that :-)

Ms.T: and second. you know what i... love about you most? your feelings really are so deep and so truthful. they really are

chessman: they drive bliss crazy

Ms.T: no, they don't, honey

chessman: and now she's got real reasons to hate me. i'm kinda panicking here

Ms.T: don't even. she's nuts about you

chessman: oh great. oh excellent. and will you put in a good word for me?

Ms.T: lol

EXCHANGE STUDENT ROOM **UNION HIGH SCHOOL**

BoBoy: well, but really. if bridget was there, then bliss was gone. so u didn't c nuthin. hah.

bliss4u: lol. but i was there, meat-head. and ur in big trouble

BoBoy: who was there? which u was there?

bliss4u: i was. ME. the me underneath

alfonso: u dawgs r getting too deep 4 me. i just know it was the best stunt ever pulled

gothling: zackly. excellent scheming

alfonso: excellent puppeteering

gothling: excellent revenge

alfonso: sublime revenge, gurlfriend. gimme 5

gothling: up top

Ms.T: revenge for what, annie?

gothling: i don't know. just revenge on the world

✉ IM from BoBoy

BoBoy: bridget—i mean, bliss?

bliss4u: yikes. what r u doing?

BoBoy: i gotta ask u something

bliss4u: but what if T finds out ur chatting me on the side?

BoBoy: sorry, but i need 2 know. was it the u underneath talking? u know, when u were bridget and i was me?

bliss4u: oh, beau, please

BoBoy: was it? because i thought that was the real thing. i totally thought so. i get these... feelings sometimes

bliss4u: i know u do. ur practically psychic sometimes

BoBoy: so was i right?

bliss4u: oh, it's so confusing. really beau, i can't talk about it

BoBoy: <sigh> k. i know, not yr fault. going away now

bliss4u: no, listen, listen. because there may never be another time to say this

BoBoy: say what?

bliss4u: beau honey, when i was bridget, i did. i really really liked u. it surprised me how much

BoBoy: aw. that helps, bliss. thanks

bliss4u: but i can't keep being bridget, u know

BoBoy: i know. it's ok

bliss4u: thanks. but beau?

BoBoy: yes ma'am?

bliss4u: we can still talk sometimes, can't we?

chessman: annie, what revenge on the world? what's the world done? what have i done to you? ever??

BoBoy: or me. i never did nothing, annie

gothling: look. ur blowing this out of proportion. this was all just a bet between me and my gurls

chessman: a bet... about what?

gothling: oh, they were so sick in luv, and i thought they needed a reality check

BoBoy: k, i just threw up in my mouth a little

chessman: you hated the idea that they were in love??

Ms.T: you're not making this better by dodging your guilt, beau

BoBoy: but what am i guilty of?

bliss4u: wait! i know this one! >;)

alfonso: lol, bridget

BoBoy: owww...

chessman: seriously, bliss and T. if you set up a false scenario, you can't claim what happens there is real

bliss4u: oh, get out. u guys totally cheated on us, and that's REAL enuf

BoBoy: man, this is so unfair... u came on 2 us 2 MAKE us cheat

Ms.T: zackly. and you went for it, romeo. i am SO mad at you, even if i did set you up chessman: know what? i say we take this to bliss's mom. i don't think she'll say it's our fault at all

bliss4u: 4get about it

BoBoy: **excellent. T's mom too. she's on my side 4 everything**

Ms.T: lol. you're grounded from my mom as of right now. she has no judgment when it comes to you

gothling: **anyway, all this proves that i was right. guys r all alike**

chessman: oh annie, that is so boring

BoBoy: **so contumelious**

alfonso: u really believe this, annabelle?

gothling: **dude, ur a fine 1 to talk**

alfonso: no that's my point. u think they're the same as me?

gothling: **sure i do**

Ms.T: ok. hold on. in the 1st place, johnson, let the record show that YOU are not as bad as you pretend. and in the 2nd place, mitch and beau are in deep doo doo because they said THEY were so pure

gothling: **zackly. guys r all like this. maybe they mean well, but their minds wander**

⊟ IM from chessman

chessman: i wasn't THAT easy, was i?

Ms.T: my american darling, i nearly despaired of *ever* winning you ;-)

chessman: lol... no wait. that isn't funny

Ms.T: but i am so mad at beau. did you see how quickly he went for bliss?

✉ IM from BoBoy

BoBoy: so, bliss. how mad do u think T is?

bliss4u: get real. she adores u

BoBoy: well, how do i get her back?

bliss4u: just say u made a mistake. she'll be fine

BoBoy: how about mitch? should i tell him 2 gravel?

bliss4u: lol. yes, tell him 2 gravel

EXCHANGE STUDENT ROOM **UNION HIGH SCHOOL**

alfonso:	ok ok. so annie's inflicted her wisdom. guys r all alike
gothling:	**thank u**
alfonso:	i won't argue with how the creator made us. all guys love all women
BoBoy:	scuse me, um, <cough> all women, but ESPECIALLY our own woman
Ms.T:	i wonder what he means by that.... anyone? anyone?
bliss4u:	what happened 2 his nerdy friend, is what i wonder

chessman: \<sigh\> i'm here, ms. bliss

bliss4u: and?

chessman: well, i feel like i just flunked all
            my classes. you guys played a great
            scam on us

bliss4u: funny. i was sure there'd be an apology
            somewhere

chessman: there is, there is...

            ok, bliss, i began to lose hope.
            i thought you had another guy, and
            then i let down my guard. i doubted
            you, and i'm sorry

bliss4u: hmmmph. i don't know...

**gothling: not that i really care, but i should remind certain
            people of the terms of their bet**

bliss4u: get out. i will NOT take him back. not until
            he's been punished

chessman: say what?

**gothling: lol. no, bliss. i don't think that's an option.
            u lost...**

bliss4u: i put this 2 my gurls. should i take him back?
            does he deserve it?

Ms.T: well... he just now groveled. and actually, he
            resisted a loooong time...

chessman: i shouldn't have doubted. won't
            happen again, bliss

Ms T: ...a MUCH longer time than SOME people

**BoBoy: yeah. me too, T. i know i'm a bonehead. lesson
            learned**

Ms.T: boy, i am going 2 pound on you so bad

BoBoy: yess!

gothling: **okokok, let's don't get all weepy**

alfonso: can i just say 1 thing?

gothling: **what is it, partner?**

alfonso: just thinking about trust and faith from the guy's side. when u mess with someone's head like that, u do make it sorta hard 4 them 2 trust u in the future

gothling: **oh please**

alfonso: no, really. he'll always ask, is this the girl i love, or is this the one who scammed me?

gothling: **sweetie. peaches. she's both**

bliss4u: i don't get it

Ms T: peaches... <groan>

gothling: **gurl, if u can only love a perfect guy, ur freakin nuts. and he's crazy too, if he thinks u have only 1 face**

Ms.T: one mask, you mean?

gothling: **it's the same thing. we've all got lots. the job of yr sweetheart is 2 luv them all**

BoBoy: **even the contumelious ones?**

chessman: well, <ahem> er, bridget, i've always been fascinated with England, what what. do you, um... have any plans for tonight?

bliss4u: shall we have a spot of tea at my place? we can talk about how grounded ur... maybe play a little chess?

chessman: i'll just get my board

Ms.T: look at that. she stole my american husband!

BoBoy: **tatiana, <ahem> i'm not much of a gypsy, but i, um...**

Ms.T: but you haff a certain feeling for me,
             i thinking

BoBoy: yes, ma'am, i surely do

Ms.T: is destiny, my darling. do not fight it

CHAPTER 24

pure poetry

⊯ IM from alfonso

JUNE 18 7:30 PM

alfonso: ahem...

gothling: johnson, sup?

alfonso: despinetta, my love

gothling: how's my favorite puppeteer?

alfonso: well. <ahem> annie, i've gotta put this 2 u 1 last time, or i'll never be able 2 face myself in the morning

gothling: why am i suddenly on my guard, i wonder?

alfonso: ur not an easy person 2 get along with, but honestly... well, the truth is i just can't imagine trying with anyone else anymore

gothling: oh, here we go again

alfonso: and don't tell me we're not talking about this

gothling: J, honey, if i needed a guy, u would definitely be on the list. like on page 50

alfonso: annie, get real. u don't need a guy—u need me

gothling: i couldn't trust u, johnson. how obvious is that?

alfonso: i know. i know i deserve that

gothling: so there it is

alfonso: well, no, it doesn't end there. because honestly, gurlfriend, i'm going 2 have trouble trusting u 2

gothling: oh really?

alfonso: are u kidding? we've just been tooling our best friends

gothling: true. and i feel terrible about that... NOT

alfonso: but in case u haven't noticed. about women, i am totally, totally a different person

gothling: r u?

alfonso: u don't know me yet. u can take the chance

gothling: dude, i just don't believe in new leaf stuff. changing stripes and all that

alfonso: eww. listen, if we're going 2 be together, you'll HAVE 2 stop mixing metaphors

gothling: lol. u do amuse me... but no, johnson, we're NOT going 2 be together. i'm telling u, i been there. ate that t-shirt

alfonso: oh, stop. just stop with all this "afraid to love again" stuff

gothling: gimme a break. yr life's a country song. u got a string of broken hearts from here 2 nashville, cowboy

alfonso: and how bout yr life, my frozen queen? u watch other people, but u've forgotten the thrill of yr own feelings

gothling: arrggh. will u stop with this?

alfonso: no, in a word. i won't. listen 2 yr feelings

gothling: look, fool, i don't trust feelings. it's that simple

alfonso: ok, that sounds true, at least

gothling: thank u

alfonso: and what R yr feelings? tell the truth

gothling: oh, u make me so mad

alfonso: that's a start, luv. but why r u mad?

gothling: no. no way will u get me 2 put it in writing

alfonso: aight. we'll go with that 4 now

gothling: fine

alfonso: fine

gothling: fine

alfonso: how about this: i finished yr poem

gothling: my poem? really?

alfonso: yeah, really

gothling: u really wrote me a poem

alfonso: it's like the hardest thing i've ever done. pure poetry

gothling: u really did?

alfonso: and i don't want u making fun of it

gothling: i won't. i won't

alfonso: of course u will. but i don't care

gothling: so where is it? and it's about me?

alfonso: it's sort of about us—not in a sick way

gothling: course not

alfonso: it's a little edgy, a little dark

gothling: show it 2 me. show it 2 me

alfonso: but it's got good structure, a good controlling image. i like it. u probably won't

gothling: are u gonna SHOW it 2 me?

alfonso: oh. right. sorry

ok, close yr eyes

gothling: lol. what's the title?

alfonso: here u go

"A Masked Ball" (for Annie)

Behind the castle, from a deepening sky,
two crows in old tuxedos slide down
the breeze like down a ballroom banister.
They dance alone, to the tune of their own
rough noise. They peck, they scavenge
sticks and strings for toys. Black ribbons.
Worthless shiny things.

Do you think in heaven they have set aside
a room for crows like you and me to whom
the world is only a museum of masks
and rumpled souls ready to be shaken
out and tried? And will we like what we
have seen, when our curiosity is satisfied?

Will we like who we've become behind our
capes and masks and sad lone ranger
eyes?

gothling: johnson, i like this

alfonso: it's a sonnet. did u catch that?

gothling: i like it very much

alfonso: k, i messed up the count in 2 lines, and
the rhymes aren't all where they should be

gothling: it's beautiful. i love it

alfonso: but it's almost a sonnet. it's the best i
can... what? u do?

gothling: i love it

alfonso: oh, gag me, i'm so relieved

gothling: maybe ur not such a chump...

alfonso: awww

gothling: u really r a poet, aren't u?

alfonso: well, when properly inspired...

gothling: awww

alfonso: well

gothling: yeah?

alfonso: well, that's all i wanted

gothling: what is?

alfonso: just 2 give u the poem

gothling: hush, i'm reading it again

alfonso: right. k

gothling: right

alfonso: so that's it then

gothling: shh

alfonso: except. um. so, annie?

gothling: hm?

alfonso: so u got any plans 2nite?

gothling: what?

alfonso: i was just heading 2 the mall...

gothling: oh u idiot

alfonso: was that a yes?? it was! it WAS!

gothling: well... buy me a lone ranger mask?

alfonso: we'll buy a pair

gothling: k, pick me up b4 i change my mind

alfonso: YES!

gothling: but johnson

alfonso: annabelle?

gothling: don't think i'll never test u... ;-)

YOUR UNCLE JERRY'S BLOG

Under Construction

19 JUNE

Your Uncle Jerry is currently taking leave of his senses.
Peace and joy.

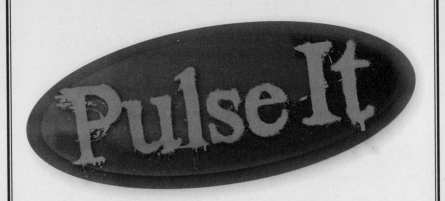
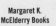 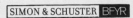

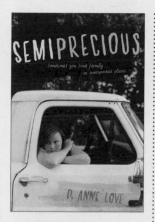
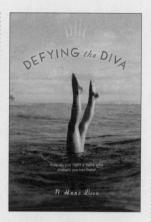
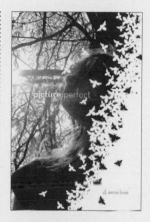

Sometimes all you have to go on is blind faith.

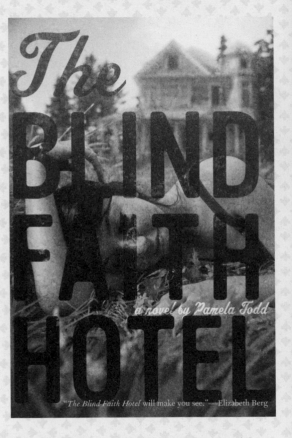

The Blind Faith Hotel will make you see." —Elizabeth Berg

WINNER OF THE 2009 GREEN EARTH BOOK AWARD FOR YOUNG ADULT FICTION

Fourteen-year-old Zoe wonders how she'll survive when her mother decides to move from the northwest coast to the midwest—leaving Zoe's father behind.

Miserable and away from the ocean she loves, Zoe loses her bearings completely. A shoplifting episode lands her in a work program at a local nature preserve, amidst what look to her like endless weeds. But the work there starts to stabilize Zoe, and when she meets a boy who shares her love of wild things, it seems she might be home after all. Until a disastrous fire threatens everything she has come to care about . . .

From Margaret K. McElderry Books · Published by Simon & Schuster · TEEN.SimonandSchuster.com

Love. Drama. High school.

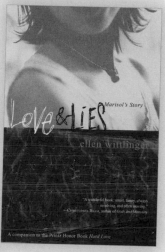

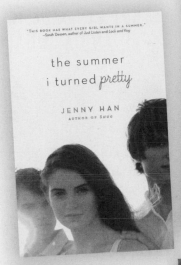

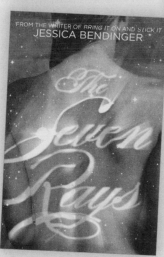

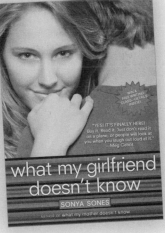

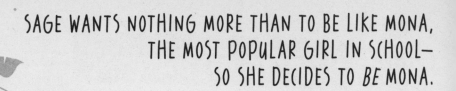

SAGE WANTS NOTHING MORE THAN TO BE LIKE MONA,
THE MOST POPULAR GIRL IN SCHOOL—
SO SHE DECIDES TO *BE* MONA.

BUT CAN SAGE SUCCEED?
AND AT WHAT COST?

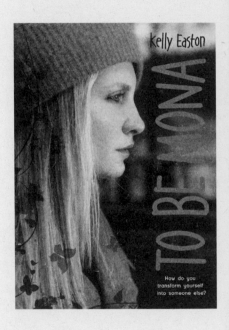

"Teens . . . will recognize themselves
in these pages."—*Kirkus Reviews*

"Easton handles difficult issues such as popularity,
a bipolar parent, poverty, and weight in a sensitive
and frequently comical fashion."—*Booklist*

FROM MARGARET K. McELDERRY BOOKS
PUBLISHED BY SIMON & SCHUSTER
TEEN.SimonandSchuster.com